I0066439

REFERENCE EDITION

ENDOCRINE BOARD REVIEW

Serge A. Jabbour, MD, Program Chair
Professor and Division Director
Division of Endocrinology
Sidney Kimmel Medical College
Thomas Jefferson University

Richard J. Auchus, MD, PhD
Professor of Internal Medicine
Division of Metabolism, Endocrinology
and Diabetes
University of Michigan Medical School

Carolyn B. Becker, MD
Associate Professor of Medicine and
Master Clinician Educator
Division of Endocrinology, Diabetes and
Hypertension
Brigham and Women's Hospital

Andrea D. Coviello, MD
Associate Professor of Medicine
Division of Endocrinology, Metabolism,
and Nutrition
Duke University School of Medicine

Frances J. Hayes, MB BCh, BAO
Clinical Director
Endocrine Division
Massachusetts General Hospital

Laurence Katznelson, MD
Professor of Neurosurgery and Medicine
Division of Endocrinology
Stanford University

Michelle F. Magee, MD
Associate Professor of Medicine
Georgetown University School of
Medicine

Kathryn A. Martin, MD
Professor of Medicine
Division of Endocrinology, Metabolism
and Molecular Medicine
Massachusetts General Hospital

Elizabeth N. Pearce, MD, MSc
Associate Professor
Endocrinology, Diabetes & Nutrition
Section
Boston University Medical Center

Abbie L. Young, MS, CGC, ELS(D)
Medical Editor

Endocrine Society
2055 L Street NW, Suite 600, Washington, DC 20036
1-888-ENDOCRINE • www.endocrine.org

ENDOCRINE
SOCIETY

ENDOCRINE
SOCIETY
Hormone Science to Health

The Endocrine Society is the world's largest, oldest, and most active organization working to advance the clinical practice of endocrinology and hormone research. Founded in 1916, the Society now has more than 18,000 global members across a range of disciplines. The Society has earned an international reputation for excellence in the quality of its peer-reviewed journals, educational resources, meetings, and programs that improve public health through the practice and science of endocrinology.

Visit us at:
education.endocrine.org
endocrine.org

Other Publications:
https://www.endocrine.org/
publications

The statements and opinions expressed in this publication are those of the individual authors and do not necessarily reflect the views of the Endocrine Society. The Endocrine Society is not responsible or liable in any way for the currency of the information, for any errors, omissions, or inaccuracies, or for any consequences arising therefrom. With respect to any drugs mentioned, the reader is advised to refer to the appropriate medical literature and the product information currently provided by the manufacturer to verify appropriate dosage, method and duration of administration, and other relevant information. In all instances, it is the responsibility of the treating physician or other health care professional, relying on independent experience and expertise, as well as knowledge of the patient, to determine the best treatment for the patient.

PERMISSIONS: For permission to reuse material, please visit the Copyright Clearance Center (CCC) at www.copyright.com or call 978-750-8400. CCC is a not-for-profit organization that provides licenses and registration for a variety of uses.

Copyright © 2019 by the Endocrine Society, 2055 L Street NW, Suite 600, Washington, DC 20036. All rights reserved. No part of this publication may be reproduced, stored in a retrieval system, posted on the Internet, or transmitted in any form, by any means, electronic, mechanical, photocopying, recording, or otherwise, without written permission of the publisher.

TRANSLATIONS AND LICENSING: Rights to translate and reproduce Endocrine Society publications internationally are extended through a licensing agreement on full or partial editions. To request rights for a local edition, please visit: https://www.endocrine.org/publications/ or licensing@endocrine.org.

ISBN: 978-1-879225-62-6
Library of Congress Control Number: 2019951422

On the Cover: © Shutterstock. Student taking notes and doing assignments in a college library. (By Jacob Lund).

OVERVIEW

Endocrine Board Review (EBR) 11th Edition (2019) is a board examination preparation book designed for endocrine fellows who have completed or are nearing completion of their fellowship and are preparing to sit for the board certification exam, and for practicing endocrinologists in search of a comprehensive self-assessment of endocrinology, either to prepare for recertification or to update their practice. EBR consists of approximately 240 case-based, American Board of Internal Medicine (ABIM) style, multiple-choice questions. Each section follows the ABIM Endocrinology, Diabetes, and Metabolism Certification Examination blueprint, covering the breadth and depth of the certification and recertification examinations. Each case is discussed in detail with detailed answer explanations and references provided.

The EBR 11th Edition (2019) reference book is intended primarily for consultation and self-assessment of knowledge relating to endocrinology. As a reference book, educational credits are not available upon completion of the multiple-choice questions included. For information on educational products that include educational credit, please visit endocrine.org/store.

LEARNING OBJECTIVES

Upon completion of this educational activity, learners will be able to demonstrate enhanced medical knowledge and clinical skills across all major areas of endocrinology; apply knowledge and skills in diagnosing, managing, and treating a wide spectrum of endocrine disorders; and successfully complete the board examination for certification or recertification in the subspecialty of endocrinology, diabetes, and metabolism.

TARGET AUDIENCE

This activity should be of substantial interest to endocrinologists, internists, and endocrine fellows preparing for the board examination or recertification; or endocrinologists and other health care practitioners seeking a review in endocrinology.

STATEMENT OF INDEPENDENCE

The Endocrine Society has a policy of ensuring that the content and quality of this educational activity are balanced, independent, objective, and scientifically rigorous. The scientific content of this activity was developed under the supervision of the Endocrine Society's EBR faculty. There are no commercial supporters of this activity and no commercial entities have had an influence over the planning of this activity.

DISCLOSURE POLICY

The faculty, committee members, and staff who are in position to control the content of this activity are required to disclose to the Endocrine Society and to learners any relevant financial relationship(s) of the individual or spouse/partner that have occurred within the last 12 months with any commercial interest(s) whose products or services are related to the content. Financial relationships are defined by remuneration in any amount from the commercial interest(s) in the form of grants; research support; consulting fees; salary; ownership interest (eg, stocks, stock options, or ownership interest excluding diversified mutual funds); honoraria or other payments for participation in speakers' bureaus, advisory boards, or boards of directors; or other financial benefits. The intent of this disclosure is not to prevent planners with relevant financial relationships from planning or delivery of content, but rather to provide learners with information that allows them to make their own judgments of whether these financial relationships may have influenced the educational activity with regard to exposition or conclusion.

The Endocrine Society has reviewed all disclosures and resolved or managed all identified conflicts of interest, as applicable.

The faculty reported the following relevant financial relationship(s) during the content development process for this activity:

Richard J. Auchus, MD, PhD, has served as a consultant to Adrenas Therapeutics, Corcept Therapeutics, Janssen Pharmaceuticals, Novartis Pharmaceuticals, Quest Diagnostics, Selenity Therapeutics, and Strongbridge Biopharma; and has conducted research for Neurocrine Biosciences, Novartis Pharmaceuticals, Spruce Biosciences, and Strongbridge Biopharma.

Carolyn B. Becker, MD, receives royalties from *UpToDate* as a chapter author.

Andrea D. Coviello, MD, has served as a consultant and speaker to Novo Nordisk and has received research support from Allergan, Bristol-Myers Squibb, and Regeneron.

Serge A. Jabbour, MD, has served as a consultant to AstraZeneca, Eli Lilly, and Janssen.

Laurence Katznelson, MD, has received research support from Novartis and has served as an advisory board member to Chiasma and Pfizer.

Michelle F. Magee, MD, has had her institution receive research support from Lilly, Mytonomy, and Sanofi; has served as a speaker for PRIMED and Mytonomy; and has served as a consultant to Mytonomy.

Kathryn A. Martin, MD, has served as a physician editor for *UpToDate.*

The following faculty reported no relevant financial relationships: Frances J. Hayes, MB BCh, BAO, and Elizabeth N. Pearce, MD, MSc.

The medical editor for this activity reported no relevant financial relationships: Abbie L. Young, MS, CGC, ELS(D).

Endocrine Society staff associated with the development of content for this activity reported no relevant financial relationships.

DISCLAIMERS

The information presented in this activity represents the opinion of the faculty and is not necessarily the official position of the Endocrine Society.

Use of professional judgment:

The educational content in this activity relates to basic principles of diagnosis and therapy and does not substitute for individual patient assessment based on the health care provider's examination of the patient and consideration of laboratory data and other factors unique to the patient. Standards in medicine change as new data become available.

Drugs and dosages:

When prescribing medications, the physician is advised to check the product information sheet accompanying each drug to verify conditions of use and to identify any changes in drug dosage schedule or contraindications.

POLICY ON UNLABELED/OFF-LABEL USE

The Endocrine Society has determined that disclosure of unlabeled/off-label or investigational use of commercial product(s) is informative for audiences and therefore requires this information to be disclosed to the learners at the beginning of the presentation. Uses of specific therapeutic agents, devices, and other products discussed in this educational activity may not be the same as those indicated in product labeling approved by the Food and Drug Administration (FDA). The Endocrine Society requires that any discussions of such "off-label" use be based on scientific research that conforms to generally accepted standards of experimental design, data collection, and data analysis. Before recommending or prescribing any therapeutic agent or device, learners should review the complete prescribing information, including indications, contraindications, warnings, precautions, and adverse events.

ACKNOWLEDGEMENT OF COMMERCIAL SUPPORT

The activity is not supported by educational grant(s) or other funds from any commercial supporters.

Publication Date: August 2019

Contents

Laboratory Reference Ranges

Lipid Values

High-density lipoprotein (HDL) cholesterol

    Optimal ----------------------------- >60 mg/dL (>1.55 mmol/L)

    Normal ------------------------ 40-60 mg/dL (1.04-1.55 mmol/L)

    Low --------------------------------- <40 mg/dL (<1.04 mmol/L)

Low-density lipoprotein (LDL) cholesterol

    Optimal -------------------------- <100 mg/dL (<2.59 mmol/L)

    Low ------------------------- 100-129 mg/dL (2.59-3.34 mmol/L)

    Borderline-high --------------- 130-159 mg/dL (3.37-4.12 mmol/L)

    High ----------------------- 160-189 mg/dL (4.14-4.90 mmol/L)

    Very high ------------------------- ≥190 mg/dL (≥4.92 mmol/L)

Non-HDL cholesterol

    Optimal -------------------------- <130 mg/dL (<3.37 mmol/L)

    Borderline-high --------------- 130-159 mg/dL (3.37-4.12 mmol/L)

    High -------------------------------- ≥240 mg/dL (≥6.22 mmol/L)

Total cholesterol

    Optimal -------------------------- <200 mg/dL (<5.18 mmol/L)

    Borderline-high --------------- 200-239 mg/dL (5.18-6.19 mmol/L)

    High -------------------------------- ≥240 mg/dL (≥6.22 mmol/L)

Triglycerides

    Optimal -------------------------- <150 mg/dL (<1.70 mmol/L)

    Borderline-high -------------- 150-199 mg/dL (1.70-2.25 mmol/L)

    High ----------------------- 200-499 mg/dL (2.26-5.64 mmol/L)

    Very high ------------------------- ≥500 mg/dL (≥5.65 mmol/L)

Lipoprotein (a) ----------------------------- ≤30 mg/dL (≤1.07 µmol/L)

Apolipoprotein B ------------------------ 50-110 mg/dL (0.5-1.1 g/L)

Hematologic Values

Erythrocyte sedimentation rate ------------------------------ 0-20 mm/h

Haptoglobin -------------------------- 30-200 mg/dL (300-2000 mg/L)

Hematocrit ------------------------------- 41%-50% (0.41-0.51) (male);

    35%-45% (0.35-0.45) (female)

Hemoglobin A$_{1c}$ ----------------------- 4.0%-5.6% (20-38 mmol/mol)

Hemoglobin --------------------- 13.8-17.2 g/dL (138-172 g/L) (male);

    12.1-15.1 g/dL (121-151 g/L) (female)

International normalized ratio ---------------------------------- 0.8-1.2

Mean corpuscular volume (MCV) -------------- 80-100 µm^3 (80-100 fL)

Platelet count --------------------- 150-450 x 10^3/µL (150-450 x 10^9/L)

Protein (total) ------------------------------- 6.3-7.9 g/dL (63-79 g/L)

Reticulocyte count -------- 0.5%-1.5% of red blood cells (0.005-0.015)

White blood cell count ------------- 4500-11,000/µL (4.5-11.0 x 10^9/L)

Thyroid Values

Thyroglobulin ----------------- 3-42 ng/mL (3-42 µg/L) (after surgery and

    radioactive iodine treatment: <1.0 ng/mL [<1.0 µg/L])

Thyroglobulin antibodies ---------------------- ≤4.0 IU/mL (≤4.0 kIU/L)

Thyrotropin (TSH) ------------------------------------- 0.5-5.0 mIU/L

Thyrotropin-receptor antibodies (TRAb) --------------------- ≤1.75 IU/L

Thyroid-stimulating immunoglobulin ---------- ≤120% of basal activity

Thyroperoxidase (TPO) antibodies ------------- <2.0 IU/mL (<2.0 kIU/L)

Thyroxine (T$_4$) (free) --------------- 0.8-1.8 ng/dL (10.30-23.17 pmol/L)

Thyroxine (T$_4$) (total) ------------- 5.5-12.5 µg/dL (94.02-213.68 nmol/L)

Free thyroxine (T$_4$) index --- 4-12

Triiodothyronine (T$_3$) (free) ------------ 2.3-4.2 pg/mL (3.53-6.45 pmol/L)

Triiodothyronine (T$_3$) (total) ----------- 70-200 ng/dL (1.08-3.08 nmol/L)

Triiodothyronine (T$_3$), reverse ---------- 10-24 ng/dL (0.15-0.37 nmol/L)

Triiodothyronine uptake, resin ----------------------------- 25%-38%

Radioactive iodine uptake ---- 3%-16% (6 hours); 15%-30% (24 hours)

Endocrine Values

Serum

Aldosterone ------------------------- 4-21 ng/dL (111.0-582.5 pmol/L)

Alkaline phosphatase -------------------- 50-120 U/L (0.84-2.00 µkat/L)

Alkaline phosphatase (bone-specific) ----------- ≤20 µg/L (adult male);

    ≤14 µg/L (premenopausal female); ≤22 µg/L (postmenopausal female)

Androstenedione -------- 65-210 ng/dL (2.27-7.33 nmol/L) (adult male);

    80-240 ng/dL (2.79-8.38 nmol/L) (adult female)

Antimullerian hormone ------------- 0.7-19.0 ng/mL (5.0-135.7 pmol/L)

    (male, >12 years); 0.9-9.5 ng/mL (6.4-67.9 pmol/L) (female, 13-45 years);

    <1.0 ng/mL (<7.1 pmol/L) (female, >45 years)

Calcitonin -------------------- <16 pg/mL (<4.67 pmol/L) (basal, male);

    <8 pg/mL (<2.34 pmol/L) (basal, female);

    ≤130 pg/mL (≤37.96 pmol/L) (peak calcium infusion, male);

    ≤90 pg/mL (≤26.28 pmol/L) (peak calcium infusion, female)

Carcinoembryonic antigen --------------------- <2.5 ng/mL (<2.5 µg/L)

Chromogranin A ------------------------------ <93 ng/mL (<93 µg/L)

Corticosterone --------- 53-1560 ng/dL (1.53-45.08 nmol/L) (>18 years)

Corticotropin (ACTH) ------------------- 10-60 pg/mL (2.2-13.2 pmol/L)

Cortisol (8 AM) ----------------------- 5-25 µg/dL (137.9-689.7 nmol/L)

Cortisol (4 PM) ----------------------- 2-14 µg/dL (55.2-386.2 nmol/L)

C-peptide -------------------------- 0.9-4.3 ng/mL (0.30-1.42 nmol/L)

C-reactive protein ------------------- 0.8-3.1 mg/L (7.62-29.52 nmol/L)

Cross-linked N-telopeptide of type 1 collagen ---------- 5.4-24.2 nmol

    BCE/mmol creat (male); 6.2-19.0 nmol BCE/mmol creat collagen (female)

Dehydroepiandrosterone sulfate (DHEA-S)

	Female	Male
Age 18-29 years	44-332 µg/dL (1.19-9.00 µmol/L)	89-457 µg/dL (2.41-12.38 µmol/L)
Age 30-39 years	31-228 µg/dL (0.84-6.78 µmol/L)	65-334 µg/dL (1.76-9.05 µmol/L)
Age 40-49 years	18-244 µg/dL (0.49-6.61 µmol/L)	48-244 µg/dL (1.30-6.61 µmol/L)
Age 50-59 years	15-200 µg/dL (0.41-5.42 µmol/L)	35-179 µg/dL (0.95-4.85 µmol/L)
Age ≥60 years	15-157 µg/dL (0.41-4.25 µmol/L)	25-131 µg/dL (0.68-3.55 µmol/L)

Deoxycorticosterone ------------------- <10 ng/dL (<0.30 nmol/L) (>18 years)

1,25-Dihydroxyvitamin D$_3$ ------------ 16-65 pg/mL (41.6-169.0 pmol/L)

Estradiol --------------------- 10-40 pg/mL (36.7-146.8 pmol/L) (male);

    10-180 pg/mL (36.7-660.8 pmol/L) (follicular, female);

    100-300 pg/mL (367.1-1101.3 pmol/L) (midcycle, female);

    40-200 pg/mL (146.8-734.2 pmol/L) (luteal, female);

    <20 pg/mL (<73.4 pmol/L) (postmenopausal, female)

Estrone --------------------- 10-60 pg/mL (37.0-221.9 pmol/L) (male);

17-200 pg/mL (62.9-739.6 pmol/L) (premenopausal female);

7-40 pg/mL (25.9-147.9 pmol/L) (postmenopausal female)

α-Fetoprotein ------------------------------------- <6 ng/mL (<6 µg/L)

Follicle-stimulating hormone (FSH) -----------------------------------

1.0-13.0 mIU/mL (1.0-13.0 IU/L) (male);

<3.0 mIU/mL (<3.0 IU/L) (prepuberty, female);

2.0-12.0 mIU/mL (2.0-12.0 IU/L) (follicular, female);

4.0-36.0 mIU/mL (4.0-36.0 IU/L) (midcycle, female);

1.0-9.0 mIU/mL (1.0-9.0 IU/L) (luteal, female);

>30 mIU/mL (>30 IU/L) (postmenopausal, female)

Free fatty acids ---------------------- 10.6-18.0 mg/dL (0.4-0.7 nmol/L)

Gastrin ------------------------------------- <100 pg/mL (<100 ng/L)

Growth hormone (GH) -------- 0.01-0.97 ng/mL (0.01-0.97 µg/L) (male);

0.01-3.61 ng/mL (0.01-3.61 µg/L) (female)

Homocysteine ------------------------------ ≤1.76 mg/L (≤13 µmol/L)

β-Human chorionic gonadotropin (β-hCG) ---------------------------

<3.0 mIU/mL (<3.0 IU/L) (nonpregnant female);

>25 mIU/mL (>25 IU/L) indicates a positive pregnancy test

β-Hydroxybutyrate ------------------------ <3.0 mg/dL (<288.2 µmol/L)

17-Hydroxypregnenolone ------------- 29-189 ng/dL (0.87-5.69 nmol/L)

17α-Hydroxyprogesterone ---- <220 ng/dL (<6.67 nmol/L) (adult male);

<80 ng/dL (<2.42 nmol/L) (follicular, female);

<285 ng/dL (<8.64 nmol/L) (luteal, female);

<51 ng/dL (<1.55 nmol/L) (postmenopausal, female)

25-Hydroxyvitamin D ---------- <20 ng/mL (<49.9 nmol/L) (deficiency);

21-29 ng/mL (52.4-72.4 nmol/L) (insufficiency); 30-80 ng/mL

(74.9-199.7 nmol/L) (optimal levels); >80 ng/mL (>199.7 nmol/L)

(toxicity possible)

Inhibin B ------------------------------ 15-300 pg/mL (15-300 ng/L)

Insulinlike growth factor 1 (IGF-1)

	Female	Male
Age 18 years	162-541 ng/mL (21.2-70.9 nmol/L)	170-640 ng/mL (22.3-83.8 nmol/L)
Age 19 years	138-442 ng/mL (18.1-57.9 nmol/L)	147-527 ng/mL (19.3-69.0 nmol/L)
Age 20 years	122-384 ng/mL (16.0-50.3 nmol/L)	132-457 ng/mL (17.3-59.9 nmol/L)
Age 21-25 years	116-341 ng/mL (15.2-44.7 nmol/L)	116-341 ng/mL (15.2-44.7 nmol/L)
Age 26-30 years	117-321 ng/mL (15.3-42.1 nmol/L)	117-321 ng/mL (15.3-42.1 nmol/L)
Age 31-35 years	113-297 ng/mL (14.8-38.9 nmol/L)	113-297 ng/mL (14.8-38.9 nmol/L)
Age 36-40 years	106-277 ng/mL (13.9-36.3 nmol/L)	106-277 ng/mL (13.9-36.3 nmol/L)
Age 41-45 years	98-261 ng/mL (12.8-34.2 nmol/L)	98-261 ng/mL (12.8-34.2 nmol/L)
Age 46-50 years	91-246 ng/mL (11.9-32.2 nmol/L)	91-246 ng/mL (11.9-32.2 nmol/L)
Age 51-55 years	84-233 ng/mL (11.0-30.5 nmol/L)	84-233 ng/mL (11.0-30.5 nmol/L)
Age 56-60 years	78-220 ng/mL (10.2-28.8 nmol/L)	78-220 ng/mL (10.2-28.8 nmol/L)
Age 61-65 years	72-207 ng/mL (9.4-27.1 nmol/L)	72-207 ng/mL (9.4-27.1 nmol/L)
Age 66-70 years	67-195 ng/mL (8.8-25.5 nmol/L)	67-195 ng/mL (8.8-25.5 nmol/L)
Age 71-75 years	62-184 ng/mL (8.1-24.1 nmol/L)	62-184 ng/mL (8.1-24.1 nmol/L)
Age 76-80 years	57-172 ng/mL (7.5-22.5 nmol/L)	57-172 ng/mL (7.5-22.5 nmol/L)
>Age 80 years	53-162 ng/mL (6.9-21.2 nmol/L)	53-162 ng/mL (6.9-21.2 nmol/L)

Insulinlike growth factor binding protein 3 ---------------- 2.5-4.8 mg/L

Insulin ------------------------------ 1.4-14.0 µIU/mL (9.7-97.2 pmol/L)

Islet-cell antibody assay --------- 0 Juvenile Diabetes Foundation units

Luteinizing hormone (LH) -------- 1.0-9.0 mIU/mL (1.0-9.0 IU/L) (male);

<1.0 mIU/mL (<1.0 IU/L) (prepuberty, female);

1.0-18.0 mIU/mL (1.0-18.0 IU/L) (follicular, female);

20.0-80.0 mIU/mL (20.0-80.0 IU/L) (midcycle, female);

0.5-18.0 mIU/mL (0.5-18.0 IU/L) (luteal, female);

>30 mIU/mL (>30 IU/L) (postmenopausal, female)

Metanephrines (plasma fractionated)

Metanephrine --------------------------- <99 pg/mL (<0.50 nmol/L)

Normetanephrine ----------------------- <165 pg/mL (<0.90 nmol/L)

75-g oral glucose tolerance test blood glucose values -----------------

60-100 mg/dL (3.3-5.6 mmol/L) (fasting);

<200 mg/dL (<11.1 mmol/L) (1 hour);

<140 mg/dL (<7.8 mmol/L) (2 hour);

between 140-200 mg/dL (7.8-11.1 mmol/L) is considered impaired

glucose tolerance or prediabetes. Greater than 200 mg/dL (11.1 mmol/L)

is a sign of diabetes mellitus.

50-g oral glucose tolerance test for gestational diabetes --------------

<140 mg/dL (<7.8 mmol/L) (1 hour)

100-g oral glucose tolerance test for gestational diabetes ------------

<95 mg/dL (<5.3 mmol/L) (fasting);

<180 mg/dL (<10.0 mmol/L) (1 hour);

<155 mg/dL (<8.6 mmol/L) (2 hour);

<140 mg/dL (<7.8 mmol/L) (3 hour)

Osteocalcin ---------------------------- 9.0-42.0 ng/mL (9.0-42.0 µg/L)

Parathyroid hormone, intact (PTH) ----------- 10-65 pg/mL (10-65 ng/L)

Parathyroid hormone–related protein (PTHrP) ------------- <2.0 pmol/L

Progesterone ----------------------- ≤1.2 ng/mL (≤3.8 nmol/L) (male);

≤1.0 ng/mL (≤3.2 nmol/L) (follicular, female);

2.0-20.0 ng/mL (6.4-63.6 nmol/L) (luteal, female);

≤1.1 ng/mL (≤3.5 nmol/L) (postmenopausal, female);

>10.0 ng/mL (>31.8 nmol/L) (evidence of ovulatory adequacy)

Proinsulin ------------------------- 26.5-176.4 pg/mL (3.0-20.0 pmol/L)

Prolactin ----------------------- 4-23 ng/mL (0.17-1.00 nmol/L) (male);

4-30 ng/mL (0.17-1.30 nmol/L) (nonlactating female);

10-200 ng/mL (0.43-8.70 nmol/L) (lactating female)

Prostate-specific antigen (PSA) ---- <2.0 ng/mL (<2.0 µg/L) (≤40 years);

<2.8 ng/mL (<2.8 µg/L) (≤50 years);

<3.8 ng/mL (<3.8 µg/L) (≤60 years);

<5.3 ng/mL (<5.3 µg/L) (≤70 years);

<7.0 ng/mL (<7.0 µg/L) (≤79 years);

<7.2 ng/mL (<7.2 µg/L) (≥80 years)

Renin activity, plasma, sodium replete, ambulatory ------------- 0.6-4.3 ng/mL per h

Renin, direct concentration --------------- 4-44 pg/mL (0.1-1.0 pmol/L)

Sex hormone–binding globulin (SHBG) ----------------- 1.1-6.7 μg/mL
(10-60 nmol/L) (male); 2.2-14.6 μg/mL (20-130 nmol/L) (female)

α-Subunit of pituitary glycoprotein hormones --------- <1.2 ng/mL (<1.2 μg/L)

Testosterone (bioavailable) ----------- 0.8-4.0 ng/dL (0.03-0.14 nmol/L)
(20-50 years, female on oral estrogen);
0.8-10.0 ng/dL (0.03-0.35 nmol/L)
(20-50 years, female not on oral estrogen);
83.0-257.0 ng/dL (2.88-8.92 nmol/L) (male 20-29 years);
72.0-235.0 ng/dL (2.50-8.15 nmol/L) (male 30-39 years);
61.0-213.0 ng/dL (2.12-7.39 nmol/L) (male 40-49 years);
50.0-190.0 ng/dL (1.74-6.59 nmol/L) (male 50-59 years);
40.0-168.0 ng/dL (1.39-5.83 nmol/L) (male 60-69 years)

Testosterone (free) ---------- 9.0-30.0 ng/dL (0.31-1.04 nmol/L) (male);
0.3-1.9 ng/dL (0.01-0.07 nmol/L) (female)

Testosterone (total) ---------- 300-900 ng/dL (10.4-31.2 nmol/L) (male);
8-60 ng/dL (0.3-2.1 nmol/L) (female)

Vitamin B$_{12}$ ------------------------- 180-914 pg/mL (133-674 pmol/L)

Chemistry Values

Alanine aminotransferase ------------------ 10-40 U/L (0.17-0.67 μkat/L)
Albumin ------------------------------------ 3.5-5.0 g/dL (35-50 g/L)
Amylase ------------------------------ 26-102 U/L (0.43-1.70 μkat/L)
Aspartate aminotransferase --------------- 20-48 U/L (0.33-0.80 μkat/L)
Bicarbonate --------------------------- 21-28 mEq/L (21-28 mmol/L)
Bilirubin (total) ----------------------- 0.3-1.2 mg/dL (5.1-20.5 μmol/L)
Blood gases
Po$_2$, arterial blood ---------------- 80-100 mm Hg (10.6-13.3 kPa)
Pco$_2$, arterial blood ------------------ 35-45 mm Hg (4.7-6.0 kPa)
Blood pH -- 7.35-7.45
Calcium --------------------------- 8.2-10.2 mg/dL (2.1-2.6 mmol/L)
Calcium (ionized) ------------------ 4.60-5.08 mg/dL (1.2-1.3 mmol/L)
Carbon dioxide ------------------------ 22-28 mEq/L (22-28 mmol/L)
CD$_4$ cell count ----------------------- 500-1400/μL (0.5-1.4 x 10^9/L)
Chloride --------------------------- 96-106 mEq/L (96-106 mmol/L)
Creatine kinase ----------------------- 50-200 U/L (0.84-3.34 μkat/L)
Creatinine ----------------- 0.7-1.3 mg/dL (61.9-114.9 μmol/L) (male);
0.6-1.1 mg/dL (53.0-97.2 μmol/L) (female)
Ferritin ---------------------------- 15-200 ng/mL (33.7-449.4 pmol/L)
Folate ----------------------------------- ≥4.0 ng/mL (≥4.0 μg/L)
Glucose ----------------------------- 70-99 mg/dL (3.9-5.5 mmol/L)
γ-Glutamyltransferase --------------------- 2-30 U/L (0.03-0.50 μkat/L)
Iron ------------------------- 50-150 μg/dL (9.0-26.8 μmol/L) (male);
35-145 μg/dL (6.3-26.0 μmol/L) (female)
Lactate dehydrogenase ------------------ 100-200 U/L (1.7-3.3 μkat/L)
Lactic acid ------------------------ 5.4-20.7 mg/dL (0.6-2.3 mmol/L)
Lipase ---------------------------- 10-73 U/L (0.17-1.22 μkat/L)
Magnesium ------------------------- 1.5-2.3 mg/dL (0.6-0.9 mmol/L)
Osmolality ---------------------- 275-295 mOsm/kg (275-295 mmol/kg)

Phosphate ------------------------- 2.3-4.7 mg/dL (0.7-1.5 mmol/L)
Potassium --------------------------- 3.5-5.0 mEq/L (3.5-5.0 mmol/L)
Prothrombin time --- 8.3-10.8 s
Serum urea nitrogen --------------------- 8-23 mg/dL (2.9-8.2 mmol/L)
Sodium --------------------------- 136-142 mEq/L (136-142 mmol/L)
Transferrin saturation --------------------------------------- 14%-50%
Troponin I --------------------------------- <0.6 ng/mL (<0.6 μg/L)
Tryptase ---------------------------------- <11.5 ng/mL (<11.5 μg/L)
Uric acid ------------------------- 3.5-7.0 mg/dL (208.2-416.4 μmol/L)

Urine

Albumin ------------------- 30-300 μg/mg creat (3.4-33.9 μg/mol creat)
Albumin-to-creatinine ratio ---------------------------- <30 mg/g creat
Aldosterone ---------------- 3-20 μg/24 h (8.3-55.4 nmol/d) (should be
<12 μg/24 h [<33.2 nmol/d] with oral sodium loading—confirmed with
24-hour urinary sodium >200 mEq)
Calcium ----------------------------- 100-300 mg/24 h (2.5-7.5 mmol/d)
Catecholamine fractionation
Normotensive normal ranges:
Dopamine ------------------------- <700 μg/24 h (<4567 nmol/d)
Epinephrine ----------------------- <35 μg/24 h (<191 nmol/d)
Norepinephrine --------------------- <170 μg/24 h (<1005 nmol/d)
Citrate ------------------------ 320-1240 mg/24 h (16.7-64.5 mmol/d)
Cortisol ------------------------------- 4-50 μg/24 h (11-138 nmol/d)
Cortisol following dexamethasone suppression test (low-dose: 2 day,
2 mg daily) ------------------------------ <10 μg/24 h (<27.6 nmol/d)
Creatinine --------------------------- 1.0-2.0 g/24 h (8.8-17.7 mmol/d)
Glomerular filtration rate (estimated) ---------- >60 mL/min per 1.73 m^2
5-Hydroxyindole acetic acid ----------- 2-9 mg/24 h (10.5-47.1 μmol/d)
Iodine (random) --- >100 μg/L
17-Ketosteroids ---------- 6.0-21.0 mg/24 h (20.8-72.9 μmol/d) (male);
4.0-17.0 mg/24 h (13.9-59.0 μmol/d) (female)
Metanephrine fractionation
Metanephrine ------------------------- <400 μg/24 h (<2028 nmol/d)
Normetanephrine --------------------- <900 μg/24 h (<4914 nmol/d)
Total metanephrine ------------------- <1000 μg/24 h (<5260 nmol/d)
Osmolality ------------------- 150-1150 mOsm/kg (150-1150 mmol/kg)
Oxalate ---------------------------------- <40 mg/24 h (<456 mmol/d)
Phosphate ----------------------- 0.9-1.3 g/24 h (29.1-42.0 mmol/d)
Potassium --------------------------- 17-77 mEq/24 h (17-77 mmol/d)
Sodium ----------------------------- 40-217 mEq/24 h (40-217 mmol/d)
Uric acid ------------------------------- <800 mg/24 h (<4.7 mmol/d)

Saliva

Cortisol (salivary), midnight ------------------ <0.13 μg/dL (<3.6 nmol/L)

Semen

Semen analysis ------------------ >20 million sperm/mL; >50% motility

COMMON ABBREVIATIONS USED IN ENDOCRINE BOARD REVIEW

ACTH = corticotropin

ACE inhibitor = angiotensin-converting enzyme inhibitor

ALT = alanine aminotransferase

AST = aspartate aminotransferase

BMI = body mass index

CNS = central nervous system

CT = computed tomography

DHEA = dehydroepiandrosterone

DHEA-S = dehydroepiandrosterone sulfate

DNA = deoxyribonucleic acid

DPP-4 inhibitor = dipeptidyl-peptidase 4 inhibitor

DXA = dual-energy x-ray absorptiometry

FDA = Food and Drug Administration

FGF-23 = fibroblast growth factor 23

FNA = fine-needle aspiration

FSH = follicle-stimulating hormone

GH = growth hormone

GHRH = growth hormone–releasing hormone

GLP-1 receptor agonist = glucagonlike peptide 1 receptor agonist

GnRH = gonadotropin-releasing hormone

hCG = human chorionic gonadotropin

HDL = high-density lipoprotein

HIV = human immunodeficiency virus

HMG-CoA reductase inhibitor = 3-hydroxy-3-methylglutaryl coenzyme A reductase inhibitor

IGF-1 = insulinlike growth factor 1

LDL = low-density lipoprotein

LH = luteinizing hormone

MCV = mean corpuscular volume

MIBG = *meta*-iodobenzylguanidine

MRI = magnetic resonance imaging

NPH insulin = neutral protamine Hagedorn insulin

PCSK9 inhibitor = proprotein convertase subtilisin/kexin 9 inhibitor

PET = positron emission tomography

PSA = prostate-specific antigen

PTH = parathyroid hormone

PTHrP = parathyroid hormone–related protein

SGLT-2 inhibitor = sodium-glucose cotransporter 2 inhibitor

SHBG = sex hormone–binding globulin

T_3 = triiodothyronine

T_4 = thyroxine

TPO antibodies = thyroperoxidase antibodies

TRH = thyrotropin-releasing hormone

TRAb = thyrotropin-receptor antibodies

TSH = thyrotropin

VLDL = very low-density lipoprotein

ENDOCRINE
BOARD
REVIEW

Adrenal Board Review

Richard J. Auchus, MD, PhD

1 A 27-year-old woman was diagnosed at birth with classic 21-hydroxylase deficiency and has been adherent to treatment with hydrocortisone and fludrocortisone acetate her entire life. She had vaginal reconstruction at age 19 years and has been using dilators periodically since then. For the last 18 months, she has been sexually active and wants to have children, but she has not conceived despite optimally timed intercourse. She currently takes hydrocortisone, 10 mg upon waking and 5 mg with both lunch and her evening meal, plus fludrocortisone acetate, 0.1 mg with breakfast. She has regular monthly menses and shaves her upper lip and chin once a month. Home urine testing documents monthly ovulation.

On physical examination, she has no moon facies, no striae or facial plethora, no acne, and a trace of shaved stubble.

Which of the following is the key laboratory parameter to monitor when adjusting her glucocorticoid therapy?

    A. Follicular-phase androstenedione
    B. Follicular-phase progesterone
    C. Postmorning dose 17-hydroxyprogesterone
    D. Periovulatory testosterone
    E. Luteal-phase 17-hydroxyprogesterone

2 A 45-year-old woman presents with resistant hypertension. She developed hypokalemia while taking amlodipine and hydrochlorothiazide. Lisinopril and potassium chloride supplements (80 mEq daily) were added, with eventual resolution of the hypokalemia but without normalization of blood pressure. She has also gained 22 lb (10 kg) over the last 2 years and now has diet-controlled diabetes mellitus.

On physical examination, she has mild dermal atrophy and three 1-cm bruises on her arms and legs from minimal trauma. Proximal muscle strength is normal. Her blood pressure is 148/95 mm Hg, and she has no dorsocervical fat pad or striae.

Laboratory test results:
    Serum sodium = 138 mEq/L (136-142 mEq/L)
      (SI: 138 mmol/L [136-142 mmol/L])
    Serum potassium = 3.6 mEq/L (3.5-5.0 mEq/L)
      (SI: 3.6 mmol/L [3.5-5.0 mmol/L])
    Serum glucose = 157 mg/dL (70-99 mg/dL)
      (SI: 8.7 mmol/L [3.9-5.5 mmol/L])
    Serum aldosterone = 13 ng/dL (4-21 ng/dL)
      (SI: 361 pmol/L [111-583 pmol/L])
    Plasma renin activity = <0.6 ng/mL per h
      (0.6-4.3 ng/mL per h)
    Serum creatinine = 0.8 mg/dL (0.6-1.1 mg/dL)
      (SI: 70.7 μmol/L [53.0-97.2 μmol/L])
    Plasma metanephrines, normal

Abdominal CT with contrast demonstrates a 3.8-cm left adrenal mass and an atrophic right adrenal gland (*see image, arrows*).

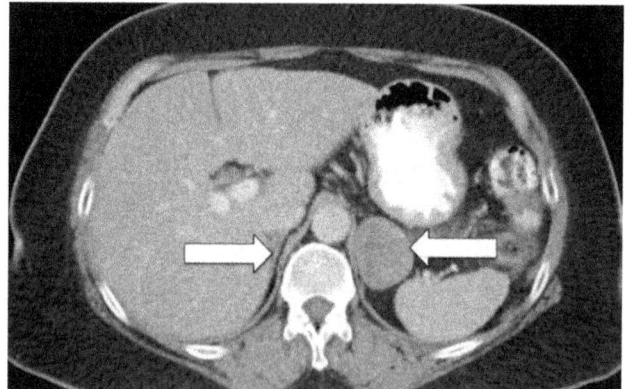

The patient is referred to you for further evaluation and recommendations.

Which of the following is the best next step?

A. Prescribe spironolactone, 50 mg daily
B. Recommend left adrenalectomy
C. Biopsy the left adrenal gland
D. Schedule adrenal venous sampling to measure aldosterone and cortisol
E. Measure serum cortisol after 1-mg dexamethasone

3 A 46-year-old woman with no notable medical history has developed paroxysms of nausea and hypertension over the past 6 months. During one such episode, she went to the emergency department and was subsequently hospitalized for a blood pressure of 200/110 mm Hg. An evaluation for a suspected pheochromocytoma is in progress, and the patient has not yet received adrenergic blockade.

Which of the following treatments for nausea is contraindicated in this patient?

A. Metoclopramide
B. Meclizine
C. Lorazepam
D. Ranitidine
E. Ondansetron

4 You are asked to provide consultation for a 28-year-old man with possible adrenal insufficiency. He was seen in the emergency department 10 days ago for unexplained hypotension following a party, and an etiology was not identified. He recovered with fluid resuscitation and a single dose of dexamethasone, 10 mg intravenously. He received no further glucocorticoids and takes no medication or nutritional supplements. Since discharge, he has had some intermittent malaise and fatigue but no hypotension, and his appetite is normal. He comes to a clinic appointment today at 4 PM, and the question posed is whether he suffers from adrenal insufficiency as the cause of his hypotensive episode.

Which laboratory test result obtained at this time will conclusively exclude adrenal insufficiency?

A. Serum cortisol concentration = 5 µg/dL (4-11 µg/dL) (SI: 138 nmol/L [110-304 nmol/L])
B. Salivary cortisol concentration = 0.1 µg/dL (0.01-0.2 µg/dL) (SI: 2.8 nmol/L [0.3-5.5 nmol/L])
C. Plasma ACTH concentration = 10 pg/mL (6-48 pg/mL) (SI: 2.2 pmol/L [1.3-10.6 pmol/L])
D. Serum DHEA-S concentration = 360 µg/dL (38-523 µg/dL) (SI: 9.8 µmol/L [1.0-14.2 µmol/L])

5 A 54-year-old man has a 2.2-cm mass in the left adrenal gland incidentally noted on CT performed to evaluate hematuria. The mass is homogeneous, the density is 30 Hounsfield units before contrast, and there is 30% washout at 15 minutes. His blood pressure is 122/78 mm Hg, and he reports no symptoms of sweating, palpitations, or headache. He takes no medications, but he has a positive family history of hypertension developing after age 50 years.

Screening laboratory test results:
Plasma metanephrine = 670 pg/mL (<99 pg/mL) (SI: 3.4 nmol/L [<0.5 nmol/L])
Plasma normetanephrine = 641 pg/mL (<165 pg/mL) (SI: 3.5 nmol/L [<0.9 nmol/L])
Serum cortisol after 1 mg dexamethasone = 0.5 µg/dL (SI: 13.8 nmol/L)

The CT image before contrast is shown (*see image*).

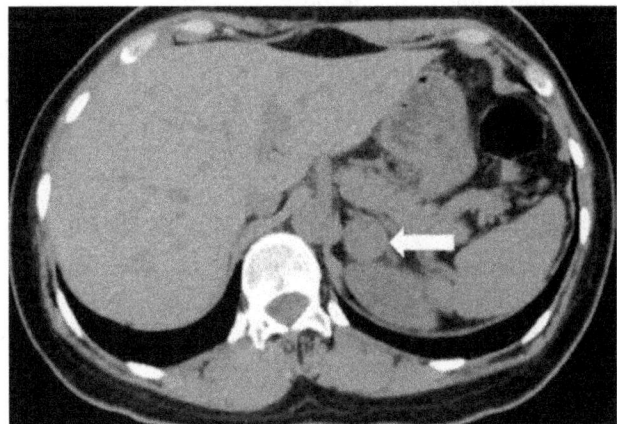

Which of the following is the most appropriate next step in this patient's management?
 A. Administer α-adrenergic blockade and refer for left adrenalectomy
 B. Measure plasma renin activity and serum aldosterone
 C. Perform adrenal MRI
 D. Repeat the CT in 12 months
 E. Perform adrenal biopsy

6 A 51-year-old man is status post right open adrenalectomy for a 6-cm adrenocortical carcinoma that was causing Cushing syndrome. The pathology specimen showed high-grade tumor with vascular invasion, but no inferior vena cava thrombosis or lymph nodes were positive for tumor. Postoperatively, he was treated with hydrocortisone, 20 mg upon waking and 10 mg in the afternoon, and he recovered well with some resolution of cushingoid features. After 4 weeks, adjuvant mitotane was added and titrated up to 1 g 4 times daily. At a clinic visit 6 weeks later, his serum mitotane value is now at therapeutic goal, but he reports nausea, anorexia, and fatigue. His blood pressure is 125/82 mm Hg without an orthostatic drop.

Laboratory test results:
 Serum mitotane = 16.4 mg/L (therapeutic goal >14 mg/L)
 Serum potassium = 4.2 mEq/L (3.5-5.0 mEq/L)
 (SI: 4.2 mmol/L [3.5-5.0 mmol/L])
 Plasma ACTH = <2 pg/mL (10-60 pg/mL)
 (SI: <0.4 pmol/L [2.2-13.2 pmol/L])
 Serum total testosterone = 480 ng/dL (300-900 ng/dL) (SI: 16.7 nmol/L [10.4-31.2 nmol/L])
 SHBG = 11.5 µg/mL (1.1-6.7 µg/mL) (SI: 102 nmol/L [10-60 nmol/L])

Which of the following is the best next step in this patient's management?
 A. Add fludrocortisone, 0.1 mg daily
 B. Reduce the mitotane dosage to 0.5 g 4 times daily
 C. Change the hydrocortisone dosage to 20 mg 3 times daily
 D. Add testosterone enanthate, 100 mg weekly
 E. Add anastrozole, 1 mg daily

7 A 32-year-old woman has a history of Cushing disease status post surgery 3 years ago with subsequent improvement in her diabetes mellitus and hypertension. She has noted weight gain, poor sleep, irregular menses, and worsening glycemia for the past 6 months. Her medications include amlodipine, 10 mg daily, and metformin, 1500 mg daily.

On physical examination, her blood pressure is 145/85 mm Hg. She has facial plethora and moderate supraclavicular fat pads.

Laboratory test results:
 Fasting glucose = 205 mg/dL (70-99 mg/dL)
 (SI: 11.4 mmol/L [3.9-5.5 mmol/L])
 Potassium = 2.7 mEq/L (3.5-5.0 mEq/L)
 (SI: 2.7 mmol/L [3.5-5.0 mmol/L])
 Serum cortisol (8 AM) = 18 µg/dL (5-25 µg/dL)
 (SI: 497 nmol/L [138-690 nmol/L])
 Hemoglobin A_{1c} = 8.5% (4.0%-5.6%)
 (69 mmol/mol [20-38 mmol/mol])
 Plasma ACTH = 65 pg/mL (10-60 pg/mL)
 (SI: 14.3 pmol/L [2.2-13.2 pmol/L])
 Late-night salivary cortisol = 0.32 µg/dL
 (<0.13 µg/dL) (SI: 8.8 nmol/L [<3.6 nmol/L])
 Urinary free cortisol = 360 µg/24 h (4-50 µg/24 h)
 (SI: 994 nmol/d [11-138 nmol/d])
 Serum hCG (qualitative), negative

Pituitary MRI shows only postoperative changes. After a discussion of treatment options, you plan to begin mifepristone, 300 mg daily.

Before starting mifepristone, you should first treat her to achieve which of the following?
 A. Normal blood pressure
 B. Normal fasting glucose
 C. Normal serum potassium
 D. Normal plasma triglycerides
 E. No additional treatment is required

8 A 68-year-old man is diagnosed with primary aldosteronism after having difficult-to-control hypertension with intermittent hypokalemia for at least 10 years and microalbuminuria for the last 2 years. Adrenal venous sampling demonstrates bilateral hyperaldosteronism, and you begin medical therapy with eplerenone, 50 mg daily, added to amlodipine, 10 mg daily. Over 6 weeks, his blood pressure falls from 158/96 mm Hg to 135/88 mm Hg, and you increase the eplerenone dosage to 50 mg twice daily. After another 8 weeks, his blood pressure is 125/82 mm Hg.

Laboratory test results (baseline before eplerenone):
Serum potassium = 3.1 mEq/L (3.5-5.0 mEq/L)
(SI: 3.1 mmol/L [3.5-5.0 mmol/L])
Serum creatinine = 1.4 mg/dL (0.7-1.3 mg/dL)
(SI: 123.8 μmol/L [61.9-114.9 μmol/L])
Serum aldosterone = 28 ng/dL (4-21 ng/dL)
(SI: 777 pmol/L [111-583 pmol/L])
Plasma renin activity = <0.6 ng/mL per h
(0.6-4.3 ng/mL per h)

Laboratory test results (after 8 weeks taking eplerenone, 50 mg twice daily):
Serum potassium = 4.4 mEq/L (3.5-5.0 mEq/L)
(SI: 4.4 mmol/L [3.5-5.0 mmol/L])
Serum creatinine = 1.8 mg/dL (0.7-1.3 mg/dL)
(SI: 159.1 μmol/L [61.9-114.9 μmol/L])
Serum aldosterone = 33 ng/dL (4-21 ng/dL)
(SI: 915 pmol/L [111-583 pmol/L])
Plasma renin activity = 1.3 ng/mL per h
(0.6-4.3 ng/mL per h)

Repeated testing 2 weeks later shows equivalent results.

On the basis of these results, which of the following changes would you make to his blood pressure therapy?
  A. Reduce the eplerenone dosage to 50 mg daily
  B. Change eplerenone to spironolactone, 100 mg daily
  C. Discontinue amlodipine
  D. Discontinue eplerenone and add atenolol, 50 mg daily
  E. No changes

9 A 38-year-old woman is referred for evaluation of adrenal nodularity. She reports weight gain of 11 lb (5 kg), poor sleep, and easy bruising over the last 2 years.

On physical examination, her blood pressure is 144/92 mm Hg. She has moderate facial plethora with rounding, dermal atrophy, and disproportionate supraclavicular fat pads. She cannot rise from a squat, and she has several 2- to 3-cm bruises on her legs.

Laboratory test results:
Serum cortisol after 1 mg dexamethasone = 4.0 μg/dL (SI: 110.4 nmol/L)
Serum DHEA-S = 110 μg/dL (31-228 μg/dL)
(SI: 3.0 μmol/L [0.8-6.8 μmol/L])
Hemoglobin A_{1c} = 7.3% (4.0%-5.6%)
(56 mmol/mol [20-38 mmol/mol])
Plasma ACTH = 5 pg/mL (10-60 pg/mL)
(SI: 1.1 pmol/L [2.2-13.2 pmol/L])
Urinary free cortisol = 62 μg/24 h (4-50 μg/24 h)
(SI: 171 nmol/d [11-138 nmol/d])

Abdominal CT shows bilateral adrenal nodularity, 4 x 3 cm on the right side and 2 x 2 cm on the left side (*see image*).

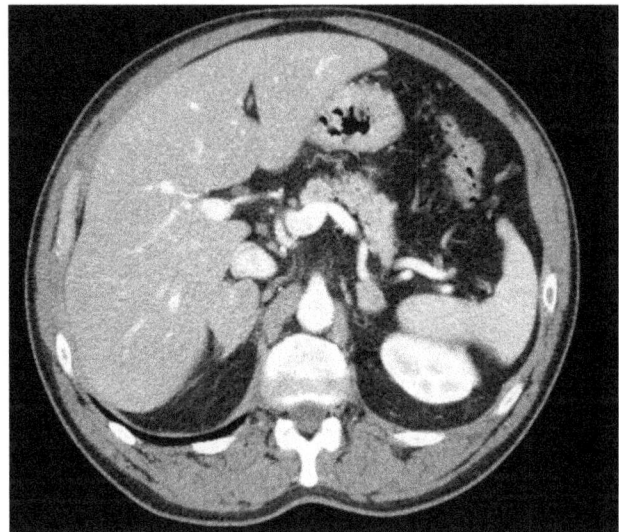

Which of the following would you recommend as the best next step in this patient's management?
  A. Observation
  B. Pasireotide
  C. Laparoscopic right adrenalectomy
  D. MRI of the adrenal glands
  E. Spironolactone and metformin

10 A 55-year-old woman presents with weight gain, easy bruising, muscle weakness, and hypertension treated with candesartan. Her symptoms have been worsening over at least 4 years.

Laboratory test results demonstrate ACTH-dependent Cushing syndrome:

Late-night salivary cortisol = 0.62 µg/dL
(<0.13 µg/dL) (SI: 17.1 nmol/L [<3.6 nmol/L])
Urinary free cortisol = 425 µg/24 h (4-50 µg/24 h)
(SI: 1173 nmol/d [11-138 nmol/d])
Basal plasma ACTH = 51 pg/mL (10-60 pg/mL)
(SI: 11.2 pmol/L [2.2-13.2 pmol/L])

After inferior petrosal sinus sampling and MRI, she undergoes transsphenoidal surgery. The morning after surgery, her cortisol value is 2.5 µg/dL (69.0 nmol/L). Candesartan is discontinued, and she is discharged on a regimen of hydrocortisone, 10 mg 3 times daily with meals.

She returns today 4 weeks after surgery. She describes diffuse muscle aches, fatigue, anorexia, and sleeping 10 to 12 hours a day. She feels worse than before the surgery.

On physical examination, her blood pressure is 120/80 mm Hg and pulse rate is 70 beats/min without orthostatic changes. Her cushingoid features are beginning to resolve, and she has lost 8 lb (3.6 kg).

Laboratory test results in clinic:

Serum sodium = 136 mEq/L (136-142 mEq/L)
(SI: 136 mmol/L [136-142 mmol/L])
Serum potassium = 4.4 mEq/L (3.5-5.0 mEq/L)
(SI: 4.4 mmol/L [3.5-5.0 mmol/L])
Fasting glucose = 80 mg/dL (70-99 mg/dL)
(SI: 4.4 mmol/L [3.9-5.5 mmol/L])
Serum cortisol (8 AM) before first dose of
hydrocortisone = <0.5 µg/dL (5-25 µg/dL)
(SI: <13.8 nmol/L [137.9-389.7 nmol/L])
DHEA-S = <15 µg/dL (18-244 µg/dL)
(SI: <0.4 µmol/L [0.5-6.6 µmol/L])
Basal plasma ACTH = <4 pg/mL (10-60 pg/mL)
(SI: <0.9 pmol/L [2.2-13.2 pmol/L])

Surgical pathology reveals a pituitary adenoma with Crooke hyaline change, and immunohistochemistry for ACTH is positive.

Which of the following is responsible for this patient's symptoms?

A. Insufficient hydrocortisone dosage
B. Insufficient mineralocorticoid replacement
C. Recurrent Cushing disease
D. Adrenal androgen deficiency
E. Adrenal medulla dysfunction

11 A 21-year-old woman is referred for evaluation of unwanted facial hair, acne, and irregular menses. She developed pubic hair and body odor at age 5 years and was the tallest girl in her class until she stopped growing at age 11 years. She developed acne and facial hair at age 12 years and menarche was at age 14 years. Her menses have always been irregular, and she has not menstruated for 8 months.

On physical examination, the patient has coarse terminal hairs and shaved stubble on her chin, upper lip, and sides of her face. She has acne on her forehead. Findings on pelvic examination, including external genitalia, are normal. She has no moon facies, dermal atrophy, myopathy, striae, or acanthosis nigricans. Her blood pressure is 120/80 mm Hg, and BMI is 23 kg/m².

Screening laboratory test results (sample drawn at 1 PM in the follicular phase):

Serum cortisol = 6.0 µg/dL (2-14 µg/dL)
(SI: 166 nmol/L [55-386 nmol/L])
Serum DHEA-S = 680 µg/dL (44-332 µg/dL)
(SI: 18.4 µmol/L [1.2-9.0 µmol/L])
Serum 17-hydroxyprogesterone = 300 ng/dL
(<80 ng/dL [follicular]) (SI: 9.1 nmol/L
[<2.4 nmol/L])
Serum total testosterone = 75 ng/dL (8-60 ng/dL)
(SI: 2.6 nmol/L [0.3-2.1 nmol/L])
SHBG = 1.0 µg/mL (2.2-14.6 µg/mL)
(SI: 8.9 nmol/L [20-130 nmol/L])
Serum prolactin = 10 ng/mL (4-30 ng/mL)
(SI: 0.4 nmol/L [0.2-1.3 nmol/L])
Serum glucose = 70 mg/dL (70-99 mg/dL)
(SI: 3.9 mmol/L [3.9-5.5 mmol/L])

Which of the following is the most appropriate next step in this patient's evaluation?
  A. Cosyntropin-stimulation test measuring 17-hydroxyprogesterone and cortisol
  B. Cosyntropin-stimulation test measuring DHEA and cortisol
  C. Adrenal-directed CT
  D. Plasma ACTH measurement
  E. No further testing

12 A 57-year-old man sees you for an annual visit for management of hypothyroidism. He has been on a stable levothyroxine dosage for 9 years and previously had normal blood pressure at each visit. He is not taking any other prescription medications.

On physical examination, he is a healthy-appearing, overweight, middle-aged man. His blood pressure today, however, is 162/102 mm Hg, pulse rate is 74 beats/min, and BMI is 26.0 kg/m^2. His thyroid gland is small and firm, and other physical examination findings are normal.

Routine laboratory test results:
  Sodium = 141 mEq/L (136-142 mEq/L)
    (SI: 141 mmol/L [136-142 mmol/L])
  Potassium = 2.8 mEq/L (3.5-5.0 mEq/L)
    (SI: 2.8 mmol/L [3.5-5.0 mmol/L])
  TSH = 1.2 mIU/L (0.5-5.0 mIU/L)
  Serum cortisol after 1 mg dexamethasone = <0.2 µg/dL
    (SI: <5.5 nmol/L)

After receiving these results, you take a thorough dietary history. The patient admits that he is now taking a daily weight-loss supplement containing extract of authentic licorice.

Which of the following biochemical profiles do you expect to find in this patient?

Answer	Plasma Renin Activity	Serum Aldosterone
A.	↑	↑
B.	↓	↑
C.	↑	↓
D.	↓	↓
E.	Normal	Normal

13 A 33-year-old woman underwent surgery for Cushing disease 2 years ago. She had normalization of urinary free cortisol but did not experience adrenal insufficiency and stopped hydrocortisone 6 weeks postoperatively. Over the last 6 months, she has noted weight gain, easy bruising, and poor sleep.

Laboratory test results:
  Midmorning serum cortisol = 28 µg/dL
    (5-25 µg/dL) (SI: 773 nmol/L [138-690 nmol/L])
  Plasma ACTH = 50 pg/mL (10-60 pg/mL)
    (SI: 11.0 pmol/L [2.2-13.2 pmol/L])
  Serum potassium = 3.8 mEq/L (3.5-5.0 mEq/L)
    (SI: 3.8 mmol/L [3.5-5.0 mmol/L])
  Serum glucose = 180 mg/dL (70-99 mg/dL)
    (SI: 10.0 mmol/L [3.9-5.5 mmol/L])
  Urinary free cortisol = 90 µg/24 h (4-50 µg/24 h)
    (SI: 249 nmol/d [11-138 nmol/d])

After discussing options, you decide to treat her with metyrapone, 500 mg 4 times daily, for inoperable Cushing disease. She returns in 2 weeks with slight weight loss and feels modestly better, but her serum cortisol level is unchanged. You increase her metyrapone dosage to 750 mg 4 times daily. She returns 2 weeks later complaining of severe fatigue, anorexia, myalgias, and poor sleep.

Laboratory test results while taking metyrapone (performed on hospital autoanalyzer):
  Serum cortisol 2 hours after morning metyrapone dose = 25 µg/dL (SI: 690 nmol/L)
  Serum potassium = 3.5 mEq/L (SI: 3.5 mmol/L)
  Serum glucose = 46 mg/dL (SI: 2.6 mmol/L)

Which of the following tests will help you to adjust the metyrapone dosage?
  A. Late-night salivary cortisol measurement
  B. Serum DHEA-S measurement
  C. Plasma renin activity measurement
  D. Cosyntropin-stimulation test
  E. Serum cortisol and 11-deoxycortisol measurements by tandem mass spectrometry

14 A 57-year-old woman was diagnosed with a pancreatic gastrinoma 10 years ago, when she presented with duodenal ulcers and abdominal pain. At the time of the resection, CT demonstrated a 1.3-cm pancreatic primary tumor and a single 4-cm hepatic metastasis. She underwent resection of the primary tumor and liver metastasis and was treated with depot octreotide, 30 mg every 4 weeks. Pathology showed a well-differentiated neuroendocrine tumor with a Ki-67 index (reflecting mitotic rate) of 1%. She remained well, but serial imaging demonstrated gradual appearance of multiple liver metastases (all <1 cm) with slight interval growth each year. In the 3 months since her last CT, she abruptly developed hypertension and hypokalemia, diabetes mellitus, poor sleep, muscle weakness, and depression.

On physical examination, her blood pressure is 167/96 mm Hg. She has a flat affect with slow response to commands, 2+ bilateral pedal edema, and muscle weakness.

Laboratory test results:
Serum potassium = 2.8 mEq/L (3.5-5.0 mEq/L)
  (SI: 2.8 mmol/L [3.5-5.0 mmol/L])
Serum cortisol (random) = 120 μg/dL (5-25 μg/dL)
  (SI: 3311 nmol/L [138-390 nmol/L])
Plasma ACTH = 750 pg/mL (10-60 pg/mL)
  (SI: 165.0 pmol/L [2.2-13.2 pmol/L])
Fasting serum gastrin = 95 pg/mL (<100 pg/mL)
  (SI: 95 ng/L [<100 ng/L])
Serum albumin = 4.1 g/dL (3.5-5.0 g/dL)
  (SI: 41 g/L [35-50 g/L])
Hemoglobin A_{1c} = 8.2% (4.0%-5.6%)
  (66 mmol/mol [20-38 mmol/mol])

On repeated CT, the liver metastases are not measurably changed from the scan 3 months ago. The adrenal glands are somewhat thickened but have no tumors.

Which of the following is the most appropriate next step in this patient's management?
A. Biopsy a liver metastasis
B. Perform bilateral adrenalectomy
C. Increase the depot octreotide dosage to 30 mg every 3 weeks
D. Refer to oncology for anthracycline-based chemotherapy
E. Perform liver MRI with gadolinium contrast

15 A 27-year-old woman with a history of systemic lupus erythematosus presents to the emergency department for evaluation of a 4-day history of nausea, vomiting, fatigue, and orthostasis. She was diagnosed with lupus 2 years ago when she presented with nephritis and arthralgias. She received a 12-week course of prednisone up to 60 mg daily. Since then, she has been maintained on alternate-day prednisone, 5 mg daily, with control of her arthralgias and normal renal function. She was well until 8 weeks ago, when she developed deep venous thrombosis in her right leg and antiphospholipid syndrome was diagnosed. Warfarin was added and titrated to achieve an INR in the target range. She became acutely ill 4 days ago with flank pain, but no fever or dysuria, and she has been unable to take her pills for the past 4 days.

Laboratory test results:
Sodium = 121 mEq/L (136-142 mEq/L)
  (SI: 121 mmol/L [136-142 mmol/L])
Potassium = 6.4 mEq/L (3.5-5.0 mEq/L)
  (SI: 6.4 mmol/L [3.5-5.0 mmol/L])
Plasma ACTH = 1330 pg/mL (10-60 pg/mL)
  (SI: 292.6 pmol/L [2.2-13.2 pmol/L])
Serum aldosterone = <2 ng/dL (4-21 ng/dL)
  (SI: <551 pmol/L [111-583 pmol/L])
Plasma direct renin = 350 pg/mL (4-44 pg/mL)
  (SI: 8.3 pmol/L [0.1-1.0 pmol/L])
Serum cortisol (8 AM) = <0.5 μg/dL (5-25 μg/dL)
  (SI: 14 nmol/L [138-390 nmol/L])

Which of the following tests will reveal the cause of her adrenal insufficiency?
A. Serum DHEA-S measurement
B. Pituitary MRI
C. Urine synthetic glucocorticoid screen for prednisone
D. Serum 21-hydroxylase antibody assessment
E. Adrenal CT

16 A 52-year-old man with hypertension and hypokalemia is completing evaluation for primary aldosteronism.

Screening laboratory test results:
Sodium = 147 mEq/L (136-142 mEq/L)
  (SI: 147 mmol/L [136-142 mmol/L])
Potassium = 3.2 mEq/L (3.5-5.0 mEq/L)
  (SI: 3.2 mmol/L [3.5-5.0 mmol/L])

Serum aldosterone = 24 ng/dL (4-21 ng/dL)
(SI: 666 pmol/L [111-583 pmol/L]) (repeated
measurement = 26 ng/dL [SI: 721 pmol/L])

Plasma renin activity = <0.6 ng/mL per h
(0.6-4.3 ng/mL per h) (repeated
measurement = <0.6 ng/mL per h)

CT with fine cuts of the adrenal demonstrates normal-appearing glands.

He undergoes adrenal venous sampling with continuous infusion of cosyntropin at 50 mcg per hour. The results are shown (*see table*).

Measurement	Right Adrenal Vein	Left Adrenal Vein	Inferior Vena Cava
Aldosterone	3000 ng/dL (SI: 83,220 pmol/L)	456 ng/dL (SI: 12,649 pmol/L)	40 ng/dL (SI: 1109 pmol/L)
Cortisol	750 µg/dL (SI: 20,691 nmol/L)	120 µg/dL (SI: 3311 nmol/L)	20 µg/dL (SI: 552 nmol/L)
Aldosterone-to-Cortisol Ratio	4.0	3.8	2.0

How do you interpret the results of the adrenal venous sampling study?

A. Unsuccessful study: unable to localize

B. Successful study: left adrenal gland is the source (left adenoma)

C. Successful study: both adrenal glands are sources (bilateral hyperaldosteronism)

D. Unsuccessful study: however, there is enough information to localize the source to the right adrenal (right adenoma)

E. Insufficient information to interpret whether the study was successful

17 You are asked to evaluate a 67-year-old woman with a right adrenal mass that was incidentally discovered on an annual surveillance CT performed for a medical history of colon cancer. She was treated with partial colectomy and adjuvant chemotherapy 6 years ago. The adrenal mass measures 2.2 cm in maximal diameter with a precontrast attenuation value of 25 Hounsfield units and 30% contrast washout at 10 minutes. The mass was not visible on CT 1 year ago.

On physical examination, her blood pressure is 123/84 mm Hg and pulse rate is 70 beats/min. She is clinically well and has no cushingoid features.

Laboratory test results:

Serum glucose = 90 mg/dL (70-99 mg/dL)
(SI: 5.0 mmol/L [3.9-5.5 mmol/L])

Serum potassium = 4.0 mEq/L (3.5-5.0 mEq/L)
(SI: 4.0 mmol/L [3.5-5.0 mmol/L])

Plasma metanephrine = <39 pg/mL (<99 pg/mL)
(SI: <0.2 nmol/L [<0.5 nmol/L])

Plasma normetanephrine = <147 pg/mL
(<165 pg/mL) (SI: 0.8 nmol/L [<0.9 nmol/L])

Serum cortisol after 1-mg dexamethasone =
0.8 µg/dL (SI: 22.1 nmol/L)

Which of the following is the best next step?

A. Perform ^{18}F-fluorodeoxyglucose PET

B. Perform MRI of the adrenal mass with in-phase and out-of-phase images

C. Refer for laparoscopic right adrenalectomy

D. Perform another CT in 1 year

E. Measure serum aldosterone and plasma renin activity

18 A 24-year-old woman is new to your practice for follow-up of adrenal insufficiency. She had adrenal crisis at birth and has been treated with hydrocortisone and fludrocortisone acetate her entire life. At age 12 years, she experienced breast budding and progressed to Tanner stage 3 breast development. She then had spontaneous menses 3 times over the next year but not since, and she has been given cyclic estrogen and progestin, with menstrual bleeding occurring monthly since age 16 years. She has limited knowledge about her adrenal insufficiency—just that her adrenal glands were very large when she was diagnosed as an infant.

On physical examination, she is a well-appearing young woman without syndromic features. Her blood pressure is 116/72 mm Hg, and pulse rate is 74 beats/min. She has mild hyperpigmentation of the palmar creases, Tanner stage 5 breasts, scant pubic hair without virilization, and a normal thyroid gland.

Which of the following patterns would you predict for her laboratory test results?

Answer	Progesterone	17-Hydroxyprogesterone	Androstenedione
A.	↑	↑	↑
B.	↑	↑	↓
C.	↓	↓	↓
D.	↓	↓	↑

19 A 26-year-old man is referred by his primary care physician for management of classic 21-hydroxylase deficiency. The patient was diagnosed at birth and received treatment with hydrocortisone and fludrocortisone throughout childhood. He stopped all medications at age 22 years until he had an adrenal crisis 6 months ago and nearly died. At hospital discharge, he agreed to take prednisone, 7.5 mg daily, and fludrocortisone acetate, 0.1 mg daily. He has been adherent to this regimen and states that he feels better now than when he was untreated.

On physical examination, he appears healthy and has no cushingoid features. He is a short, muscular young man with a blood pressure of 116/81 mm Hg and pulse rate of 66 beats/min.

Laboratory test results:
  Serum sodium = 135 mEq/L (136-142 mEq/L)
    (SI: 135 mmol/L [136-142 mmol/L])
  Serum potassium = 4.2 mEq/L (3.5-5.0 mEq/L)
    (SI: 4.2 mmol/L [3.5-5.0 mmol/L])
  Plasma renin activity = 2.4 ng/mL per h
    (0.6-4.3 ng/mL per h)
  Serum androstenedione = 880 ng/dL (65-210 ng/dL)
    (SI: 30.7 nmol/L [2.3-7.3 nmol/L])
  Serum total testosterone = 420 ng/dL
    (300-900 ng/dL) (SI: 14.6 nmol/L
    [10.4-31.2 nmol/L])

Which of the following is the most important test to order next?
  A. Serum aldosterone measurement
  B. Adrenal MRI
  C. Serum 17-hydroxyprogesterone measurement
  D. Testicular ultrasonography
  E. Semen analysis

20 A 28-year-old man is diagnosed with autoimmune adrenal insufficiency and hypothyroidism. He presented with a 25-lb (11.4 kg) weight loss and adrenal crisis during a gastrointestinal illness. He was discharged from the hospital taking hydrocortisone, 20 mg upon waking in the morning and 10 mg in the early afternoon, as well as levothyroxine, 125 mcg daily. He regained most of his lost weight over the next 6 months and remained well without additional crises. For convenience, his glucocorticoid was changed to methylprednisolone, 6 mg upon waking. He has continued to slowly regain his lost weight, but he now experiences a generalized feeling of fatigue throughout the day, which does not improve shortly after taking the methylprednisolone. He has even tried dividing his daily dose (3 mg upon waking and 3 mg in the early afternoon), but he did not experience relief from the fatigue following either dose.

On physical examination, his blood pressure is 104/66 mm Hg and pulse rate is 88 beats/min. He has no purple striae, facial rounding, dermal atrophy, vitiligo, or bruises.

Laboratory test results:
  Sodium = 138 mEq/L (136-142 mEq/L)
    (SI: 138 mmol/L [136-142 mmol/L])
  Potassium = 4.9 mEq/L (3.5-5.0 mEq/L)
    (SI: 4.9 mmol/L [3.5-5.0 mmol/L])
  Plasma ACTH = 400 pg/mL (10-60 pg/mL)
    (SI: 88.0 pmol/L [2.2-13.2 pmol/L])
  Plasma renin activity = 13.4 ng/mL per h
    (0.6-4.3 ng/mL per h)
  Serum TSH = 2.2 mIU/L (0.5-5.0 mIU/L)

Which of the following changes do you recommend in his management?
  A. Administer methylprednisolone, 4 mg upon waking and 2 mg at bedtime
  B. Switch methylprednisolone to hydrocortisone, 20 mg upon waking
  C. Add fludrocortisone acetate, 0.1 mg daily
  D. Switch methylprednisolone to dexamethasone, 1 mg upon waking
  E. Reassure him that no changes are necessary

21 An 84-year-old man is referred by an oncologist for evaluation of nonsuppressible testosterone. Prostate cancer was diagnosed 3 years ago, and he received local radiotherapy followed by degarelix (long-acting GnRH antagonist, androgen-deprivation therapy). His PSA concentration remained less than 1.0 ng/mL (<1.0 µg/L) for 2 years, but over the last year it has risen to 15.0 ng/mL (15.0 µg/L). A ^{99}Tc bone scan shows bone metastases, and subsequent CT shows bilateral 5- to 7-cm adrenal masses (*see image, arrows*). In retrospect, the masses were present (but slightly smaller) on baseline CT 3 years ago.

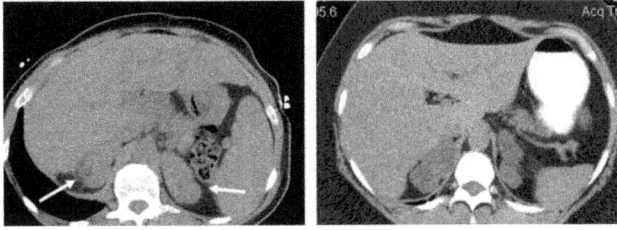

Laboratory test results:

Serum LH = <0.8 mIU/mL (1.0-9.0 mIU/mL)
(SI: <0.8 IU/L [1.0-9.0 IU/L])

Serum FSH = <0.2 mIU/mL (1.0-13.0 mIU/mL)
(SI: <0.2 IU/L [1.0-13.0 mIU/mL])

Serum total testosterone = 120 ng/dL (300-900
ng/dL) (SI: 4.2 nmol/L [10.4-31.2 nmol/L])

LH, FSH, and total testosterone are measured again
1 week later and similar values are documented. The
following test results are also obtained:

Serum androstenedione = 340 ng/dL (65-210
ng/dL) (SI: 11.9 mmol/L [2.3-7.3 mmol/L])

Plasma ACTH = 70 pg/mL (10-60 pg/mL)
(SI: 15.4 pmol/L [2.2-13.2 pmol/L])

Serum aldosterone = 3 ng/dL (4-21 ng/dL)
(SI: 83 pmol/L [111-583 pmol/L])

Plasma renin activity = 1.8 ng/mL per h
(0.6-4.3 ng/mL per h)

Serum DHEA-S = 90 µg/dL (25-131 µg/dL)
(SI: 2.4 µmol/L [0.7-3.6 µmol/L])

Plasma metanephrine = 39 pg/mL (<99 pg/mL)
(SI: <0.2 nmol/L [<0.5 nmol/L])

Plasma normetanephrine = 202 pg/mL
(<165 pg/mL) (SI: 1.1 nmol/L [<0.9 nmol/L])

Serum cortisol:

Baseline 8 AM = 11 µg/dL (5-25 µg/dL)
(SI: 303 nmol/L [138-390 nmol/L])

After 1 mg dexamethasone = <1 µg/dL
(SI: <28 nmol/L)

On physical examination, he is a well-appearing elderly
man in minimal pain. His blood pressure is 106/72 mm
Hg and pulse rate is 84 beats/min. Both testes are 4 to
6 mL, firm, and slightly irregular.

**Which of the following diagnostic studies would
provide a diagnosis?**

A. ^{123}I-MIBG SPECT-CT
B. Serum 17-hydroxyprogesterone measurement
C. Adrenal biopsy
D. Serum SHBG measurement
E. Adrenal MRI with in-phase and out-of-phase
images

22 A 67-year-old woman presents with weakness
and edema of 6 months' duration.

On physical examination, she has large supraclavicular and mild dorsocervical fat pads with slight
facial plethora and 1+ bilateral pitting edema. She has
several ecchymoses on the arms and legs, significant
dermal atrophy, and no striae. She is alert and con-
versant with moderately reduced proximal and distal
muscle strength.

Laboratory test results:

Potassium = 3.3 mEq/L (3.5-5.0 mEq/L)
(SI: 3.3 mmol/L [3.5-5.0 mmol/L])

Plasma ACTH = values in the range of 50-80 pg/mL
(10-60 pg/mL) (SI: values in the range of
11.0-17.6 pmol/L [2.2-13.2 pmol/L])

Urinary free cortisol = 85 µg/24 h (4-50 µg/24 h)
(SI: 235 nmol/d [11-138 nmol/d])

Serum cortisol after dexamethasone = 17 µg/dL
(SI: 469 nmol/L)

MRI of the pituitary (T1-weighted image with gadolinium contrast) is interpreted as normal (*see image*):

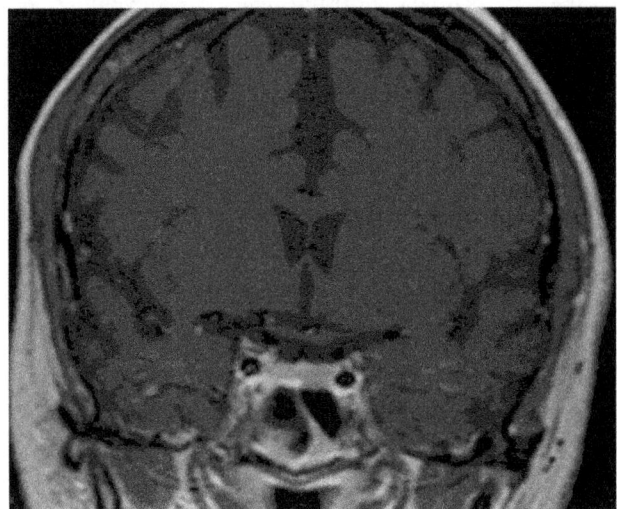

CT of the chest/abdomen/pelvis shows enlarged adrenal glands and a 9-mm vascular mass in the pancreas, interpreted as being consistent with a neuroendocrine tumor (*see image, arrow*).

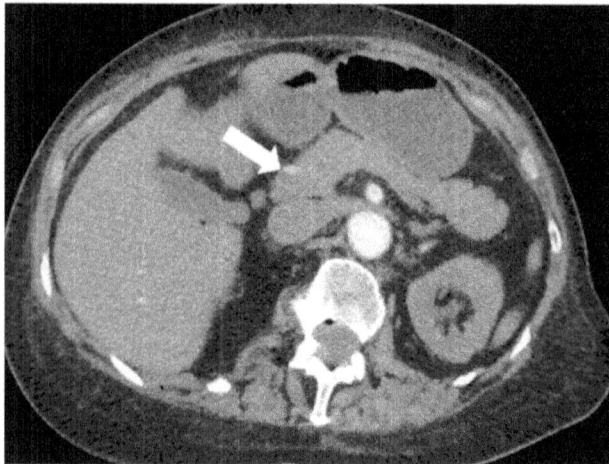

She is referred to you for further management.

Which of the following is the best next step in this patient's evaluation and management?

A. ^{111}In-DTPA-pentetreotide (octreotide) SPECT-CT

B. Serum cortisol measurement after 8 mg dexamethasone

C. ^{18}F-fluorodeoxyglucose PET-CT

D. 3 specimens for measurement of late-night salivary cortisol

E. Inferior petrosal sinus sampling

23 A 53-year-old man is referred for evaluation of primary aldosteronism. He developed resistant hypertension in his late 40s and was found to be hypokalemic 6 months ago on routine blood testing.

Screening laboratory test results:
Sodium = 147 mEq/L (136-142 mEq/L)
(SI: 147 mmol/L [136-142 mmol/L])
Potassium = 3.2 mEq/L (3.5-5.0 mEq/L)
(SI: 3.2 mmol/L [3.5-5.0 mmol/L])
Serum aldosterone = 33 ng/dL (4-21 ng/dL)
(SI: 915 pmol/L [111-583 pmol/L])
Plasma renin activity = <0.6 ng/mL per h
(0.6-4.3 ng/mL per h)

On the third day of a high-salt diet:
Urinary sodium = 280 mEq/24 h (280 mmol/d)
Urinary aldosterone = 40 µg/24 h (111 nmol/d)

CT with fine cuts of the adrenals shows minor irregularities in both glands but no conclusive tumors. Adrenal venous sampling was delayed for 4 months, and his serum potassium and blood pressure were controlled with spironolactone, 25 mg daily. He was told to stop the spironolactone 2 weeks before adrenal venous sampling.

He undergoes adrenal venous sampling with continuous infusion of cosyntropin at 50 mcg per h. As he is leaving the interventional radiology suite, however, he informs the staff that he forgot to stop the spironolactone, and he took his last dose the previous day. A week later, you receive the laboratory results (*see table*).

Measurement	Right Adrenal Vein	Left Adrenal Vein	Inferior Vena Cava
Aldosterone	300 ng/dL (SI: 8322 pmol/L)	8000 ng/dL (SI: 221,920 pmol/L)	44 ng/dL (SI: 1221 pmol/L)
Cortisol	300 µg/dL (SI: 8276 nmol/L)	800 µg/dL (SI: 22,070 nmol/L)	22 µg/dL (SI: 607 nmol/L)
Aldosterone-to-Cortisol Ratio	1.0	10.0	2.0

How do you interpret the results of the adrenal venous sampling study?

A. Unable to interpret the study and must repeat 2 weeks after stopping spironolactone

B. Left adrenal gland is the source (left adenoma)

C. Both adrenal glands are sources (bilateral, idiopathic hyperaldosteronism)

D. Right adrenal gland is the source (right adenoma)

E. Unsuccessful study, failure to access right adrenal vein

24 A 48-year-old woman has a whole-body MRI at a wellness center as part of an executive physical evaluation. The study found a 1.5-cm right adrenal tumor. She self-refers herself to your clinic to ask what she should do about the tumor. You do not have the films, but the report states that the mass has "loss of signal on out-of-phase images and low signal on T2-weighted images."

On physical examination, her blood pressure is normal, and she has no cushingoid stigmata. You tell her that based on current guidelines, you recommend screening for cortisol and catecholamine production with a 1-mg overnight dexamethasone suppression test and 24-hour urinary metanephrines.

Which feature of this case most conclusively favors that the mass is a benign cortical adenoma?

A. The size of the mass
B. Normal blood pressure
C. The fact that the tumor was found incidentally
D. MRI imaging characteristics
E. Absence of cushingoid stigmata

25 An 18-year-old man is referred for follow-up of adrenal insufficiency, which he developed at age 13 years. He takes hydrocortisone, 15 mg upon waking and 5 mg in the early afternoon, plus fludrocortisone acetate, 0.2 mg daily. He also takes fluconazole, 150 mg once weekly, for recurrent episodes of oral thrush since age 10 years. An older sibling died suddenly at age 5 of unknown causes.

On physical examination, his height is 64 in (162.6 cm) and weight is 110 lb (50 kg) (BMI = 18.9 kg/m²). He has thin nails and brown horizontal bands on his teeth without oral thrush (*see image*). His blood pressure is 115/75 mm Hg, and pulse rate is 70 beats/min. He has no hyperpigmentation or vitiligo.

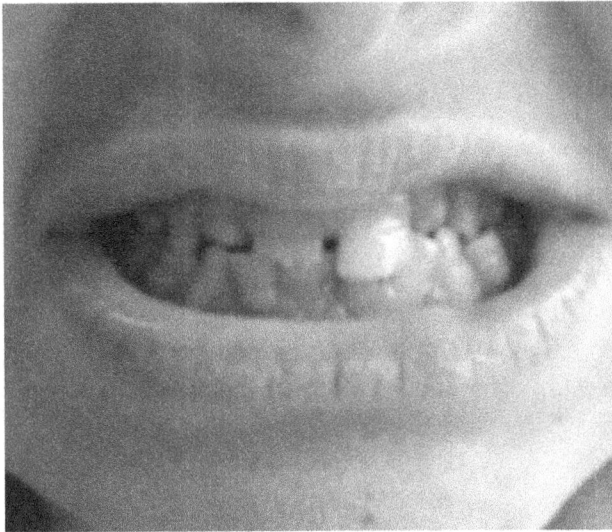

Laboratory test results (sample drawn at 9 AM):
Serum sodium = 142 mEq/L (136-142 mEq/L)
(SI: 142 mmol/L [136-142 mmol/L])
Serum potassium = 3.9 mEq/L (3.5-5.0 mEq/L)
(SI: 3.9 mmol/L [3.5-5.0 mmol/L])
Plasma ACTH = 250 pg/mL (10-60 pg/mL)
(SI: 55.0 pmol/L [2.2-13.2 pmol/L])
Plasma direct renin = 33 pg/mL (30-40 pg/mL)
(SI: 0.8 pmol/L [0.7-1.0 pmol/L])

Serum 21-hydroxylase antibodies = 70 U/mL
(<1 U/mL)

Which of the following other endocrinopathies is he most at risk to develop?

A. Hypothyroidism
B. Type 1 diabetes mellitus
C. Gonadal failure
D. Hypoparathyroidism
E. Graves disease

Calcium & Bone Board Review

Carolyn B. Becker, MD

1 A 40-year-old woman is noted to have serum calcium levels that are mildly but consistently elevated over several months of observation (range, 10.3-10.9 mg/dL [SI: 2.6-2.7 mmol/L]) (reference range, 8.2-10.2 mg/dL [SI: 2.1-2.6 mmol/L]). She notes some achiness and fatigue that she attributes to a stressful job. A recent DXA ordered by her gynecologist shows Z-scores of –1.5 at the spine and –1.2 at the hip. She has never had a fracture. No family history is available.

Laboratory test results:
PTH = 69 pg/mL (10-65 pg/mL) (SI: 69 pg/mL [10-65 ng/L])
25-Hydroxyvitamin D = 33 ng/mL (30-80 ng/mL [optimal]) (SI: 82.4 nmol/L [74.9-199.7 nmol/L])
TSH, normal
Creatinine, normal

Which of the following is the best next step in this patient's management?
A. Urinary calcium-to-creatinine clearance ratio
B. DXA of the one-third distal radius
C. Referral to a parathyroid surgeon
D. Sestamibi parathyroid scanning
E. Continued annual monitoring

2 You are evaluating a 35-year-old man who presents with low-trauma bilateral midshaft femur fractures treated surgically with rods by the orthopedist last week. His medical history is positive for 3 previous metatarsal fractures and poor dentition. His mother was diagnosed with osteoporosis in her 60s.

On physical examination, 2 teeth are missing and there are scars from recent femur surgery. Stature is normal, as are findings on testicular examination.

DXA reveals Z-scores of –3.5 at the lumbar spine, –4.0 at the total hip, and –3.8 at the femoral neck.

Preliminary laboratory test results show:
Calcium = 9.8 mg/dL (8.2-10.2 mg/dL) (SI: 2.5 mmol/L [2.1-2.6 mmol/L])
PTH = 35 pg/mL (10-65 pg/mL) (SI: 35 ng/L [10-65 ng/L])
Phosphate = 2.4 mg/dL (2.3-4.7 mg/dL) (SI: 0.8 mmol/L [0.7-1.5 mmol/L])
25-Hydroxyvitamin D = 32 ng/mL (30-80 ng/mL [optimal]) (SI: 79.9 nmol/L [74.9-199.7 nmol/L])

Measuring which of the following is key to this patient's diagnosis?
A. 24-Hour urinary calcium excretion
B. Serum C-telopeptide
C. Serum alkaline phosphatase
D. Serum 1,25-dihydroxyvitamin D
E. Serum FGF-23

3 A 50-year-old man with renal failure due to poorly controlled type 1 diabetes mellitus has been on hemodialysis for 15 years. He underwent 3.5-gland parathyroidectomy 10 years ago because of tertiary hyperparathyroidism. After temporary remission, his hyperparathyroidism returned. He comes to you now because of multiple fragility fractures over the past 2 years, including vertebral, hip, and wrist fractures.

DXA reveals T-scores of –2.5, –2.8, and –3.0 at the lumbar spine, femoral neck, and one-third distal radius, respectively. His long-term medications include cinacalcet, 90 mg twice daily, and calcitriol, 1.0 mcg twice daily.

Laboratory test results:
Serum calcium = 8.1 mg/dL (8.2-10.2 mg/dL) (SI: 2.0 mmol/L [2.1-2.6 mmol/L])
Albumin = 3.8 g/L (3.5-5.0 g/dL) (SI: 38 g/L [35-50 g/dL])
Phosphate = 5.2 mg/dL (2.3-4.7 mg/dL) (SI: 1.7 mmol/L [0.7-1.5 mmol/L])

Creatinine = 8.4 mg/dL (0.7-1.3 mg/dL)
(SI: 742.6 µmol/L [61.9-114.9 µmol/L])
25-Hydroxyvitamin D = 24 ng/mL (30-80 ng/mL
[optimal]) (SI: 59.9 nmol/L [74.9-199.7 nmol/L])
PTH = 75 pg/mL (10-65 pg/mL) (SI: 75 ng/L
[10-65 ng/L])
Alkaline phosphatase = 48 U/L (50-120 U/L)
(SI: 0.80 µkat/L [0.84-2.00 µkat/L])

Which of the following is the best next step in this patient's management?
A. Arrange for surgical removal of the remaining parathyroid tissue
B. Treat with denosumab
C. Treat with pamidronate
D. Stop cinacalcet
E. Stop calcitriol

4 A 20-year-old man is seen because of hypercalcemia, nephrocalcinosis, recurrent kidney stones, and low bone density. He had his first stone in childhood and has had frequent recurrent bilateral stones since then. Findings on recent chest x-ray are negative and CT shows bilateral nonobstructing stones and nephrocalcinosis. Prior stone analysis revealed 100% calcium phosphate. He takes no medications or supplements. Family history is negative for known calcium or renal disorders.

DXA shows Z-scores of –2.3 at the spine and –3.0 at the total hip.

Laboratory test results:
Calcium = 10.9 mg/dL (8.2-10.2 mg/dL)
(SI: 2.7 mmol/L [2.1-2.6 mmol/L])
Intact PTH = <10 pg/mL (10-65 pg/mL)
(SI: <10 ng/L [10-65 ng/L])
Phosphate = 4.5 mg/dL (2.3-4.7 mg/dL)
(SI: 1.5 mmol/L [0.7-1.5 mmol/L])
25-Hydroxyvitamin D = 40 ng/mL (30-80 ng/mL
[optimal]) (SI: 99.8 nmol/L [74.9-199.7 nmol/L])
1,25-Dihydroxyvitamin D = 95 pg/mL
(16-65 pg/mL) (SI: 247.0 pmol/L
[41.6-169.0 pmol/L])
Urinary calcium (good collection) = 450 mg/24 h
(100-300 mg/24 h) (SI: 11.3 mmol/d
[2.5-7.5 mmol/d])
Angiotensin-converting enzyme, normal

Which of the following is the most likely diagnosis?
A. Renal leak hypercalciuria
B. 24,25-Dihydroxyvitamin D deficiency
C. Sarcoidosis
D. Elevated vitamin D–binding protein
E. Vitamin D resistance

5 A 75-year-old man is admitted to the hospital with lethargy, altered mental status, nausea, and vomiting.

On physical examination, he is barely arousable. His blood pressure is 98/60 mm Hg, and pulse rate is 120 beats/min. He has dry mucosa, no lymphadenopathy or neck masses, and no organomegaly.

Chest x-ray in the emergency department reveals a 3-cm spiculated mass in the right upper lung lobe with destruction of an adjacent rib.

Laboratory tests results:
Total calcium = 16.5 mg/dL (8.2-10.2 mg/dL)
(SI: 4.1 mmol/L [2.1-2.6 mmol/L])
Ionized calcium = 7.08 mg/dL (4.60-5.08 mg/dL)
(SI 1.8 mmol/L [1.2-1.3 mmol/L])
Creatinine = 2.2 mg/dL (0.7-1.3 mg/dL)
(SI: 194.5 µmol/L [61.9-114.9 µmol/L])
Intact PTH = <10 pg/mL (10-65 pg/mL)
(SI: <10 ng/L [10-65 ng/L])
25-Hydroxyvitamin D = 23 ng/dL (30-80 ng/mL
[optimal]) (SI: 57.4 nmol/L [74.9-199.7 nmol/L])
1,25-Dihydroxyvitamin D = 12 pg/mL
(16-65 pg/mL) (SI: 31.2 pmol/L
[41.6-169.0 pmol/L])

He receives vigorous intravenous saline hydration (2 L in the first hour followed by 150 cc/h); calcitonin, 4 units/kg subcutaneously every 6 hours; and zoledronic acid, 4 mg intravenously over 30 minutes. Two days later, he is more alert and responsive.

Laboratory test results:
Serum calcium (corrected for albumin) =
12.2 mg/dL (SI: 3.1 mmol/L)
Creatinine = 1.8 mg/dL (SI: 159.1 µmol/L)

Which of the following is the best next step in this patient's management?

A. Stop calcitonin and continue current intravenous hydration

B. Increase the rate of hydration and add furosemide

C. Give denosumab, 120 mg subcutaneously

D. Give another dose of zoledronic acid, 4 mg intravenously

E. Begin intravenous methylprednisolone, 20 mg every 8 hours

6 A 45-year-old woman with longstanding symptomatic primary hyperparathyroidism undergoes resection of a large parathyroid adenoma. Because of concerns about bleeding, she is kept overnight in the hospital.

Preoperative serum laboratory results:

Calcium = 12.5 mg/dL (8.2-10.2 mg/dL)
(SI: 3.1 mmol/L [2.1-2.6 mmol/L])

Phosphate = 2.2 mg/dL (2.3-4.7 mg/dL)
(SI: 0.7 mmol/L [0.7-1.5 mmol/L])

25-Hydroxyvitamin D = 18 ng/mL (30-80 ng/mL [optimal]) (SI: 44.9 nmol/L [74.9-199.7 nmol/L])

Intact PTH = 558 pg/mL (10-65 pg/mL)
(SI: 558 ng/L [10-65 ng/L])

Alkaline phosphatase = 382 U/L (50-120 U/L)
(SI: 6.38 µkat/L [0.84-2.00 µkat/L])

On the morning after surgery, she describes perioral numbness, muscle twitching, and distal paresthesias. She has markedly positive Chvostek and Trousseau signs.

Postoperative serum laboratory results:

Calcium = 6.2 mg/dL (SI: 1.6 mmol/L)
Albumin = 3.8 g/dL (SI: 38 g/L)
Phosphate = 2.0 mg/dL (SI: 0.6 mmol/L)
Magnesium = 1.8 mg/dL (1.5-2.3 mg/dL)
(SI: 0.7 mmol/L [0.6-0.9 mmol/L])

Which of the following is the best next step in this patient's management?

A. Elemental calcium, 1000 mg 3 times daily, and calcitriol, 1 mcg twice daily by mouth

B. Ergocalciferol, 100,000 IU x1 dose; elemental calcium, 1000 mg 3 times daily; and calcitriol, 1 mcg twice daily by mouth

C. Elemental calcium, 500 mg 3 times daily; calcitriol, 1 mcg twice daily by mouth; and recombinant human PTH, 80 mcg subcutaneously daily

D. Calcium gluconate, 2 ampules (186 mg elemental calcium) in 50 cc D5W over 20 minutes intravenously, followed by elemental calcium, 1 mg/mL at 50 mL/h

E. Calcium gluconate, 4 ampules (372 mg elemental calcium) in 50 cc D5W over 20 minutes intravenously, followed by elemental calcium, 2 mg/mL at 100 mL/h

7 A 58-year-old woman is referred because of a spontaneous painful vertebral fracture in her thoracic spine. Radiographs confirm a severe compression fracture at T10 and radiographic osteopenia.

The patient entered menopause 5 years ago and did not take hormone therapy. Her main health issue is degenerative disc disease and painful osteoarthritis in her lower spine, hips, and knees for which she has received numerous injections over the past several years. Her last injection was 2 weeks ago.

Her only current medications are calcium and vitamin D supplements.

Her mother had a hip fracture at age 83 years.

On physical examination, she is obese. Her blood pressure 130/85 mm Hg. She has a round face with slight ruddiness; thin, lightly pigmented striae on her abdomen; mild kyphosis; and marked tenderness over the lower thoracic spine.

DXA documents the lowest T-score to be –3.8 at L1-L4 (a decrease of 30% since baseline DXA 3 years ago).

Laboratory testing documents normal results on complete blood cell count, chemistry screen, calcium, phosphate, alkaline phosphatase, 25-hydroxyvitamin D, and intact PTH. Results of serum and urine protein electrophoresis are normal.

Urine results (adequate collection):

Calcium = 275 mg/24 h (SI: 6.9 mmol/d)

Free cortisol = <4 µg/24 h (<11.0 nmol/d)
(undetectable)

Which of the following is the most likely cause of her severe osteoporosis?
    A. Postmenopausal bone loss
    B. Cyclical Cushing syndrome
    C. Pseudo-Cushing syndrome
    D. Exogenous glucocorticoid exposure
    E. Surreptitious hydrocortisone administration

8 A 79-year-old woman is diagnosed with osteoporosis after falling and breaking her right wrist. DXA shows T-scores of –2.8, –2.9, and –3.5 at the lumbar spine, left femoral neck, and left one-third distal radius, respectively.

Laboratory test results:

Serum calcium = 11.2 mg/dL (8.2-10.2 mg/dL)
(SI: 2.8 mmol/L [2.1-2.6 mmol/L])

Serum creatinine = 1.8 mg/dL (0.6-1.1 mg/dL)
(SI: 159.1 µmol/L [53.0-97.2 µmol/L])

Estimated glomerular filtration rate = 27 mL/min per 1.73 m^2 (>60 mL/min per 1.73 m^2)

25-Hydroxyvitamin D = 16 ng/mL (30-80 ng/mL [optimal]) (SI: 39.9 nmol/L [74.9-199.7 nmol/L])

PTH = 176 pg/mL (10-65 pg/mL) (10-65 pg/mL)
(SI: 176 ng/L [10-65 ng/L])

She refuses to consider parathyroid surgery but is willing to take medication.

Which of the following would you recommend for her bone health now?
    A. Raloxifene, 60 mg orally daily
    B. Alendronate, 70 mg orally each week
    C. Cinacalcet, 30 mg orally twice daily
    D. Cholecalciferol, 1000 IU orally daily
    E. Denosumab, 60 mg subcutaneously every 6 months

9 A 22-year-old woman comes to you for follow-up of hypoparathyroidism. She initially presented at age 3 years with a seizure and severe hypocalcemia. Since then, she has been maintained on calcium and calcitriol. She has also been treated for intermittent oral candidiasis and fungal infections of her fingernails and toenails since childhood. Otherwise, she feels well.

On physical examination, she has some tinea of the nails and negative Chvostek and Trousseau signs.

In addition to measuring calcium, phosphate, and renal function, which of the following should be measured now?
    A. Antiphospholipid antibodies
    B. Glutamic acid decarboxylase (GAD-65) antibodies
    C. 21-Hydroxylase antibodies
    D. Tissue transglutaminase antibodies
    E. TPO antibodies

10 A 54-year-old woman is referred for management of osteoporosis. She entered menopause 2 years ago, takes adequate calcium and vitamin D, exercises regularly, and has no toxic habits. She has no history of fractures. Family history is positive for hip fracture in her mother and estrogen receptor–positive breast cancer in both her mother and an older sister. The patient had a breast lump removed 5 years ago that showed cellular atypia but no malignancy.

A recent screening DXA showed a lumbar spine T-score of –2.6, femoral neck T-score of –1.8, and total hip T-score of –1.4. Vertebral fracture assessment shows no vertebral deformities.

Findings on physical examination are unremarkable and a laboratory evaluation for secondary causes of osteoporosis is normal. A fasting 8-AM serum C-telopeptide level is 275 pg/mL (104-1008 pg/mL).

Which of the following would you recommend for this patient?
    A. Oral bisphosphonate
    B. Zoledronate
    C. Denosumab
    D. Anabolic therapy
    E. Raloxifene

11 A 71-year-old man develops severe back pain after bending to lift up his grandchild. His medical history is notable for prostate cancer treated with surgery and external beam pelvic irradiation. Current medications are calcium, 500 mg daily, and vitamin D, 1000 IU daily. He has a history of heavy tobacco and alcohol use (stopped 3 years ago).

On physical examination, his BMI is 25 kg/m^2. He has tenderness over the L1 vertebra.

Screening DXA at age 70 (last year) revealed T-scores of –1.5 (L1-L4) and –1.8 (femoral neck) with FRAX scores well below treatment thresholds. Results from extensive blood and urine tests for secondary causes of fracture are negative.

Other laboratory test results:
Serum PSA = <4 ng/mL (<7.0 ng/mL) (SI: <4 µg/L [<7.0 µg/L])
Serum testosterone (8 AM) = 290 ng/dL (300-900 ng/dL) (SI: 10.1 nmol/L [10.4-31.2 nmol/L])

Which of the following is the best next step?
A. Perform DXA again and recalculate FRAX scores
B. Begin anabolic therapy (teriparatide or abaloparatide)
C. Begin an oral bisphosphonate
D. Refer for kyphoplasty and biopsy of L1
E. Begin treatment with transdermal testosterone

12 A 38-year-old man is referred to you by his primary care physician because of hypophosphatemia. The patient notes a history of joint deformities and fractures beginning in childhood, but he has had no recent fractures or bone pain. He has regular dental check-ups and has no notable dental issues at this time, although he had major dental problems in the past. His main concerns now are back pain and stiff joints that restrict his activities, including walking. Radiographs from his primary care physician show calcification of several tendons and ligaments including the Achilles tendons, as well as calcifications of interspinous ligaments (*see images*).

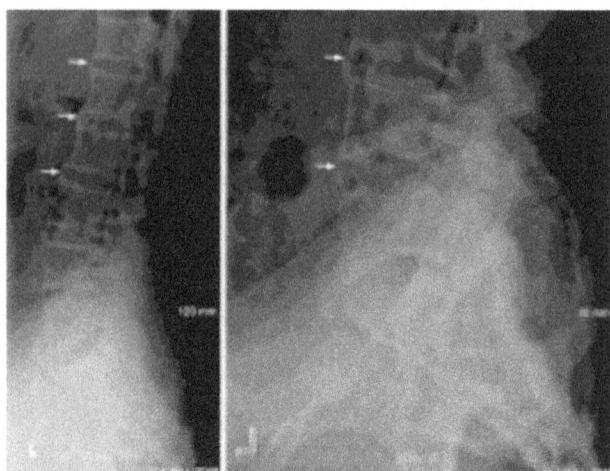

On physical examination, he has short stature, genu varum (bow-leggedness), and restricted movement at his ankles, spine, wrists, and shoulders. Sclerae are white.

Laboratory test results:
Calcium = 8.5 mg/dL (8.2-10.2 mg/dL) (SI: 2.1 mmol/L [2.1-2.6 mmol/L])
Albumin, normal
Phosphate = 1.3 mg/dL (2.3-4.7 mg/dL) (SI: 0.4 mmol/L [0.7-1.5 mmol/L])
25-Hydroxyvitamin D = 32 ng/mL (30-80 ng/mL [optimal]) (SI: 79.9 nmol/L [62.4-199.7 nmol/L])
1,25-Dihydroxyvitamin D = 30 pg/mL (16-65 pg/mL) (SI: 78.0 pmol/L [41.6-169.0 pmol/L])
Intact PTH = 75 pg/mL (10-65 pg/mL) (SI: 75 ng/L [10-65 ng/L])
Alkaline phosphatase = 184 U/L (50-120 U/L) (SI: 3.07 µkat/L [0.84-2.00 µkat/L])
Renal tubular reabsorption of phosphate, low

Which of the following would you recommend for this patient?
A. Calcitriol plus oral phosphate
B. Calcitriol only
C. Oral phosphate only
D. Cinacalcet
E. Physical therapy

13 A 63-year-old man is referred for management of bone health. He recently started prednisone, 15 mg daily, for a diffuse dermatitis that did not respond well to topical agents, and has derived tremendous benefit from this. Attempts to lower the steroid dosage have resulted in return of his rash. The dermatologist plans to continue prednisone for up to 6 months. The patient is otherwise in excellent health, consumes adequate calcium and vitamin D, and exercises regularly. He has no personal or family history of fractures.

DXA documents that the patient's lowest T-score is –1.8 at the femoral neck. A vertebral fracture assessment of the spine is negative for fractures. The FRAX calculator reveals a 10-year absolute risk for major osteoporotic fracture of 12% and a risk for hip fracture of 2.7%. The thresholds for starting pharmacologic treatment in the United States are 20% for major osteoporotic fracture and 3% for hip fracture.

Laboratory test results are normal, including vitamin D measurement.

Which of the following is the best next step?
A. Measure fasting 8-AM serum C-telopeptide
B. Measure serum procollagen type 1 N-terminal propeptide
C. Adjust the FRAX scores upward for both major osteoporotic and hip fracture risks
D. Begin an oral bisphosphonate
E. Begin anabolic therapy

14 A 75-year-old postmenopausal woman with multiple sclerosis is referred because of severe osteoporosis. She is not aware of any fractures, but she has fallen twice in the past year and has also lost height. She currently takes no medications for her neurologic disease. She takes adequate calcium and vitamin D.

DXA reveals T-scores of –3.0 at the lumbar spine (L1, L3), –2.8 at the femoral neck, and –2.6 at the total hip. Vertebral fracture assessment shows moderate compression fractures at T10, L2, and L4.

On physical examination, she is alert and mentally intact. She has moderate kyphosis without tenderness, brisk reflexes, poor balance, and a slightly unstable gait. She walks with a cane.

Laboratory test results, including serum calcium, phosphate, creatinine, PTH, TSH, serum protein electrophoresis, and 25-hydroxyvitamin D, are normal. Fasting serum C-telopeptide is 658 pg/mL (104-1008 pg/mL).

You refer her to physical therapy for muscle strengthening and gait and balance training.

In addition, which of the following would be the optimal therapy for improving her bone mineral density?
A. An oral bisphosphonate
B. Teriparatide
C. An oral bisphosphonate combined with teriparatide
D. Denosumab
E. Denosumab combined with teriparatide

15 An 82-year-old woman with severe osteoporosis presents for follow-up. She had been on oral bisphosphonates with poor adherence for years. For the past 5 years, she switched to denosumab, 60 mg subcutaneously every 6 months. She has a history of hip, humeral, and vertebral fractures, but she has done very well on denosumab. Current T-scores are –3.0 at lumbar spine (previously –3.5) and –3.2 at the total hip (previously –3.7). She asks if she can take a "drug holiday" for the next 12 to 18 months.

What do you predict will happen over the next 12 to 18 months if she goes on the drug holiday?

Answer	Bone Mineral Density at the Lumbar Spine	Bone Mineral Density at the Femoral Neck and Total Hip	Markers of Bone Turnover
A.	Decrease	Decrease	Increase
B.	No change	No change	No change
C.	Decrease	No change	Increase
D.	No change	Decrease	Increase

16 You are called to see a 36-year-old woman with hypercalcemia. She comes to the emergency department following 24 hours of nausea, vomiting, and abdominal pain. Her medical history is notable for heavy alcohol use and severe gastroesophageal reflux disease. She takes no prescription medications but does take several over-the-counter therapies "for her stomach."

On physical examination, she is afebrile and lethargic with very dry mucous membranes and epigastric tenderness.

Findings on chest x-ray and abdominal CT are normal.

Initial laboratory test results:
Calcium = 14.8 mg/dL (8.2-10.2 mg/dL) (SI: 3.7 mmol/L [2.1-2.6 mmol/L])
Phosphate = 3.5 mg/dL (2.3-4.7 mg/dL) (SI: 1.1 mmol/L [0.7-1.5 mmol/L])
Potassium = 3.0 mEq/L (3.5-5.0 mEq/L) (SI: 3.0 mmol/L [3.5-5.0 mmol/L])
Bicarbonate = 39 mEq/L (21-28 mEq/L) (SI: 39 mmol/L [21-28 mmol/L])
Serum urea nitrogen = 50 mg/dL (8-23 mg/dL) (SI: 17.9 mmol/L [2.9-8.2 mmol/L])
Creatinine = 3.5 mg/dL (0.6-1.1 mg/dL) (SI: 309.4 µmol/L [53.0-97.2 µmol/L])
Intact PTH = <10 pg/mL (10-65 pg/mL) (SI: <10 ng/L [10-65 ng/L])
Other labs, pending

After 48 hours of nothing-by-mouth and vigorous intravenous hydration, her condition is dramatically improved and her serum calcium normalizes.

Which of the following diagnoses best explains her clinical presentation?
   A. Milk-alkali syndrome
   B. Pancreatitis
   C. Dehydration
   D. Vitamin D intoxication
   E. Acute renal failure

17 A 48-year-old woman with nephrotic syndrome is found to have the following laboratory results:
   Serum calcium = 7.0 mg/dL (8.2-10.2 mg/dL)
      (SI: 2.0 mmol/L [2.1-2.6 mmol/L])
   Serum creatinine = 0.9 mg/dL (0.6-1.1 mg/dL)
      (SI: 79.6 µmol/L [53.0-97.2 µmol/L])
   Phosphate = 2.7 mg/dL (2.3-4.7 mg/dL)
      (SI: 0.9 mmol/L [0.7-1.5 mmol/L])

She reports no paresthesias or muscle cramps. On physical examination, she has 2+ pitting edema up to her mid-thighs and negative Trousseau and Chvostek signs.

Serum measurement of which of the following would be most useful to explain the laboratory findings?
   A. Intact PTH
   B. 25-Hydroxyvitamin D
   C. 1,25-Dihydroxyvitamin D
   D. Magnesium
   E. Ionized calcium

18 You are called to see a 65-year-old man in the emergency department who is brought in because of a seizure. The patient started outpatient chemotherapy for an aggressive lymphoma 3 days ago and was doing well until he developed nausea, vomiting, and weakness the day before admission. This morning, his wife found him unresponsive with tonic-clonic movements.

On physical examination, he is lethargic. He is afebrile, blood pressure is 100/60 mm Hg, and pulse rate is 120 beat/min and irregular. He has positive Chvostek and Trousseau signs, diffuse lymphadenopathy, and splenomegaly. Electrocardiography shows atrial fibrillation with peaked T-waves.

Laboratory test results (serum):
   Sodium = 130 mEq/L (136-142 mEq/L)
      (SI: 130 mmol/L [136-142 mmol/L])
   Potassium = 8.4 mEq/L (3.5-5.0 mEq/L)
      (SI: 8.4 mmol/L [3.5-5.0 mmol/L])
   Calcium = 5.4 mg/dL (8.2-10.2 mg/dL)
      (SI: 1.4 mmol/L [2.1-2.6 mmol/L])
   Uric acid = 17 mg/dL (3.5-7.0 mg/dL)
      (SI: 1011.2 µmol/L [208.2-416.4 µmol/L])
   Creatinine = 15 mg/dL (0.7-1.3 mg/dL)
      (SI: 1326 µmol/L [61.9-114.9 µmol/L])
   Bicarbonate = 10 mEq/L (21-28 mEq/L)
      (SI: 10 mmol/L [21-28 mmol/L])
   Creatine kinase = 550 U/L (50-200 U/L) (SI: 9.2 µkat/L [0.84-3.34 µkat/L])

Which of the following is the most likely cause of his severe hypocalcemia?
   A. Acute rhabdomyolysis
   B. Splenic sequestration of calcium
   C. Hyperphosphatemia
   D. Acute renal failure
   E. Severe metabolic acidosis

19 A 40-year-old woman who recently immigrated from the Middle East is referred to you for evaluation of muscle and bone pain, fatigue, weakness, spontaneous fractures, and difficulty walking. After removing her burqa (full outer garment and veil), physical examination reveals diffuse bony tenderness, proximal muscle weakness, and antalgic (waddling) gait.

DXA documents T-scores of –3 to –4 at all sites.

Laboratory test results:
   Electrolytes and renal function, normal
   Calcium (corrected for albumin) = 8.0 mg/dL
      (8.2-10.2 mg/dL) (SI: 2.0 mmol/L
      [2.1-2.6 mmol/L])
   Phosphate = 2.1 mg/dL (2.3-4.7 mg/dL)
      (SI: 0.7 mmol/L [0.7-1.5 mmol/L])
   Alkaline phosphatase = 325 U/L (50-120 U/L)
      (SI: 5.43 µkat/L [0.84-2.00 µkat/L])
   Intact PTH = 138 pg/mL (10-65 pg/mL)
      (SI: 138 ng/L [10-65 ng/L])
   25-Hydroxyvitamin D = <10 ng/mL (30-80 ng/mL
      [optimal]) (SI: 25.0 nmol/L [74.9-199.7 nmol/L])

Which of the following histomorphometric findings would you expect to see on a bone biopsy of her iliac crest?
  A. Large areas of unmineralized osteoid
  B. Thin, widely separated trabecular plates and microarchitectural damage
  C. Excessive bone resorption with disorganized, dysregulated bone formation
  D. Excessive bone resorption, fibrosis, and osteoclast-lined cysts containing pigmented blood products

20 A 31-year-old woman presents with back pain and stiffness 3 months after delivering her first child. She had an uncomplicated pregnancy and delivery and is still breastfeeding. She has no history of fractures, but her mother has osteoporosis.

On physical examination, she is thin (BMI = 21 kg/m^2). She has spinal tenderness and paraspinal muscle spasm. Radiographs show mild to moderate compression fractures at T11, L1, and L2.

DXA documents Z-scores of –3.5 at the lumbar spine, –2.8 at the femoral neck, and –1.9 at the total hip. Findings from an extensive laboratory evaluation are normal except for a 25-hydroxyvitamin D value of 18 ng/mL (30-80 ng/mL [optimal]) (SI: 44.9 nmol/L [74.9-199.7 nmol/L]).

In addition to starting calcium and vitamin D, which of the following would you recommend for this patient immediately?
  A. Teriparatide
  B. An oral bisphosphonate
  C. Denosumab
  D. Cessation of breastfeeding
  E. A fentanyl patch for pain relief

21 A 30-year-old woman is transitioning to you for management of osteogenesis imperfecta. She was diagnosed in childhood and until several years ago, her care was managed by a pediatric endocrinologist in another city. During childhood, she sustained several long-bone fractures that were initially attributed to an active lifestyle. After mild osteogenesis imperfecta was eventually diagnosed, she was treated with intravenous pamidronate for a few years. Her last fracture was at age 15 years. Currently, she has regular menses and a healthy lifestyle.

On physical examination, she is a well-appearing woman without any dysmorphic features. Her height is 65 in (165.1 cm). Sclerae appear bluish. She has no joint deformities or laxity. Her dentition appears normal.

Laboratory test results are normal, including complete blood cell count, complete chemistry panel, TSH, 25-hydroxyvitamin D, 1,25-dihydroxyvitamin D, and PTH. DXA documents Z-scores of –2.0 at the lumbar spine, –1.5 at the femoral neck, and –1.4 at the total hip.

Which of the following would you recommend now?
  A. A complete dental examination
  B. A formal hearing test
  C. Echocardiography
  D. Gynecology referral for a tubal ligation
  E. A restart of bisphosphonate therapy

22 A 52-year-old man is urgently referred to you because of hypocalcemia. He first noted the onset of occasional paresthesias and muscle cramping about 2 months ago, and the symptoms have not resolved despite taking extra calcium carbonate supplements. Four months ago, he underwent Roux-en-Y gastric bypass surgery for class 3 obesity and has already lost 60 lb (27.3 kg). Before surgery, his serum calcium level was 8.8 mg/dL (8.2-10.2 mg/dL) (SI: 2.2 mmol/L [2.1-2.6 mmol/L]) and he was asymptomatic.

In addition to bariatric surgery, his surgical history is notable for a subtotal thyroidectomy 10 years ago to treat a large multinodular goiter.

On physical examination, BMI is 40 kg/m^2. He has a mildly positive Chvostek sign and negative Trousseau sign. He has a well-healed neck scar and no palpable thyroid nodules or goiter.

Laboratory test results:
  Serum calcium (corrected for albumin) = 7.7 mg/dL (8.2-10.2 mg/dL) (SI: 1.9 mmol/L [2.1-2.6 mmol/L])
  Serum phosphate = 4.9 mg/dL (2.3-4.7 mg/dL) (SI: 1.6 mmol/L [0.7-1.5 mmol/L])
  Intact PTH = 28 pg/mL (10-65 pg/mL) (SI: 28 ng/L [10-65 ng/L])
  25-Hydroxyvitamin D = 10 ng/mL (30-80 ng/mL [optimal]) (SI: 25.0 nmol/L [74.9-199.7 nmol/L])
  Urinary calcium excretion = <50 mg/24 h (100-300 mg/24 h) (SI: <1.3 mmol/d [2.5-7.5 mmol/d])
  Serum magnesium = 1.5 mEq/L (1.5-2.2 mEq/L) (SI: 0.6 mmol/L [0.6-0.9 mmol/L])

In addition to optimizing calcium supplementation, which of the following would you recommend for this patient?

A. Ergocalciferol, 50,000 IU weekly
B. Cholecalciferol, 5000 IU daily
C. Cholecalciferol, 5000 IU daily, plus calcitriol, 0.5 mcg twice daily
D. Calcitriol, 0.5 mcg twice daily
E. Magnesium gluconate, 500 mg orally 3 times daily

23 A 73-year-old woman comes to see you for a second opinion regarding her skeletal health. She is currently due for her fifth annual infusion of zoledronate for treatment of severe osteoporosis. She did not tolerate oral bisphosphonates. The patient has had no thigh or groin pain and has tolerated the zoledronate infusions very well with an excellent bone mineral density response. However, she worries that the medication is building "bad bone" and that continuing it will cause her "femurs to crack." In an effort to address her concerns, you order a test.

Which of the following test results would be most concerning for an impending atypical femur fracture?

A. A fasting 8-AM C-telopeptide level <200 pg/mL (postmenopausal reference range = 104-1008 pg/mL)
B. Plain radiographs of the femurs showing cortical thinning of both femoral shafts
C. A radionuclide bone scan showing increased activity on the medial surface of one or both femurs
D. Plain radiographs showing a transverse linear lucency extending medially through a thickened lateral cortex on one or both femurs
E. An iliac crest bone biopsy showing increased numbers of giant, multinucleated osteoclasts

24 A 62-year-old woman is referred to you for management of primary hyperparathyroidism. She was noted to have serum calcium concentration of 10.7 mg/dL (8.2-10.2 mg/dL) (SI: 2.7 mmol/L [2.1-2.6 mmol/L]) on a routine chemistry panel. A previous serum calcium measurement from 2 years ago

was 10.0 mg/dL (2.5 mmol/L). She feels well and has no symptoms of hypercalcemia. She has no history of fractures or kidney stones.

Her medical history is notable for mild hypertension. Current medications are hydrochlorothiazide, 12.5 mg daily (for the last 4 years), and cholecalciferol, 1000 IU daily. Her family history is noncontributory.

On physical examination, her blood pressure is 120/72 mm Hg.

Laboratory test results:
Serum calcium = 11.0 mg/dL (8.2-10.2 mg/dL) (SI: 2.8 mmol/L [2.1-2.6 mmol/L])
Albumin, normal
Creatinine, normal
Phosphate = 3.0 mg/dL (2.3-4.7 mg/dL) (SI: 10.0 mmol/L [0.7-1.5 mmol/L])
Intact PTH = 60 pg/mL (10-65 pg/mL) (SI: 60 ng/L [10-65 ng/L])
25-Hydroxyvitamin D = 35 ng/mL (30-80 ng/mL [optimal]) (SI: 87.4 nmol/L [74.9-199.7 nmol/L])
Urinary calcium (adequate collection) = 105 mg/24 h (100-300 mg/24 h) (SI: 2.6 mmol/d [2.5-7.5 mmol/d])

Which of the following is the best next step?

A. Calculate the calcium-to-creatinine clearance ratio
B. Order DXA, including one-third distal radius
C. Measure 1,25-dihydroxyvitamin D
D. Measure calcium and PTH after stopping hydrochlorothiazide for 3 months
E. Order sestamibi parathyroid scan

25 A 60-year-old postmenopausal woman is found to have osteoporosis on DXA scan with the lowest T-score of –2.8 at the femoral neck. She has no history of fractures, but her mother had a hip fracture at age 75 years. A workup for secondary causes of osteoporosis shows a normal serum calcium concentration but elevated PTH concentration. She has taken cholecalciferol, 1000 IU daily, for many years, along with at least 1000 mg elemental calcium daily (diet plus a supplement).

Laboratory test results:

Serum total calcium (3 measurements) = 9.5 mg/dL, 9.8 mg/dL, and 9.7 mg/dL (8.2-10.2 mg/dL) (SI: 2.38 mmol/L, 2.45 mmol/L, 2.43 mmol/L [2.1-2.6 mmol/L])

Ionized calcium, normal

Intact PTH (3 measurements) = 87 pg/mL, 78 pg/mL, and 85 pg/mL (10-65 pg/mL) (SI: 87 ng/L, 78 ng/L, 85 ng/L [10-65 ng/L])

Urinary calcium = 180 mg/24 h (100-300 mg/24 h) (SI: 4.5 mmol/d [2.5-7.5 mmol/d])

Serum creatinine = 0.8 mg/dL (0.6-1.1 mg/dL) (SI: 70.7 μmol/L [53.0-97.2 μmol/L])

Phosphate = 2.6 mg/dL (2.3-4.7 mg/dL) (SI: 0.8 mmol/L [0.7-1.5 mmol/L])

25-Hydroxyvitamin D = 48 ng/mL (30-80 ng/mL [optimal]) (SI: 119.8 nmol/L [74.9-199.7 nmol/L])

Which of the following is the most appropriate next step?
A. Perform DXA of the one-third distal radius
B. Perform preoperative parathyroid imaging
C. Perform renal ultrasonography
D. Double the calcium supplementation and measure calcium and PTH again in 3 months
E. Measure serum calcium and PTH again in 6 months

26 A 25-year-old woman is sent to you following unsuccessful parathyroid surgery. She presented after passage of a kidney stone and was noted to be hypercalcemic. Preoperative imaging was not definitive, so she underwent bilateral neck exploration. The surgeon found and removed 2 enlarged parathyroid adenomas and biopsied 2 normal-appearing glands, yet she remains hypercalcemic.

Current postoperative laboratory test results:

Serum calcium = 11.5 mg/dL (8.2-10.2 mg/dL) (SI: 2.9 mmol/L [2.1-2.6 mmol/L])

Intact PTH = 110 pg/mL (10-65 pg/mL) (SI: 110 ng/L [10-65 ng/L])

25-Hydroxyvitamin D = 22 ng/mL (30-80 ng/mL [optimal]) (SI: 54.9 nmol/L [74.9-199.7 nmol/L])

Urinary calcium excretion (adequate collection) = 425 mg/24 h (100-300 mg/24 h) (SI: 10.6 mmol/d [2.5-7.5 mmol/d])

Her medical history is notable for 2 episodes of renal colic. Her only medication is an oral contraceptive pill for secondary amenorrhea. Her father has had multiple kidney stones and also has renal insufficiency. She has no siblings.

Which of the following is the most likely diagnosis?
A. Familial isolated primary hyperparathyroidism
B. Hyperparathyroidism–jaw tumor syndrome
C. Multiple endocrine neoplasia type 1
D. Multiple endocrine neoplasia type 2

27 A 58-year-old man is taken to the emergency department after a minor motorcycle crash. He is awake and alert, but he sustained trauma to his pelvis. Findings on radiographs are shown (*see image*). A radionuclide total body scan shows increased activity throughout the pelvis and left femur.

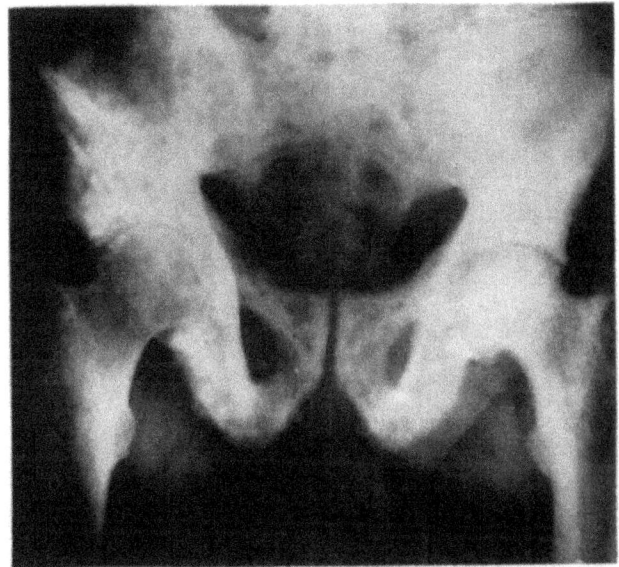

Laboratory test results document normal concentrations of serum calcium, phosphate, creatinine, 25-hydroxyvitamin D, PTH, and liver transaminases. The alkaline phosphatase concentration is 324 U/L (50-120 U/L) (SI: 5.41 μkat/L [0.84-2.00 μkat/L]).

On further questioning, the patient notes chronic pain in his left hip and pelvis, which has been getting worse over time.

Which of the following would you recommend for this patient?

   A. Alendronate, 70 mg orally weekly

   B. Zoledronate, 5 mg intravenously (1 dose)

   C. Risedronate, 35 mg orally weekly

   D. Calcitonin nasal spray, 200 IU daily

   E. Physical therapy

28 A 21-year-old woman presents with progressive massive swelling on the right side of her face and left knee swelling for the last 3 years. She has also had multiple fractures.

On physical examination, a large, firm, nontender mass is observed in the right mandible and a smaller mass is present on the left side. Knee examination reveals swelling and restricted flexion on the left side (*see images*). There are no neck masses or lymphadenopathy. The report from biopsy of the mandibular mass indicates the presence of a "giant-cell lesion."

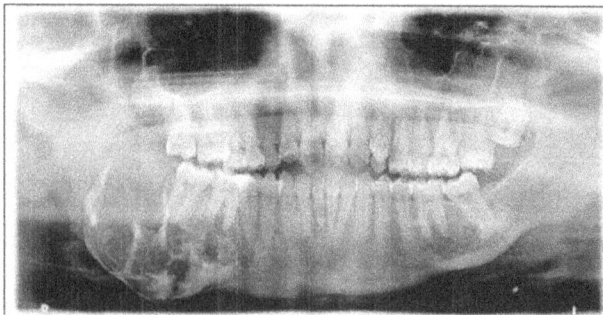

Panoramic x-ray of the jaw.

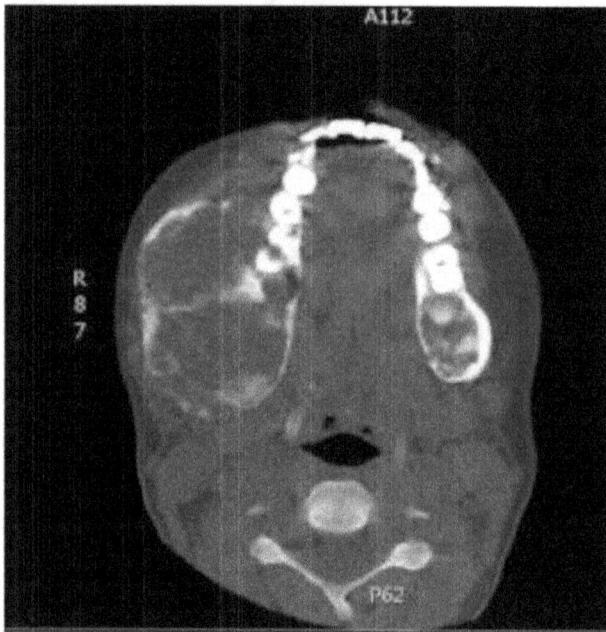

CT of the maxillofacial area.

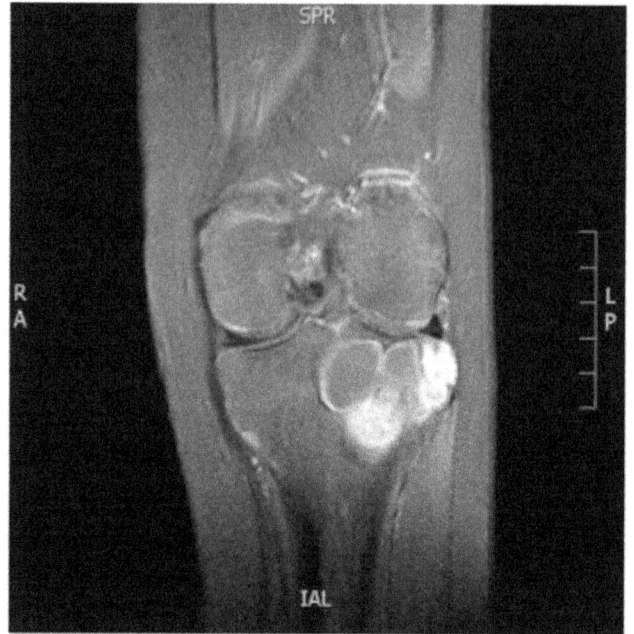

MRI of the left knee.

Laboratory test results:

   Calcium = 8.6 mg/dL (8.2-10.2 mg/dL)
     (SI: 2.2 mmol/L [2.1-2.6 mmol/L])

   Intact PTH = 1580 pg/mL (10-65 pg/mL) (SI: 1580 ng/L [10-65 ng/L])

   Alkaline phosphatase = 875 U/L (50-120 U/L)
     (SI: 14.6 μkat/L [0.84-2.00 μkat/L])

   25-Hydroxyvitamin D = <10 ng/mL (30-80 ng/mL [optimal]) (SI: 25.0 nmol/L [74.9-199.7 nmol/L])

   Serum creatinine, normal

She is treated with ergocalciferol, 50,000 IU weekly for 8 weeks. Current laboratory test results:

   Calcium = 12.1 mg/dL (8.2-10.2 mg/dL)
     (SI: 3.0 mmol/L [2.1-2.6 mmol/L])

   Intact PTH = 564 pg/mL (10-65 pg/mL) (SI: 564 ng/L [10-65 ng/L])

   25-Hydroxyvitamin D = 18.3 ng/mL (30-80 ng/mL [optimal]) (SI: 45.7 nmol/L [74.9-199.7 nmol/L])

Which of the following is this patient's most likely diagnosis?

   A. Parathyroid carcinoma

   B. Primary hyperparathyroidism with osteitis fibrosa cystica

   C. Hyperparathyroidism–jaw tumor syndrome

   D. Metastatic giant-cell tumor with ectopic PTH secretion

29 A 45-year-old transgender woman visiting from out of town is admitted to the hospital because of hypercalcemia, 30-lb (13.6-kg) weight loss, anorexia, nausea, and malaise for the past 3 months. She underwent bilateral orchiectomy 20 years ago and had bilateral breast and buttock implants 7 years ago. Her only medication is transdermal estradiol. She does not drink, smoke cigarettes, or take illicit drugs.

Findings on physical examination are notable for lethargy, dehydration, and firm masses in the buttocks and upper thighs. Findings on CT of the chest are normal. Abdominal CT shows bilateral nephrocalcinosis and nephrolithiasis.

Laboratory test results:
Serum calcium (corrected for albumin) = 15.2 mg/dL (8.2-10.2 mg/dL) (SI: 3.8 mmol/L [2.1-2.6 mmol/L])
Serum phosphate = 5.2 mg/dL (2.3-4.7 mg/dL) (SI: 1.7 mmol/L [0.7-1.5 mmol/L])
Creatinine = 3.0 mg/dL (0.6-1.1 mg/dL) (SI: 265.2 µmol/L [53.0-97.2 µmol/L])
Intact PTH = <10 pg/mL (10-65 pg/mL) (SI: <10 ng/L [10-65 ng/L])
1,25-Dihydroxyvitamin D = 105 pg/mL (16-65 pg/mL) (SI: 273 pmol/L [41.6-169.0 pmol/L])

Which of the following is this patient's most likely diagnosis?
A. Systemic sarcoidosis
B. B-cell lymphoma
C. Disseminated coccidioidomycosis
D. Leiomyosarcoma
E. Foreign-body granulomata

30 A 20-year-old homeless woman is taken to the emergency department for evaluation. She is unable to provide a clear history due to mild intellectual disability, but she does describe numbness and tingling of her hands.

On physical examination, she is short and obese. Her hand film is shown (*see image*).

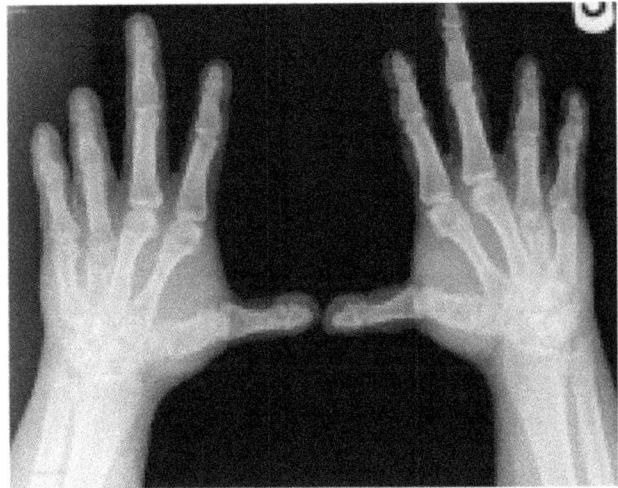

Laboratory test results:
Calcium = 6.0 mg/dL (8.2-10.2 mg/dL) (SI: 1.5 mmol/L [2.1-2.6 mmol/L])
Albumin = 3.0 g/dL (3.5-5.0 g/dL) (SI: 30 g/L [35-50 g/dL])
Phosphate = 5.9 mg/dL (2.3-4.7 mg/dL) (SI: 1.9 mmol/L [0.7-1.5 mmol/L])
PTH = 420 pg/dL (10-65 pg/mL) (SI: 420 ng/L [10-65 ng/L])
25-Hydroxyvitamin D = 16 ng/mL (30-80 ng/mL [optimal]) (SI: 39.9 nmol/L [74.9-199.7 nmol/L])
TSH = 8.0 mIU/L (0.5-5.0 mIU/L)
Free T_4 = 0.9 ng/dL (0.8-1.8 ng/dL) (SI: 11.6 pmol/L [10.30-23.17 pmol/L])

Which of the following genetic profiles is most consistent with her clinical presentation?
A. Deletion of a small segment of chromosome 22 (22q11.2 deletion syndrome)
B. Inactivating pathogenic variant in the *GNAS* gene inherited from her mother
C. Inactivating pathogenic variant in the *GNAS* gene inherited from her father
D. Activating pathogenic variant in the *CASR* gene
E. Inactivating pathogenic variant in the *AIRE* gene

Diabetes Mellitus Section 1 Board Review

Serge A. Jabbour, MD

1 A 48-year-old woman with a 6-year history of type 2 diabetes mellitus is referred for a second opinion regarding her unexplained high hemoglobin A_{1c} level. She has been treated with basal plus mealtime insulin for 3 years. She performs self-monitoring of blood glucose 6 to 8 times daily, with values ranging between 75 and 120 mg/dL (4.2-6.7 mmol/L) before meals and between 110 and 130 mg/dL (6.1-7.2 mmol/L) 2 hours after meals. She reports rare hypoglycemic episodes.

Her review of systems is notable for recent fatigue and lightheadedness. Her medications include aspirin and ramipril. For years, her hemoglobin A_{1c} level has been in the range of 6.5% to 6.9% (48-52 mmol/mol), but 4 months ago it was 7.8% (62 mmol/mol) and a recent value was 8.5% (69 mmol/mol).

Laboratory test results:
Hemoglobin = 8.9 g/dL (12.1-15.1 g/dL)
(SI: 89 g/L [121-151 g/L])
Serum creatinine = 0.8 mg/dL (0.6-1.1 mg/dL)
(SI: 70.7 μmol/L [53.0-97.2 μmol/L])
Liver function, normal
TSH, normal
Urine albumin-to-creatinine ratio = 205 mg/g creat
(<30 mg/g creat)

Which of the following is the most likely cause of her high hemoglobin A_{1c}?
A. Iron deficiency
B. Laboratory error
C. Hemolysis
D. Pregnancy
E. High nighttime blood glucose levels

2 A 31-year-old man with a 16-year history of type 1 diabetes mellitus complicated by nephropathy and retinopathy is referred for help achieving better glycemic control. His regimen consists of insulin degludec, 18 units at bedtime, and insulin lispro with meals using an insulin-to-carbohydrate ratio of 1:12. He performs self-monitoring of blood glucose 4 times daily, with values ranging between 200 and 300 mg/dL (11.1-16.7 mmol/L). His hemoglobin A_{1c} level has been between 8.5% and 10.0% (69-86 mmol/mol). His medications include lisinopril, rosuvastatin, and biotin.

Laboratory test results:
Hemoglobin A_{1c} = 9.0% (4.0%-5.6%)
(75 mmol/mol [20-38 mmol/mol])
Serum creatinine = 2.2 mg/dL (0.7-1.3 mg/dL)
(SI: 194.5 μmol/L [61.9-114.9 μmol/L])
Urine albumin-to-creatinine ratio = 3886 mg/g creat (<30 mg/g creat)
Liver function, normal
TSH = 7.5 mIU/L (0.5-5.0 mIU/L)
Serum fructosamine = 210 μmol/L
(200-285 μmol/L)

The discrepancy between this patient's hemoglobin A_{1c} and fructosamine levels is most likely caused by which of the following?
A. Laboratory error
B. Biotin
C. Hemolysis
D. Hypothyroidism
E. Proteinuria

3 A 42-year-old man with a 22-year history of type 1 diabetes mellitus is seeing you for a follow-up visit. He has had poor glycemic control over the past few years while on insulin pump therapy. He is reluctant to increase his pump settings because of the potential for weight gain. He has tried metformin and pramlintide in the past, but he could not tolerate the gastrointestinal adverse effects. His hemoglobin A_{1c} value is now 7.8% (62 mmol/mol), and his BMI is 27 kg/m^2.

His basic metabolic panel, liver function, and TSH level are normal. You suggest off-label use of empagliflozin to lower his hemoglobin A_{1c} and reduce his weight. He asks about potential adverse effects.

You tell him that empagliflozin could increase his risk of which of the following?
   A. Hip fracture
   B. Diabetic ketoacidosis
   C. Bladder tumor
   D. Lower-limb amputations
   E. Hyperkalemia

4 A 32-year-old woman with type 1 diabetes mellitus is 6 weeks' pregnant. Her most recent hemoglobin A_{1c} value is 6.9% (52 mmol/mol). She is taking insulin detemir, 8 units in the morning and 12 units in the evening, in addition to prandial doses of insulin aspart based on an insulin-to-carbohydrate ratio of 1:10 and a sensitivity (or correction) factor of 1:40. Her overnight (3 AM) and fasting blood glucose levels range between 110 and 122 mg/dL (6.1-6.8 mmol/L), and her peak (1-hour) postprandial glucose levels range between 112 and 129 mg/dL (6.2-7.2 mmol/L).

Which of the following should you recommend during this pregnancy?
   A. Continue same regimen
   B. Change insulin-to-carbohydrate ratio to 1:8
   C. Increase morning insulin detemir to 12 units
   D. Increase evening insulin detemir to 14 units
   E. Change sensitivity (or correction) factor to 1:30

5 A 35-year-old man has a 15-year history of type 1 diabetes mellitus complicated by nonproliferative diabetic retinopathy. He is concerned about renal complications of diabetes. His most recent hemoglobin A_{1c} level is 7.8% (62 mmol/mol) on insulin glargine and mealtime insulin aspart.

Two separate measurements of his urine albumin-to-creatinine ratio are 20 and 12 mg/g creat. His estimated glomerular filtration rate is 82 mL/min per 1.73 m^2 (>60 mL/min per 1.73 m^2).

On physical examination, his blood pressure is 128/72 mm Hg and BMI is 24 kg/m^2.

Which of the following is the most effective approach to reduce future risk of clinically significant diabetic nephropathy in this patient?
   A. Start ramipril
   B. Start losartan
   C. Advise a reduction in his dietary protein intake to <0.5 g/kg per day
   D. Lower his hemoglobin A_{1c} to <7.0% (<53 mmol/mol)
   E. Lower his blood pressure to <120/70 mm Hg

6 A 19-year-old man presents for continued management of diabetes mellitus, having "aged-out" of pediatric endocrine care. Diabetes was diagnosed at age 16 years when glycosuria and moderate hyperglycemia were documented on a yearly checkup. Insulin therapy was started immediately. His current insulin dose is approximately 0.3 units/kg per day, administered as multiple daily injections, and his current hemoglobin A_{1c} level is 6.4% (46 mmol/mol) with occasional hypoglycemia. His family history is positive for diabetes in his mother, maternal grandfather, and an older sibling, all diagnosed at age 19 years or younger. His BMI is 23 kg/m^2.

Tests for glutamic acid decarboxylase antibodies, islet-cell antibodies, insulinoma-associated protein 2 antibodies, and ZnT8 antibodies are negative; he did not have antibody testing at the time of diagnosis. His serum C-peptide concentration is 1.1 ng/mL (0.4 nmol/L).

Which of the following is the optimal management of this patient's diabetes?
   A. Insulin administration via insulin pump therapy
   B. Discontinuation of insulin and initiation of dapagliflozin
   C. Discontinuation of insulin and initiation of glimepiride
   D. Discontinuation of insulin and initiation of metformin

7 A 58-year-old man with no notable medical history presents to his primary care physician after unintentionally losing 10 lb (4.5 kg) over the last few months, as well as having a 2-week history of polyuria and nocturia. His family history includes diabetes mellitus in a maternal aunt.

On physical examination, his blood pressure is 110/72 mm Hg, weight is 163 lb (74.1 kg), and BMI is

24 kg/m^2. His examination findings are unremarkable, with no localizing signs of infection.

Laboratory test results:
 Random serum glucose = 254 mg/dL
  (70-99 mg/dL) (SI: 14.1 mmol/L
  [3.9-5.5 mmol/L])
 Hemoglobin A$_{1c}$ = 8.3% (4.0%-5.6%)
  (67 mmol/mol [20-38 mmol/mol])
 Creatinine = 0.7 mg/dL (0.7-1.3 mg/dL)
  (SI: 61.9 µmol/L [61.9-114.9 µmol/L])
 Complete blood cell count, normal
 Electrolytes, normal

He is referred to you 3 months later, while he is taking metformin, 1000 mg twice daily. He has lost an additional 5 lb (2.3 kg). You review the following laboratory test results:
 Random serum glucose = 233 mg/dL
  (SI: 12.9 mmol/L)
 Hemoglobin A$_{1c}$ = 9.1% (76 mmol/mol)
 C-peptide = 0.6 ng/mL (0.9-4.3 ng/mL)
  (SI: 0.2 nmol/L [0.30-1.42 nmol/L])

Review of his twice-daily self-monitoring blood glucose log reveals most values in the range of the high 100s to low 200s (mg/dL) (5.6-11.1 mmol/L), with an average of 189 mg/dL (10.5 mmol/L).

Which of the following is the best next step to manage this patient's glycemia?
 A. Start insulin
 B. Add an SGLT-2 inhibitor
 C. Add a once-weekly GLP-1 receptor agonist
 D. Add a sulfonylurea

8 An 82-year-old woman with a 22-year history of type 2 diabetes mellitus has developed episodes of confusion and disorientation over the past few weeks. Her current diabetes treatment regimen consists of insulin degludec, 50 units at bedtime; metformin, 1000 mg twice daily; and nateglinide, 60 mg before meals. She measures her blood glucose levels 3 times daily, typically before meals. Over the past few weeks, she has had several blood glucose values less than 50 mg/dL (<2.8 mmol/L), but she has not felt any symptoms of hypoglycemia. Her hemoglobin A$_{1c}$ level is 6.2% (44 mmol/mol). You diagnose hypoglycemia unawareness.

Blood chemistries, urinalysis, and liver function tests are within normal limits.

Which of the following is the best next step in her care?

	Insulin Degludec	Nateglinide
A.	Decrease to 40 units at bedtime	Continue same dosage
B.	Decrease to 40 units at bedtime	Discontinue
C.	Replace with 50 units of insulin detemir	Discontinue
D.	Replace with 25 units of twice-daily NPH insulin	Discontinue

9 A 65-year-old man is referred by his primary care physician for a 12-year history of uncontrolled type 2 diabetes mellitus. Diet, exercise, and 3 agents (metformin, glimepiride, and canagliflozin) have been unsuccessful. One year ago, oral agents were discontinued and he was prescribed intensive insulin therapy with multiple daily injections. Currently, he is on 80 units of insulin glargine twice daily and 120 units daily of insulin lispro with meals. However, his hemoglobin A$_{1c}$ levels have ranged from 9.4% to 10.7% (79-93 mmol/mol).

On physical examination, his BMI is 46 kg/m^2 and blood pressure is 130/79 mm Hg.

Laboratory test results:
 Hemoglobin A$_{1c}$ = 9.8% (4.0%-5.6%)
  (84 mmol/mol [20-38 mmol/mol])
 Estimated glomerular filtration rate = 68 mL/min
  per 1.73 m^2 (>60 mL/min per 1.73 m^2)

Which of the following is the best next step to improve this patient's glycemic control?
 A. Add linagliptin to current insulin therapy
 B. Convert multiple daily injections to insulin pump therapy with insulin lispro
 C. Convert the insulin regimen to regular U500 insulin
 D. Switch insulin glargine to insulin degludec, 110 units in the morning and evening

10 A 36-year-old Asian American man presents to his primary care physician for an annual visit. He feels well and has no concerns. He has no known medical conditions. His only medication is a daily multivitamin. He has no known family history of diabetes mellitus and does not smoke cigarettes or drink alcohol.

On physical examination, his blood pressure is 120/70 mm Hg and BMI is 24.0 kg/m^2. The rest of his examination findings are unremarkable.

In addition to lifestyle management counseling regarding diet and physical activity, when should screening be performed with respect to his prediabetes/diabetes risk?

A. Now

B. At age 45 years

C. When symptomatic

D. Only if BMI is greater than 25 kg/m^2

11 A 17-year-old woman is referred to you for her recent diagnosis of diabetes mellitus. Her father has confirmed type 1 diabetes, and the patient, out of curiosity, checked her own blood glucose level with his glucose meter. She reported a value of 212 mg/dL (11.8 mmol/L) 2 hours after dinner. A hemoglobin A$_{1c}$ measurement was subsequently documented to be 6.9% (52 mmol/mol) and a fasting glucose value was 91 mg/dL (5.1 mmol/L). Tests for islet-cell antibodies, insulin autoantibodies, and glutamic acid decarboxylase autoantibodies were negative. The patient began a low-carbohydrate diet and has been exercising regularly for 3 months, but her repeated hemoglobin A$_{1c}$ level is now 7.4% (57 mmol/mol) and many of her postprandial glucose measurements are in the range of 200 to 250 mg/dL (11.1-13.9 mmol/L). She has no symptoms of hyperglycemia.

On physical examination, she has no skin tags or acanthosis nigricans. Her weight is 153 lb (69.5 kg) (BMI = 23 kg/m^2). You wonder whether she has type 1 diabetes.

Which of the following should you order next to help confirm the diagnosis of type 1 diabetes?

A. Fructosamine measurement

B. Zinc transporter 8 (ZnT8) antibody testing

C. Genetic testing for pathogenic variants in the *GCK* gene (glucokinase)

D. Genetic testing for pathogenic variants in the *HNF1A* gene (hepatocyte nuclear factor-1 alpha)

12 A 32-year-old woman with a 6-year history of type 1 diabetes mellitus is referred to you to establish care. She has no diabetes complications and is not planning pregnancy. Her treatment regimen consists of insulins degludec and aspart. She takes an oral contraceptive. She exercises regularly.

On physical examination, her blood pressure is 120/70 mm Hg and BMI is 27 kg/m^2.

Laboratory test results:

Hemoglobin A$_{1c}$ = 6.9% (4.0%-5.6%) (52 mmol/mol [20-38 mmol/mol])

Total cholesterol = 206 mg/dL (<200 mg/dL) (SI: 5.34 mmol/L [<5.18 mmol/L])

LDL cholesterol = 126 mg/dL (<100 mg/dL) (SI: 3.26 mmol/L [<2.59 mmol/L])

HDL cholesterol = 40 mg/dL (>60 mg/dL) (SI: 1.04 mmol/L [>1.55 mmol/L])

Triglycerides = 210 mg/dL (<150 mg/dL) (SI: 2.37 mmol/L [<1.70 mmol/L])

Serum creatinine = 0.86 mg/dL (0.6-1.1 mg/dL) (SI: 76.0 µmol/L [53.0-97.2 µmol/L])

Urinary albumin-to-creatinine ratio = 19 mg/g creat (<30 mg/g creat)

Which of the following should you advise as the best course of action?

A. Start omega-3 fatty acids (460 mg eicosapentaenoic acid and 380 mg docosahexaenoic acid), 1 g daily

B. Start atorvastatin, 10 mg daily

C. Start ramipril, 10 mg daily

D. Start fenofibrate, 145 mg daily

E. Refer to a nutritionist

13 A 28-year-old man is referred to you for a 1-year history of low libido and erectile dysfunction. He drinks 2 beers daily.

On physical examination, his BMI is 27 kg/m^2 and blood pressure is 110/60 mm Hg. He has no cushingoid features. He has a mildly enlarged, nontender liver.

Laboratory test results:

Hemoglobin A$_{1c}$ = 6.9% (4.0%-5.6%) (52 mmol/mol [20-38 mmol/mol])

Creatinine = 0.8 mg/dL (0.7-1.3 mg/dL) (SI: 70.7 µmol/L [61.9-114.9 µmol/L])

ALT = 142 U/L (10-40 U/L) (SI: 2.4 µkat/L [0.17-0.67 µkat/L])

Total testosterone = 220 ng/dL (300-900 ng/dL) (SI: 7.6 nmol/L [10.4-31.2 nmol/L])

Which of the following tests is the best next step?
  A. Glutamic acid decarboxylase antibody titer
  B. Total iron-binding capacity and serum ferritin measurements
  C. Liver ultrasonography
  D. Pituitary MRI

14 A 68-year-old man wants your opinion on how he can prevent diabetes in the future. He has a history of hypertension and dyslipidemia, both well controlled on ramipril and atorvastatin.

On physical examination, his BMI is 33 kg/m² and blood pressure is 120/60 mm Hg. He has 2+ edema in both lower extremities. Findings are otherwise unremarkable.

Recent laboratory test results:
  Plasma glucose (fasting) = 108 mg/dL
    (70-99 mg/dL) (SI: 6.0 mmol/L [3.9-5.5 mmol/L])
  2-Hour postload glucose = 165 mg/dL
    (SI: 9.2 mmol/L)
  Hemoglobin A_{1c} = 5.9% (4.0%-5.6%)
    (41 mmol/mol [20-38 mmol/mol])
  Serum creatinine, normal
  Liver function tests, normal
  TSH, normal
  Estimated glomerular filtration rate = 76 mL/min
    per 1.73 m² (>60 mL/min per 1.73 m²)

On the basis of available studies, which of the following is the best option?
  A. Once-weekly exenatide
  B. Dapagliflozin
  C. Metformin
  D. Lifestyle intervention
  E. Pioglitazone

15 A 25-year-old woman with a 10-year history of type 1 diabetes mellitus is seeing you for a follow-up visit. She has been stressed out at work for the past few months and reports having intermittent nausea for the last few days. She tells you that she feels unwell and attributes it to stress. She uses insulin pump therapy with insulin lispro at a basal rate of 1.4 units/h, an insulin-to-carbohydrate ratio of 1:10, and a sensitivity factor of 1:30. She has not been doing glucose fingerstick readings at home on a regular basis, but when she does, the values range between 70 and 250 mg/dL (3.9-13.9 mmol/L) without a real pattern. A glucose fingerstick measurement in the office today is 385 mg/dL (21.4 mmol/L).

Laboratory tests from 2 weeks ago show a hemoglobin A_{1c} value of 8.3% (67 mmol/mol) with normal basic metabolic panel, TSH, and complete blood cell count. A pregnancy test is negative.

Which of the following is the best immediate next step?
  A. Basal rate testing
  B. Diabetes education
  C. Assessment for ketones
  D. Initiation of a continuous glucose sensor
  E. Therapy for stress management

16 You are asked to see a 72-year-old man with a 30-year history of type 2 diabetes mellitus who is admitted to the hospital with severe hyperglycemia and change in mental status. The patient lives alone and was found by his neighbor in a confused state. It is unclear whether the patient has been taking his insulin and other medications.

On physical examination, the patient is lethargic and unable to answer any questions. His temperature is 100.5°F (38.1°C), blood pressure is 100/60 mm Hg, and pulse rate is 110 beats/min. His weight is 220 lb (100 kg), and BMI is 32 kg/m². Skin and mucous membranes are dry. There is no focal neurologic deficit.

Laboratory test results:
  Hemoglobin A_{1c} = 9.5% (4.0%-5.6%)
    (80 mmol/mol [20-38 mmol/mol])
  Plasma glucose = 1300 mg/dL (70-99 mg/dL)
    (SI: 72.2 mmol/L [3.9-5.5 mmol/L])
  Serum sodium = 126 mEq/L (136-142 mEq/L)
    (SI: 126 mmol/L [136-142 mmol/L])
  Serum potassium = 4.5 mEq/L (3.5-5.0 mEq/L)
    (SI: 4.5 mmol/L [3.5-5.0 mmol/L])
  Serum bicarbonate = 21 mEq/L (21-28 mEq/L)
    (SI: 21 mmol/L [21-28 mmol/L])
  Serum chloride = 106 mEq/L (96-106 mEq/L)
    (SI: 106 mmol/L [96-106 mmol/L])
  Serum creatinine = 1.9 mg/dL (0.7-1.3 mg/dL)
    (SI: 168.0 µmol/L [61.9-114.9 µmol/L])
  Arterial pH = 7.35 (7.35-7.45)
  Serum β-hydroxybutyrate = 2.6 mg/dL
    (<3.0 mg/dL) (SI: 249.8 µmol/L [<288.2 µmol/L])
  Effective serum osmolality = 324 mOsm/kg
    (275-295 mOsm/kg) (SI: 324 mmol/kg
    [275-295 mmol/kg])

Which of the following is the best next step?

	Fluids	Insulin
A.	1.5 L of 0.9% NaCl over the first hour	Intravenous insulin bolus of 10 units, then 10 units per hour
B.	1.5 L of 0.9% NaCl over the first hour	Intravenous insulin bolus of 4 units, then 2 units per hour
C.	1.5 L of 0.45% NaCl over the first hour	Intravenous insulin bolus of 10 units, then 10 units per hour
D.	1.5 L of 0.45% NaCl over the first hour	Intravenous insulin at 10 units per hour
E.	1.5 L of 3.0% NaCl over the first hour	Intravenous insulin bolus of 10 units, then 10 units per hour

17 A 69-year-old man with type 2 diabetes mellitus is seeing you for a routine follow-up visit and is accompanied by his wife. His medical history is notable for hypertension and dyslipidemia. His main concern is fatigue, which he has been experiencing for the past few months. One of his friends told him he should have testing for "adrenal fatigue." He has erectile dysfunction despite normal libido. His medications include metformin, sitagliptin, rosuvastatin, ramipril, and baby aspirin. He does not smoke cigarettes.

On physical examination, his BMI is 36 kg/m^2 and blood pressure is 120/60 mm Hg.

Laboratory test results:
Hemoglobin A_{1c} = 6.8% (4.0%-5.6%)
(51 mmol/mol [20-38 mmol/mol])
Hemoglobin = 17.0 g/dL (13.8-17.2 g/dL)
(SI: 170 g/L [138-172 g/L])
Serum sodium = 141 mEq/L (136-142 mEq/L)
(SI: 141 mmol/L [3.9-5.5 mmol/L])
Serum potassium = 4.0 mEq/L (3.5-5.0 mEq/L)
(SI: 4.0 mmol/L [3.5-5.0 mmol/L])
Serum creatinine = 0.6 mg/dL (0.7-1.3 mg/dL)
(SI: 53.0 µmol/L [61.9-114.9 µmol/L])
TSH = 3.8 mIU/L (0.5-5.0 mIU/L)
Serum cortisol (8 AM) = 12 µg/dL (5-25 µg/dL)
(SI: 331.1 nmol/L [137.9-689.7 nmol/L])
Total testosterone = 250 ng/dL (300-900 ng/dL)
(SI: 8.7 nmol/L [10.4-31.2 nmol/L])
LH = 4.0 mIU/mL (1.0-9.0 mIU/mL)
(SI: 4.0 IU/L [1.0-9.0 IU/L])
FSH = 9.0 mIU/mL (1.0-13.0 mIU/mL)
(SI: 9.0 IU/L [1.0-13.0 IU/L])

Which of the following assessments should you order next?
A. Cosyntropin-stimulation test
B. Pituitary MRI
C. Serum prolactin measurement
D. Polysomnography
E. Free T_4 measurement

18 You are evaluating a 48-year-old woman with new-onset type 2 diabetes mellitus. Non-alcoholic steatohepatitis was recently diagnosed after routine testing showed abnormal liver function. Subsequent workup, including a liver biopsy, revealed nonalcoholic steatohepatitis with pathologic evidence of steatosis, lobular inflammation, hepatocellular ballooning, and fibrosis. There was no evidence of cirrhosis.

Laboratory test results:
Hemoglobin A_{1c} = 8.0% (4.0%-5.6%)
(64 mmol/mol [20-38 mmol/mol])
Creatinine = 0.8 mg/dL (0.6-1.1 mg/dL)
(SI: 70.7 µmol/L [53.0-97.2 µmol/L])
Alanine aminotransferase = 89 U/L (10-40 U/L)
(SI: 1.5 µkat/L [0.17-0.67 µkat/L])
TSH = 2.5 mIU/L (0.5-5.0 mIU/L)

The hepatologist suggests that you prescribe an antidiabetes agent that would also improve her liver histology.

Which of the following would be the best choice?
A. Metformin
B. Dapagliflozin
C. Dulaglutide
D. Sitagliptin
E. Pioglitazone

19 A 26-year-old woman with polycystic ovary syndrome is seeing you for the first time to establish care after her previous endocrinologist left the area. She has had irregular menses since menarche, facial hirsutism, and acne. She has had a good clinical response to hormonal contraception and spironolactone. She has no concerns at this time and has no pregnancy plans.

On physical examination, her BMI is 32 kg/m^2 and blood pressure is 110/60 mm Hg. She has acanthosis nigricans on her neck.

Electrolytes, creatinine, and TSH are normal.

Which of the following is the most sensitive test to evaluate her risk for diabetes?
- A. 2-Hour oral glucose tolerance test
- B. Serum insulin measurement
- C. Hemoglobin A$_{1c}$ measurement
- D. Fasting glucose measurement
- E. Glucose-to-insulin ratio

20 An 18-year-old man is referred to you for management of type 1 diabetes mellitus, which was recently diagnosed during a hospital admission 6 weeks ago. After conversion from an intravenous insulin drip, he started basal and mealtime insulins. He is currently doing well with stable home blood glucose measurements and has no concerns.

If testing for other autoimmune conditions, which of the following antibodies will this patient most likely have?"
- A. Tissue transglutaminase antibodies
- B. Thyroid-stimulating immunoglobins
- C. 21-Hydroxylase antibodies
- D. Parathyroid gland antibodies
- E. TPO antibodies

21 A 22-year-old woman has a 10-year history of type 1 diabetes mellitus. She is referred to you for management of poor glycemic control. Her diabetes treatment regimen consists of bedtime insulin glargine, 16 units, and mealtime insulin lispro at a dose of 1 unit for every 10 g of carbohydrates. Her glycemic control was initially acceptable with hemoglobin A$_{1c}$ values around 7.0% (53 mmol/mol), but over the past few years, she has missed a few appointments and her hemoglobin A$_{1c}$ has reached 9.0% to 10.0% (75-86 mmol/mol). She has had 3 episodes of diabetic ketoacidosis in the past 8 months. Recurrent hypoglycemic events have been occurring without a specific pattern. She always forgets to bring a record of her home glucose measurements or even her glucose meter to visits. She has no symptoms. She states she has intentionally lost 8 lb (3.6 kg) over the past year. Her menses are regular on hormonal contraception. She has a family history of Graves disease.

Current medications include insulin glargine, insulin lispro, oral contraceptive, and biotin.

On physical examination, her blood pressure is 110/60 mm Hg and BMI is 22 kg/m^2. Examination findings are unremarkable.

Laboratory test results:
Hemoglobin A$_{1c}$ = 9.1% (4.0%-5.6%)
(76 mmol/mol [20-38 mmol/mol])
Estimated glomerular filtration rate = 75 mL/min per 1.73 m^2 (>60 mL/min per 1.73 m^2)
Serum sodium = 141 mEq/L (136-142 mEq/L)
(SI: 141 mmol/L [3.9-5.5 mmol/L])
Serum potassium = 3.6 mEq/L (3.5-5.0 mEq/L)
(SI: 3.6 mmol/L [3.5-5.0 mmol/L])
Serum cortisol, not done due to laboratory error
ACTH = 38 pg/mL (10-60 pg/mL) (SI: 8.4 pmol/L [2.2-13.2 pmol/L])
TSH = 2 mIU/L (0.5-5.0 mIU/L)
Tissue transglutaminase antibodies, negative

Which of the following is the best next step?
- A. Initiate insulin pump therapy
- B. Perform a cosyntropin-stimulation test
- C. Measure TSH again after stopping biotin for 5 days
- D. Refer for psychological evaluation
- E. Initiate a tricyclic antidepressant

22 A 46-year-old man presents for advice on treatment of type 2 diabetes mellitus. He has been treated with metformin for 2 years. He has dyslipidemia and longstanding hypertension with chronic kidney disease. His only medications are metformin, rosuvastatin, and lisinopril.

On physical examination, his BMI is 33 kg/m^2 and blood pressure is 138/84 mm Hg.

Laboratory test results:
Hemoglobin A$_{1c}$ = 7.8% (4.0%-5.6%)
(62 mmol/mol [20-38 mmol/mol])
Estimated glomerular filtration rate = 53 mL/min per 1.73 m^2 (>60 mL/min per 1.73 m^2)

You decide to add linagliptin. You explain to him that this drug, by increasing GLP-1 levels, will target the following pathogenetic defects:

A. Insulin resistance and β-cell dysfunction
B. Hepatic glucose output and satiety
C. Renal glucose reabsorption and satiety
D. Glucagon secretion and insulin resistance
E. Hepatic glucose output and β-cell dysfunction

23 A 42-year-old woman with type 1 diabetes mellitus and Hashimoto thyroiditis has been experiencing increasing pain and stiffness of her axial, lumbar, and cervical muscles. Her pain has become debilitating and is not relieved by aspirin. She also has spasms in her arms and legs associated with sudden movements. Her only medications are insulin degludec, insulin aspart, and levothyroxine.

On physical examination, her blood pressure is 120/70 mm Hg and BMI is 22.0 kg/m^2. The rest of her examination findings are unremarkable except for hyperreflexia and inability to bend her knees.

Laboratory results reveal:
  Hemoglobin A$_{1c}$ = 6.8% (4.0%-5.6%)
    (51 mmol/mol [20-38 mmol/mol])
  TSH = 1.2 mIU/L (0.5-5.0 mIU/L)
  Creatinine = 0.8 mg/dL (0.6-1.1 mg/dL)
    (SI: 70.7 μmol/L [53.0-97.2 μmol/L])
  Glutamic acid decarboxylase antibodies, strongly
    positive
  TPO antibodies, positive

Which of the following medications would provide the diagnosis if there is a positive therapeutic response?

A. Prednisone
B. Gabapentin
C. Amitriptyline
D. Diazepam
E. Potassium

24 A 42-year-old man with type 1 diabetes mellitus since age 21 years has been experiencing an increased frequency of early hypoglycemia and late hyperglycemia associated with certain meals. Otherwise, his home glucose values (fingerstick) are within range. He has been on insulin pump therapy for years with insulin aspart. His current hemoglobin A$_{1c}$ level is 6.9% (4.0%-5.6%) (52 mmol/mol [20-38 mmol/mol]). His hypoglycemic episodes occur mostly within an hour after eating his favorite large meal (pizza with extra cheese and ice cream). The early hypoglycemia is followed by high blood glucose values (200-300 mg/dL [11.1-16.7 mmol/L]) hours after the meal. He has gained weight in recent years, and his BMI is 28 kg/m^2.

His basal rate is 1.0 unit/h from midnight to 6 AM and 1.2 units/h from 6 AM to midnight. His mealtime boluses are 1 unit per 10 g of carbohydrate.

Which of the following is the best recommendation?

A. Change his insulin-to-carbohydrate ratio to
   1 unit per 12 g for high-fat meals
B. Split the insulin bolus into standard/extended
   for high-fat meals
C. Eat more carbohydrates with high-fat meals
D. Change insulin aspart to insulin
   aspart-niacinamide
E. Take metoclopramide with high-fat meals

25 A 25-year-old man with a 10-year history of type 1 diabetes mellitus is preparing for a 1-hour tennis game to be played at 8 AM. His usual regimen is insulin glargine, 14 units every morning, and insulin lispro with an insulin-to-carbohydrate ratio of 1:10 for meals. He eats breakfast at 7 AM. His most recent hemoglobin A$_{1c}$ value is 6.9% (4.0%-5.6%) (52 mmol/mol [20-38 mmol/mol]).

He asks for advice about his insulin regimen the morning of the tennis game, assuming on that day, his fasting glucose is in the usual range of 120 to 140 mg/dL (6.7-7.8 mmol/L).

Which of the following do you recommend?

A. Eat breakfast, take insulin glargine (14 units)
   and insulin lispro with an
   insulin-to-carbohydrate ratio of 1:20
B. Skip breakfast and morning insulins; drink 8 oz
   of orange juice before the game
C. Eat breakfast, take insulin lispro with an
   insulin-to-carbohydrate ratio of 1:10 and lower
   glargine dose to 7 units
D. Eat breakfast, take insulin lispro with an
   insulin-to-carbohydrate ratio of 1:10 and skip
   the insulin glargine dose

26 A 45-year-old man with type 2 diabetes mellitus returns for follow-up. He is currently treated with metformin and basal and mealtime insulins. At the last visit, he asked to switch his mealtime insulin from glulisine to a different formulation because of many early postprandial blood glucose spikes (30-60 minutes) after he eats high-carbohydrate meals. His hemoglobin A_{1c} level at that time was 7.5% (58 mmol/mol).

Currently, after having been on the new mealtime insulin for a few months, he is very satisfied, as his postprandial blood glucoses are within range. His hemoglobin A_{1c} level is now 7.3% (58 mmol/mol).

His current mealtime insulin has the pharmacokinetic profile shown (*see image*).

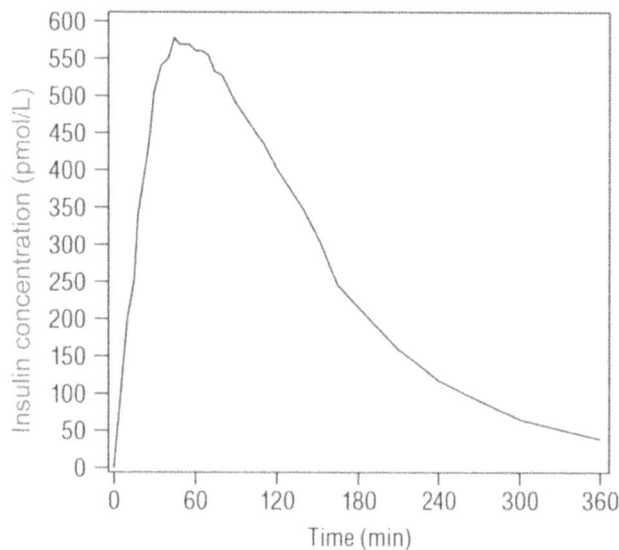

Which of the following is his current mealtime insulin?
  A. Glulisine-fatty acid
  B. Aspart-arginine
  C. Aspart-niacinamide
  D. Glulisine-glutamic acid

27 A 52-year-old woman with type 2 diabetes asks you for a prescription for the flash glucose monitoring system. Her blood glucose is well controlled on basal and mealtime insulins, and she checks her blood glucose 4 to 6 times daily. Her blood glucose values range between 90 and 130 mg/dL (5.0-7.2 mmol/L) before meals and are less than 200 mg/dL (<11.1 mmol/L) after meals. Her most recent hemoglobin A_{1c} value is 7.0% (53 mmol/mol). Her BMI is 29 kg/m^2.

Her current medications are insulin degludec, 30 units at bedtime; insulin lispro, 1 unit/8 g of carbohydrate;

metformin, 2000 mg daily; dapagliflozin, 10 mg daily; atorvastatin, 40 mg daily; ramipril, 10 mg daily; cinnamon, 2000 mg daily; vitamin C, 1000 mg daily; chromium, 1 mg daily; and occasionally acetaminophen.

The patient wears the new sensor on her arm. The next day, she sees an unusual reading of 350 mg/dL (19.4 mmol/L) on her sensor; a concomitant blood glucose fingerstick value is 110 mg/dL (6.1 mmol/L). The same discrepancy keeps happening for the next few days. The patient decides to call you for guidance.

Which of the following you do recommend?
  A. Adjust the insulin based on the sensor data, as blood glucose fingersticks are inaccurate
  B. Change the site of the sensor from the arm to the abdomen
  C. Stop cinnamon, as it can interfere with sensor glucose readings
  D. Stop acetaminophen, as it can interfere with sensor glucose readings
  E. Stop vitamin C, as it can interfere with sensor glucose readings

28 A 58-year-old man with a 4-year history of type 2 diabetes mellitus is concerned about his cardiovascular health. His diabetes has been treated with metformin. He has hypertension and dyslipidemia, both well controlled on ramipril and rosuvastatin. He has no known cardiovascular disease. His family history is notable for type 2 diabetes and hypertension but no heart disease or stroke. He does not smoke cigarettes or drink alcohol.

On physical examination, his blood pressure is 120/70 mm Hg and BMI is 30 kg/m^2. Examination findings are otherwise unremarkable.

Laboratory test results:
  Hemoglobin A_{1c} = 7.2% (4.0%-5.6%)
    (55 mmol/mol [20-38 mmol/mol])
  Estimated glomerular filtration rate, normal
  Liver function, normal
  TSH, normal
  LDL cholesterol = 65 mg/dL (<100 mg/dL)
    (SI: 1.68 mmol/L [<2.59 mmol/L])
  HDL cholesterol = 45 mg/dL (>60 mg/dL)
    (SI: 1.67 mmol/L [>1.55 mmol/L])
  Triglycerides = 145 mg/dL (<150 mg/dL)
    (SI: 1.64 mmol/L [<1.70 mmol/L])

On the basis of randomized controlled trial(s), which of the following would lead to significantly lower rates of serious vascular events in this patient?

A. Empagliflozin
B. Lixisenatide
C. Aspirin
D. Sitagliptin

29 A 68-year-old man with a 4-year history of type 2 diabetes mellitus is referred for advice on achieving better glycemic control. His medical history includes hypertension and dyslipidemia. Current medications are metformin, 500 mg twice daily; glimepiride, 4 mg daily; atorvastatin, 10 mg daily; and ramipril, 10 mg daily.

On review of systems, he has had shortness of breath on exertion and orthopnea for the past few months.

On physical examination, he has few crackles at the lung bases and 1+ bilateral pitting edema. Findings are otherwise unremarkable.

Laboratory test results:
Hemoglobin A_{1c} = 8.4% (4.0%-5.6%)
(68 mmol/mol [20-38 mmol/mol])
Estimated glomerular filtration rate = 39 mL/min per 1.73 m^2 (>60 mL/min per 1.73 m^2)
Liver function, normal
TSH, normal

Home self-glucose monitoring shows blood glucose values between 200 and 300 mg/dL (11.1-16.7 mmol/L).

Which of the following is the best next step in this patient's care?

A. Add saxagliptin, 5 mg daily
B. Increase the glimepiride dosage to 8 mg daily
C. Increase the metformin dosage to 1000 mg twice daily
D. Add insulin glargine, 10 units at bedtime
E. Add empagliflozin, 10 mg daily

30 A 62-year-old cardiologist is self-referred for diabetes management. He has had type 2 diabetes mellitus for 3 years and takes metformin, 2000 mg daily. His medical history includes hypertension, dyslipidemia, and myocardial infarction. In addition to metformin, current medications are lisinopril, rosuvastatin, metoprolol, and aspirin.

On physical examination, his blood pressure is 132/84 mm Hg and BMI is 33 kg/m^2. He has a soft systolic ejection murmur and weak pedal pulses.

Laboratory test results:
Hemoglobin A_{1c} = 8.0% (4.0%-5.6%)
(64 mmol/mol [20-38 mmol/mol])
Estimated glomerular filtration rate = 72 mL/min per 1.73 m^2 (>60 mL/min per 1.73 m^2)
Liver function, normal
TSH, normal

His primary care physician would like to add glimepiride, but the patient has declined. He wants a drug that, in randomized controlled trials, has been proven to significantly lower the risk of cardiovascular death in patients such as himself.

Which of the following agents would you add next?

A. Sitagliptin
B. Semaglutide
C. Once-weekly exenatide
D. Liraglutide
E. Canagliflozin

Diabetes Mellitus Section 2 Board Review

Michelle F. Magee, MD

31 A 54-year-old man with longstanding type 1 diabetes mellitus and peripheral vascular disease is admitted to the intensive care unit with an infected foot ulcer, cellulitis, and septic shock. He weighs 220 lb (100 kg). His condition has stabilized, and he is to begin eating meals and is to be transferred to a general surgical unit. He has been receiving continuous intravenous insulin, and glucose values have ranged from 140 mg/dL to 180 mg/dL (7.8-10.0 mmol/L). He has received 50 units of intravenous regular insulin in the past 24 hours.

It is now 9 AM. Before the intravenous insulin drip is discontinued, you order basal U100 insulin glargine, 20 units subcutaneously twice daily, with the first dose now and supplemental scale insulin for blood glucose values greater than 180 mg/dL (>10.0 mmol/L). This insulin glargine dose represents 80% of the total daily insulin dose being delivered via insulin drip—all of which was "basal" insulin, as he was not eating.

Which of the following orders will you also place in addition to that for basal insulin glargine and supplemental-scale insulin dosing?

Answer	Administer	Discontinue Insulin Drip
A.	Insulin lispro, 15 units with meals	Now
B.	Regular insulin, 10 units with meals	2 to 3 hours after the first dose of insulin glargine is administered
C.	Insulin lispro, 10 units with meals	2 to 3 hours after the first dose of insulin glargine is administered
D.	Regular insulin, 3 units 30 minutes before meals	Now

32 A 49-year-old man with stage 3 chronic kidney disease related to polycystic kidney disease has a 2-year history of type 2 diabetes mellitus treated with glipizide and liraglutide. He recently underwent segmental left colonic resection for complications related to diverticulitis. On postoperative days 1 and 2, his blood glucose climbed into the range of 250 to 300 mg/dL (13.9-16.7 mmol/L). He remains on nothing-by-mouth status in the surgical ward.

On physical examination, his temperature is 99.5°F (37.5°C), blood pressure is 142/86 mm Hg, and pulse rate is 104 beats/min. His abdomen is distended with decreased bowel sounds.

Which of the following options is the best glycemic management regimen for him now?
- A. Regular insulin sliding scale beginning at a blood glucose value greater than 150 mg/dL (>8.3 mmol/L)
- B. Aspart premixed insulin twice daily beginning at a blood glucose value greater than 180 mg/dL (>10.0 mmol/L)
- C. Reinitiation of liraglutide; hold glipizide until eating
- D. Basal insulin daily plus regular insulin every 6 hours when his blood glucose is greater than 180 mg/dL (>10.0 mmol/L) to achieve most blood glucose values between 140 and 180 mg/dL (7.8-10.0 mmol/L)
- E. Intravenous insulin infusion titrated to achieve blood glucose values between 80 and 110 mg/dL (4.4-6.1 mmol/L)

33 A 28-year-old woman with a 20-year history of type 1 diabetes mellitus is considering an isolated pancreas transplant. Her blood glucose values have been labile. Her hemoglobin A_{1c} level has ranged from 8.0% to 10.0% (64 to 86 mmol/mol), and she has hypoglycemic unawareness despite being on a sensor-augmented insulin pump. She has early nephropathy, proliferative retinopathy, gastroparesis, and peripheral neuropathy.

Laboratory test results:

Hemoglobin A_{1c} = 8.8% (4.0%-5.6%)
(73 mmol/mol [20-38 mmol/mol])
Creatinine = 1.9 mg/dL (0.6-1.1 mg/dL)
(SI: 168.0 μmol/L [53.0-97.2 μmol/L])
Urinary albumin-to-creatinine ratio = 98 mg/g
creat (<30 mg/g creat)

Which of the following outcomes can this patient expect within 5 years after a successful pancreas transplant?
A. Regression of retinopathy
B. Recovery of peripheral sensation
C. Regression of gastroparesis
D. Reduced albuminuria

34 A 34-year-old man with type 1 diabetes mellitus who is treated with multiple daily insulin injections is in the clinic waiting room. He seems confused when his name is called and is slurring his words. His fingerstick blood glucose value is 39 mg/dL (2.2 mmol/L). After being treated, he reports that despite using a continuous glucose sensor, he has been having frequent episodes of hypoglycemia without any warning symptoms and with blood glucose readings ranging from 40 to 50 mg/dL (2.2-2.8 mmol/L). He has always aimed for tight glycemic control. His hemoglobin A_{1c} level is 5.9% (41 mmol/mol), and he takes multiple daily insulin injections.

Which of the following is the most important advice to give this patient?
A. Begin a regimen of frequent small meals
B. Temporarily relax tight glucose targets
C. Switch to an insulin pump
D. See the diabetes educator to review symptoms and treatment of hypoglycemia

35 You have received a letter from an insurance company alerting you that a 47-year-old woman with a 21-year history of type 1 diabetes mellitus whom you have been caring for over many years is not taking a statin. You have had this discussion with her in the past and she is extremely reluctant to start this therapy. She has no diabetes-related complications and no specific concerns. She takes no medications other than insulin lispro, which is delivered via an insulin pump, and a daily baby aspirin.

On physical examination, her blood pressure is 131/78 mm Hg, and BMI is 24.5 kg/m^2.

Laboratory test results:

Hemoglobin A_{1c} = 7.2% (4.0%-5.6%)
(55 mmol/mol [20-38 mmol/mol])
Total cholesterol = 173 mg/dL (<200 mg/dL
[optimal]) (SI: 4.48 mmol/L [<5.18 mmol/L])
LDL cholesterol = 92 mg/dL (<100 mg/dL
[optimal]) (SI: 2.38 mmol/L [<2.59 mmol/L])
HDL cholesterol = 45 mg/dL (>60 mg/dL)
(SI: 1.17 mmol/L [>1.55 mmol/L])
Triglycerides = 178 mg/dL (<150 mg/dL [optimal])
(SI: 2.01 mmol/L [<1.70 mmol/L])
Serum creatinine = 0.86 mg/dL (0.6-1.1 mg/dL)
(SI: 76.0 μmol/L [53.0-97.2 μmol/L])
Urinary albumin-to-creatinine ratio = 8 mg/g creat
(<30 mg/g creat)

How should you advise the patient regarding the best course of action now to reduce her risk for cardiovascular disease?
A. Intensify her glycemic regimen to attain a target hemoglobin A_{1c} level <7.0% (<53 mmol/mol)
B. Recommend assessment of her coronary artery calcium score
C. Start treatment with an ACE inhibitor
D. Refer to a nutritionist for dietary instruction for weight loss and review of fat intake
E. Increase the aspirin dosage to 325 mg daily

36 A 47-year-old man presents for evaluation of hypoglycemia. He has been having increasingly frequent hyperadrenergic symptoms over the last 1 year. In the last 2 months, he has had episodes of confusion. Two weeks ago, he was taken to the emergency department following a syncopal event during which his blood glucose concentration was documented to be 39 mg/dL (2.2 mmol/L). The neuroglycopenic episodes occur during the day, and he attributes them to either small meals or eating "sweets." He has had no nocturnal or fasting episodes, and his symptoms always improve with carbohydrate intake. He has gained 18 lb (8.2 kg) over the past 6 months.

He has a history of heavy alcohol consumption, but he reports being sober for 6 months. He takes no medications and does not use illicit drugs. There is no family history of diabetes. He lives alone and works in technology.

On physical examination, his BMI is 31 kg/m^2, and he has no other notable features.

The patient returns for a blood draw after a 12-hour fast. He is asymptomatic.

Glucose = 57 mg/dL (70-99 mg/dL) (SI: 3.2 mmol/L [3.9-5.5 mmol/L])

Insulin = 14.0 µIU/mL (1.4-14.0 µIU/mL) (SI: 97.2 pmol/L [9.7-97.2 pmol/L])

C-peptide = 1.5 ng/mL (0.9-4.3 ng/mL) (SI: 0.50 nmol/L [0.30-1.42 nmol/L])

Cortisol = 21 µg/dL (5-25 µg/dL) (SI: 579.3 nmol/L [137.9-689.7 nmol/L])

TSH = 1.2 mIU/L (0.5-5.0 mIU/L)

IGF-1 = 225 ng/mL (91-246 ng/mL) (SI: 29.5 nmol/L [11.9-32.2 nmol/L])

On the basis of this patient's history and test results, which of the following is the best next management step?

A. Abdominal CT

B. Sulfonylurea screen

C. Measurement of blood alcohol and γ-glutamyl transpeptidase

D. Standard supervised 72-hour fast

E. Meal tolerance test

37 A 42-year-old woman with a 33-year history of type 1 diabetes mellitus presents for routine follow-up. She has nonproliferative retinopathy. She takes lisinopril, 5 mg daily, for proteinuria. She has been feeling fatigued.

Her insulin regimen includes insulin detemir twice daily and insulin glulisine with meals. She is having frequent episodes of hypoglycemia that are sometimes, but not always, related to skipped meals. She is not sleeping well and sometimes awakens with low blood glucose levels. She has adjusted her basal insulin dosage in 10% decrements several times, but she is still having frequent hypoglycemia. Her lifestyle regimen has not changed. She also reports becoming lightheaded when she stands up quickly.

On physical examination, her weight is 139 lb (63.2 kg) (BMI = 22 kg/m^2). When supine, her blood pressure is 124/74 mm Hg and pulse rate is 84 beats/min; when standing, her blood pressure is 91/68 mm Hg and pulse rate is 106 beats/min. Findings on cardiorespiratory examination are otherwise unremarkable. Neurologic examination reveals hyperesthesia at the foot compared with the knee on 1-g

monofilament testing and mild delayed ankle reflex recovery.

Pertinent nonfasting laboratory test results:

Serum sodium = 133 mg/dL (136-142 mEq/L) (SI: 133 mmol/L [136-142 mmol/L])

Potassium = 4.7 mEq/L (3.5-5.0 mEq/L) (SI: 4.7 mmol/L [3.5-5.0 mmol/L])

Creatinine = 0.9 mg/dL (0.6-1.1 mg/dL) (SI: 79.6 µmol/L [53.0-97.2 µmol/L])

Urinary albumin-to-creatinine ratio = 35 mg/g creat (<30 mg/g creat)

TSH = 8.2 mIU/L (0.5-5.0 mIU/L)

Hemoglobin A$_{1c}$ = 7.8% (4.0%-5.6%) (62 mmol/mol [20-38 mmol/mol])

Which of the following is the most likely cause of her orthostatic hypotension?

A. Adrenal insufficiency

B. Cardiovascular autonomic neuropathy

C. Hypothyroidism

D. Sensorimotor neuropathy

E. Salt-wasting nephropathy

38 An 82-year-old woman with a 32-year history of type 2 diabetes mellitus and hypertension is referred for glycemic management following an emergency department visit for severe hypoglycemia with loss of consciousness. Emergency medical technicians report that her initial blood glucose value was 27 mg/dL (1.5 mmol/L).

Her current home diabetes treatment regimen consists of 25 units of insulin detemir at bedtime, 9 units of rapid-acting insulin with meals, and correction doses for blood glucose values greater than 180 mg/dL (>10.0 mmol/L). She does not record the insulin doses taken. She asks you to review how and when to take correction insulin doses.

Her home blood glucose measurements are as follows:

Blood Glucose Values and Observations	Fasting	Prelunch	Predinner	Bedtime
Blood glucose values	Upper 100s mg/dL (SI: ~5.6 mmol/L)	Upper 100s mg/dL (SI: ~5.6 mmol/L)	100s mg/dL (SI: ~5.6 mmol/L)	150 to low 200s mg/dL (SI: 8.3-11.1 mmol/L)
Observations	Occasional values in the range of 68-75 mg/dL (3.8-4.2 mmol/L) or 211-274 mg/dL (11.7-15.2 mmol/L)	If lunch is late, values are 90 to low 100s mg/dL (SI: 5.0-5.6 mmol/L)	N/A	Occasional value in the range of 110-130 mg/dL (SI: 6.1-7.2 mmol/L)

On physical examination, her BMI is 19 kg/m^2 and blood pressure is 142/78 mm Hg. She has markedly reduced sensation in both feet. Her mood and affect are normal and her memory appears to be sharp.

Laboratory test results:
Hemoglobin A$_{1c}$ = 8.7% (4.0%-5.6%)
(72 mmol/mol [20-38 mmol/mol]) (estimated average glucose value 203 mg/dL [SI: 11.3 mmol/L])
Estimated glomerular filtration rate = 52 mL/min per 1.73 m^2 (<60 mL/min per 1.73 m^2)
C-peptide = 3.6 ng/mL (0.9-4.3 ng/mL) (SI: 1.2 nmol/L [0.30-1.42 nmol/L])

Which of the following would you recommend to reduce the risk for further episodes of severe hypoglycemia in this older woman?
A. Refer to a diabetes educator to help her better understand how to take her insulins
B. Reduce basal insulin to 20 units and keep meal boluses at 9 units
C. Reduce basal insulin to 20 units in the morning, stop the mealtime insulin, and start linagliptin
D. Stop the basal and meal insulins and start repaglinide with meals

39 A 19-year-old man with type 1 diabetes mellitus reports a 6-month history of diarrhea, unintentional weight loss, poor glycemic control, and a rash. On physical examination, he has no abdominal tenderness, normal sensation to 1-g monofilament testing, and a rash that is characterized by erythematous, papular, small and large blisters that burn and itch intensely (*see image*).

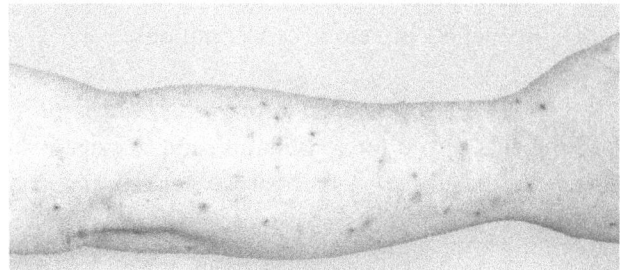

Which of the following is the best initial approach to evaluate his symptoms and rash?
A. Colonoscopy
B. Tissue transglutaminase antibody assessment
C. TPO antibody assessment
D. Upper gastrointestinal series with small-bowel follow-through
E. Skin biopsy

40 A 26-year-old man is referred for evaluation of glucosuria. He has had occasional urinary infections, which have responded to short courses of pharmacotherapy in the past. He has otherwise been healthy. He is not taking any medications. His new primary care physician documented the glucosuria when he saw him to establish care.

On physical examination, his blood pressure is 115/63 mm Hg and BMI is 21 kg/m^2.

Further laboratory testing excludes a diagnosis of diabetes and renal function is otherwise normal. You diagnose familial renal glucosuria. He asks you about the possible long-term implications of this diagnosis on his health.

Which of the following outcomes is most likely?
A. Increased risk of all-cause mortality
B. Increased risk of rapid renal function decline if he develops chronic kidney disease
C. Reduced risk of cardiovascular disease
D. A benign course

41 The mechanism of action of SGLT-2 inhibitors that provides the most prominent explanation for cardioprotection is which of the following?
- A. Diuretic effect–induced reflex activation of the sympathetic nervous system
- B. Diuretic effect of glucose reabsorption and consequent reduction in plasma volume
- C. Distal inhibition of glucose and sodium reabsorption
- D. Reduction in ketone concentrations

42 A 24-year-old man with cystic fibrosis presents to you for consultation and management of newly diagnosed cystic fibrosis–related diabetes (CFRD).

On the basis of your review of the literature and guidelines, which of the following would you recommend for treatment at this time?
- A. Metformin
- B. Glyburide
- C. Pioglitazone
- D. Insulin

43 Which action of available antihyperglycemic agents addresses the primary defect in the pathogenesis of type 2 diabetes?
- A. Increased first-phase insulin secretion from the pancreatic β cell
- B. Increased SGLT-2 receptor expression in the renal proximal convoluted tubule
- C. Reduced peripheral glucose disposal
- D. Increased gastric emptying

44 A 30-year-old man with an 11-year history of type 1 diabetes mellitus and hypertension is experiencing erectile dysfunction. He has normal libido. He is taking insulin and an ACE inhibitor.

Laboratory test results:
Hemoglobin A_{1c} = 7.8% (4.0%-5.6%)
  (62 mmol/mol [20-38 mmol/mol])
Testosterone = 487 ng/dL (300-900 ng/dL)
  (SI: 16.9 nmol/L [10.4-31.2 nmol/L])

Which of the following would you recommend to help improve his erectile dysfunction?
- A. Improve blood glucose control with a target hemoglobin A_{1c} <7.0% (<53 mmol/mol)
- B. Begin treatment with testosterone cypionate
- C. Stop taking the ACE inhibitor
- D. Begin treatment with a phosphodiesterase inhibitor

45 A 51-year-old man with type 2 diabetes mellitus, hypertension, and dyslipidemia is taking metformin and a sulfonylurea. His hemoglobin A_{1c} level is 8.1% (65 mmol/mol). He is obese, and his BMI has been as high as 38 kg/m^2. Today he reports that he has been on a low-carbohydrate, ketogenic diet and has been exercising for the past 3 months. He is excited that he has lost 8 lb (3.6 kg) and feels more energetic. More detailed review of his diet reveals that he is eating primarily high-protein, high-fat foods derived from animal products.

To help improve his glycemic control and further decrease his weight, which of the following strategies would you advise?
- A. Begin taking linagliptin and switch to a calorie-restricted, low-fat diet
- B. Begin taking semaglutide and continue his current lifestyle regimen
- C. Increase the frequency and intensity of his exercise regimen
- D. Begin taking dapagliflozin and continue the ketogenic diet

46 A 57-year-old woman returns for management of type 2 diabetes mellitus. She is taking metformin, pioglitazone, and linagliptin. She has peripheral neuropathy, background retinopathy, and declining renal function with progressive albuminuria. She has been eating out frequently and not exercising. One year ago, her 24-hour albumin excretion was 700 mg and her estimated glomerular filtration rate was 55 mL/min per 1.73 m^2. She also has longstanding hypertension treated with losartan, 100 mg daily, and amlodipine, 5 mg daily.

On physical examination, her BMI is 35 kg/m^2, weight is 211 lb (95.9 kg) (increased 6.5 lb [3 kg] in the last year), and blood pressure is 132/76 mm Hg. There is no evidence of congestive heart failure. She has 1+ ankle edema.

Laboratory test results:

Hemoglobin A_{1c} = 7.0% (4.0%-5.6%)
(53 mmol/mol [20-38 mmol/mol])

Creatinine = 1.5 mg/dL (0.6-1.1 mg/dL)
(SI: 132.6 μmol/L [53.0-97.2 μmol/L])

Sodium = 142 mEq/L (136-142 mEq/L)
(SI: 142 mmol/L [136-142 mmol/L])

Fasting glucose = 134 mg/dL (70-99 mg/dL)
(SI: 7.4 mmol/L [3.9-5.5 mmol/L])

Serum urea nitrogen = 28 mg/dL (8-23 mg/dL)
(SI: 10.0 mmol/L [2.9-8.2 mmol/L])

Potassium = 4.1 mEq/L (3.5-5.0 mEq/L)
(SI: 4.1 mmol/L [3.5-5.0 mmol/L])

Bicarbonate = 26 mEq/L (21-28 mEq/L)
(SI: 26 mmol/L [21-28 mmol/L])

TSH = 2.3 mIU/L (0.5-5.0 mIU/L)

Estimated glomerular filtration rate = 52 mL/min
per 1.73 m^2 (>60 mL/min per 1.73 m^2)

Urinary albumin = 1200 mg/24 h (<30 mg/24 h)

Urinary sodium = 11.0 g/24 h (3.4-3.8 g/24 h)

Urinary potassium = 3.0 g/24 h (2.0-2.3 g/24 h)

Which of the following is the best next step in treating her renal disease?

A. Add ramipril

B. Add spironolactone

C. Add insulin glargine

D. Institute dietary protein restriction

E. Institute dietary sodium restriction

47 A 76-year-old woman with a 29-year history of type 2 diabetes mellitus is referred for glycemic management. She has no microvascular complications, but she had a myocardial infarction 8 years ago. Her hemoglobin A_{1c} levels range from 8.5% to 9.0% (69-75 mmol/mol), and she has frequent nocturia.

She is taking glipizide, 10 mg daily, and NPH insulin, 24 units twice daily, before breakfast and her evening meal. Once-daily glucose monitoring shows fasting values ranging from 87 to 257 mg/dL (4.8-14.3 mmol/L). She reports waking overnight several times monthly with nightmares and wanting to snack. Based on her age and comorbidities, you recommend a hemoglobin A_{1c} target of 8.0% (64 mmol/mol), which correlates with blood glucose levels less than 180 mg/dL (<10 mmol/L).

Which of the following adjustments to her regimen is most likely to enable safe attainment of her new glycemic goals?

A. Increase the predinner NPH insulin dose to 28 units

B. Increase the morning and evening insulin doses to 28 units

C. Add 6 units of regular insulin before meals and stop glipizide

D. Decrease the evening dose of NPH insulin to 20 units and give it at bedtime

E. Add a bedtime snack to her regimen

48 You are referred a 32-year-old overweight woman with hypothyroidism who had gestational diabetes mellitus and is 6 weeks post partum. Gestational diabetes was diagnosed based on an abnormal result from an oral glucose tolerance test at 22 weeks' gestation. She required insulin therapy during the third trimester. The delivery was uneventful and her healthy daughter weighed 7 lb, 3 oz (3260 g).

The patient has lost 10 lb (4.5 kg) since delivery and has continued to use a low-dosage basal-bolus insulin regimen since hospital discharge. Her fasting and postmeal fingerstick blood glucose levels have been normal since she has been home. She has occasional episodes of hypoglycemia. She wonders whether she can stop insulin therapy.

Which of the following should you recommend?

A. Continue current therapy

B. Change from insulin to metformin

C. Stop insulin therapy; perform an oral glucose tolerance test in 1 month

D. Stop insulin therapy; measure hemoglobin A_{1c} in 3 months

49 You are referred a patient with new-onset diabetes mellitus. He recently received a diagnosis of myasthenia gravis. He was prescribed pyridostigmine and prednisone. On a prednisone dosage of 20 mg daily, he developed polyuria and blurred vision and was found to have a random blood glucose concentration of 327 mg/dL (18.2 mmol/L). His rheumatologist started metformin, 1000 mg daily, which the patient has been taking for several weeks. The projected course of his steroid treatment is several months.

On physical examination, his weight 172 lb (78.2 kg) and blood pressure is 126/88 mm Hg.

Which of the following is the most reasonable treatment approach?
A. Start NPH insulin, 12 units with breakfast
B. Increase the metformin dosage to 2000 mg daily
C. Increase the metformin dosage to 2000 mg daily and add sitagliptin, 100 mg daily
D. Increase the metformin dosage to 2000 mg daily and add insulin glargine, 30 units daily

50 A 69-year-old man with a history of long-standing type 1 diabetes mellitus presents for a follow-up visit. His blood glucose is managed using U100 insulin lispro delivered via a personal insulin pump and continuous glucose monitoring. He follows a low-carbohydrate and low-fat diet and exercises 5 to 6 days a week.

The basal insulin delivery rates are shown.

Time Segment	Basal Insulin Rate (units/h)
12 AM-2 AM	0.75
2 AM-9 AM	0.65
9 AM-12 PM	1.75
12 PM-12 AM	0.7

He eats breakfast at 9 AM and eats his evening meal between 6 PM and 7 PM. He administers an insulin bolus at the beginning of meals using a 1:20 insulin-to-carbohydrate ratio and takes small correction boluses as needed for hyperglycemia using a 1:60 insulin correction factor.

He has no history of severe hypoglycemia. His hemoglobin A_{1c} level is 6.9% (52 mmol/mol) today and was 6.5% (48 mmol/mol) 3 months ago. His continuous glucose monitoring daily overlay report for the week before the visit is shown.

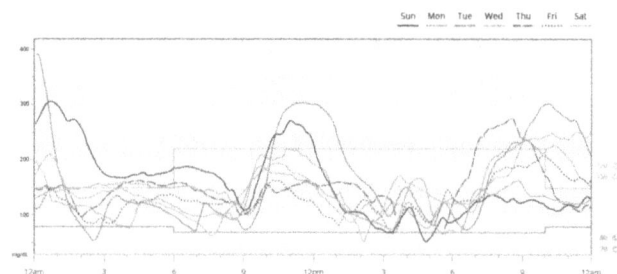

Which of the following would you recommend to help attenuate the marked postprandial glycemic excursions this patient is experiencing?
A. Advise him to take his insulin bolus 10 to 15 minutes before meals
B. Reduce the grams of carbohydrate eaten with each meal by 25%
C. Perform a basal rate test from 9 AM to 9 PM
D. Adjust his insulin-to-carbohydrate ratio to 1:6 for breakfast and the evening meal

51 A 29-year-old woman presents for management of uncontrolled diabetes. Diabetes was diagnosed 2 years ago, but she has never had good glycemic control. She was unable to tolerate metformin due to gastrointestinal adverse effects. She briefly took an SGLT-2 inhibitor, but she had recurrent yeast infections, so she stopped this therapy. Glimepiride was not effective. Six weeks ago, she began taking once-weekly dulaglutide, 1.5 mg, and her glucose values have not decreased significantly since this regimen change. Graves disease was recently diagnosed, and it is being managed with methimazole. She has been overweight since she was a teenager. She restricts her calories and exercises almost every day. She has been losing weight, but she has also been hyperthyroid. Her fasting and 2-hour postprandial glucose concentrations range from 180 to 220 mg/dL (10.0-12.2 mmol/L). She has never had diabetic ketoacidosis. She has a family history of type 2 diabetes.

On physical examination, her weight is 240.5 lb (109.3 kg) and BMI is 33.7 kg/m^2. Her blood pressure is 132/88 mm Hg, and pulse rate is 108 beats/min. There is no exophthalmos. The thyroid gland is uniformly enlarged. She has no acanthosis nigricans. The rest of the examination findings are normal.

Her hemoglobin A_{1c} level is 10.8% (95 mmol/mol).

Which of the following would you measure to help you decide the next step in improving her diabetes management?
A. Glutamic acid decarboxylase antibodies
B. Fructosamine
C. Fasting insulin
D. C-peptide

52 A 62-year-old woman has type 2 diabetes mellitus, hypertension, stage 3 chronic kidney disease, and congestive heart failure. She also has osteoarthritis of the knees and is wheelchair bound. She is referred to you following an emergency department visit with a blood glucose level of 556 mg/dL (30.9 mmol/L) and a hemoglobin A_{1c} level of 14.8% (138 mmol/mol). She needs glycemic management in preparation for knee surgery. She has symptoms of hyperglycemia. She is taking 50 units of insulin glargine U100 twice daily and 35 units of insulin lispro U100 3 times daily with meals. She misses 1 to 2 of her insulin doses 3 or more days every week.

She agrees to take all her insulin doses and check fingerstick blood glucose levels twice daily and then talk again next week. At her next appointment, you note that her glucose levels have been ranging from 371 to 601 mg/dL (20.6-33.4 mmol/L). She has been taking correction insulin doses when her glucose concentration is greater than 240 mg/dL (>13.3 mmol/L). You titrate her U100 insulin glargine up to 55 units twice daily and increase her mealtime insulin lispro dose to 40 units.

She sees you 1 week later and reports that she is taking all her prescribed insulin doses. Her point-of-care glucose value is 469 mg/dL (26.0 mmol/L). There is no evidence of infection. You observe her taking a correction dose of 40 units of U100 insulin lispro, which she does with good technique.

In addition to starting a GLP-1 receptor agonist that will work synergistically with insulin to help improve her glycemic control, which of the following recommendations would you make for glycemic management now?
    A. Recommend insulin pump therapy
    B. Increase each of her insulin doses by 20%
    C. Add an SGLT-2 inhibitor
    D. Switch to U500 regular insulin

53 A 78-year-old has had type 2 diabetes mellitus for more than 40 years and has coronary artery disease. He takes insulin glargine and empagliflozin. He was doing well until last week when he was taken to the emergency department after being found unresponsive in the early morning with a blood glucose concentration of 34 mg/dL (1.9 mmol/L). There was no evidence of myocardial infarction. His current hemoglobin A_{1c} level is 6.4% (46 mmol/mol). His family wants to know if another severe hypoglycemic episode would increase his risk of having a cardiac event.

If this patient continues to have severe hypoglycemia, for which of the following cardiac arrhythmias is he most at risk?
    A. Bradycardia
    B. Atrial flutter
    C. Complex ventricular premature beats
    D. Shortened Q-T interval

54 A 26-year-old man with type 1 diabetes mellitus had just moved out of his family home. His diabetes was treated with multiple daily insulin injections. He was found unresponsive in his apartment. Euglycemic diabetic ketoacidosis was diagnosed shortly after his arrival at the hospital where he subsequently died.

Which of the following most likely precipitated his euglycemic diabetic ketoacidosis?
    A. Adrenal insufficiency
    B. Canagliflozin
    C. Rationing his insulin
    D. Hypothyroidism

55 A 67-year-old woman with type 2 diabetes mellitus and chronic kidney disease presents with weight loss, polydipsia, and polyuria. Her hemoglobin A_{1c} level is 12.3% (111 mmol/mol), which is increased from 7.8% (62 mmol/mol) 4 months ago. A variety of oral antihyperglycemic agents were previously unsuccessful. She takes 32 units of U100 insulin glargine each evening, which she sometimes misses because she falls asleep after dinner, and 8 units of U100 insulin lispro before meals. The insulins are taken using prefilled pens. You advise her to increase her insulin doses to 38 units of U100 insulin glargine in the morning and 23 units of U100 insulin lispro before each meal and to stop drinking carbohydrate-containing beverages and to avoid sweets.

At a follow-up visit 1 week later, her blood glucose values are ranging from 266 to 394 mg/dL (14.8-21.9 mmol/L) with a mean value of 312 mg/dL (17.3 mmol/L), which does not represent much improvement despite the increased insulin dosage and a self-reported significant reduction in carbohydrate intake.

Which of the following would you advise next to improve her glycemic control?
  A. Refer her for diabetes self-management education and support
  B. Ask her to show you how she self-administers a correction insulin dose using her pen
  C. Ask her to start engaging in vigorous physical activity for at least 30 minutes each day
  D. Order diagnostic continuous glucose monitor testing

56 A 59-year-old man with newly diagnosed type 2 diabetes mellitus presents to establish care. He has no concerns. He has hyperlipidemia, hypertension, and obesity. He does not smoke cigarettes. He is taking benazepril, 20 mg daily, and atorvastatin, 40 mg daily.

On physical examination, his blood pressure is 128/78 mm Hg, pulse rate is 87 beats/min, and BMI is 30.8 kg/m^2.

Laboratory test results:
  Hemoglobin A_{1c} = 7.8% (4.0%-5.6%)
    (62 mmol/mol [20-38 mmol/mol])
  Plasma glucose (fasting) = 148 mg/dL
    (70-99 mg/dL) (SI: 8.2 mmol/L [3.9-5.5 mmol/L])
  Serum creatinine = 1.17 mg/dL (0.7-1.3 mg/dL)
    (SI: 103.4 μmol/L [61.9-114.9 μmol/L])
  Total cholesterol = 136 mg/dL (<200 mg/dL
    [optimal]) (SI: 3.52 mmol/L [<5.18 mmol/L])
  LDL cholesterol = 72 mg/dL (<100 mg/dL
    [optimal]) (SI: 1.86 mmol/L [<2.59 mmol/L])
  HDL cholesterol = 40 mg/dL (>60 mg/dL)
    (SI: 1.04 mmol/L [>1.55 mmol/L])
  Triglycerides = 180 mg/dL (<150 mg/dL [optimal])
    (SI: 2.03 mmol/L [<1.70 mmol/L])
  Urinary albumin-to-creatinine ratio = 32 mg/g
    creat (<30 mg/g creat)
  Basic metabolic panel, normal
  Complete blood cell count, normal

Using the online risk estimator of the American College of Cardiology and the American Heart Association (available at: www.cvriskcalculator.com), you determine that his 10-year calculated cardiovascular disease risk (heart disease or stroke) is 14.1%.

On the basis of his clinical presentation, laboratory test results, and 10-year atherosclerotic cardiovascular disease risk score, which of the following medications would you recommend for his glucose control?
  A. Metformin
  B. Empagliflozin
  C. Liraglutide
  D. Sitagliptin

57 A 57-year-old man with type 2 diabetes mellitus was hospitalized with a new diagnosis of congestive heart failure (ejection fraction <10%). His cardiac status is now stabilized with inotropic support. He is being evaluated for advanced heart failure therapies, and he will most likely be hospitalized for another 5 to 7 days. You are consulted for glycemic management.

He is eating well and does not report any gastrointestinal disturbances. His is receiving subcutaneous injections of insulin glargine (10 units each morning) plus a low-dose supplemental insulin scale when his blood glucose is greater than 180 mg/dL (>10.0 mmol/L). Your hospital target for blood glucose in patients on medicine units is 140 to 180 mg/dL (7.8-10.0 mmol/L).

His point-of-care blood glucose values over the past 24 hours are as follows:

Day	Time	Blood Glucose	Insulin Lispro Correction Dose
Yesterday	10:45 PM	244 mg/dL (SI: 13.5 mmol/L)	2 units
Today	07:18 AM	166 mg/dL (SI: 9.2 mmol/L)	--
Today	11:58 AM	212 mg/dL (SI: 11.8 mmol/L)	4 units
Today	05:18 PM	203 mg/dL (SI: 11.3 mmol/L)	4 units

Which of the following evidence-based therapies would you recommend as an addition to his hospital glycemic control regimen?
  A. Sitagliptin
  B. Metformin
  C. Pioglitazone
  D. Canagliflozin

58 A 67-year old woman has type 2 diabetes mellitus and congestive heart failure, which slightly limits her usual physical activity. She is comfortable at rest and can do her daily walk, although this does make her tired and induces some palptiations. She takes metformin for glycemic management. Her hemoglobin A_{1c} level is 8.1% (65 mmol/mol), and her estimated glomerular filtration rate is 58 mL/min per 1.73 m^2.

Which antihyperglycemic medication would you advise to potentially reduce her risk of hospitalizations due to heart failure?
   A. A GLP-1 receptor agonist
   B. Metformin
   C. An SGLT-2 inhibitor
   D. A thiazolidinedione

59 A 52-year-old woman with type 2 diabetes mellitus, proliferative retinopathy, painful neuropathy, hypertension, and dyslipidemia presents for a follow-up visit. She is concerned about "hives" with intense itching. They can appear anywhere on her body. She saw a dermatologist who gave her ranitidine, cetirizine, and a topical cream—none of which have helped. She had a similar episode 2 years ago following a switch from one brand of insulin to another, which resolved when she switched back to the prior brand. When she administers her insulin injections, there is no redness or itching at the shot site. She has been under a lot of stress, but her blood glucose levels are usually within the range of 90 to 180 mg/dL (5.0-10.0 mmol/L). She has not made any changes in soaps, lotions, or laundry detergent. Her dog takes flea and tick prevention medication. She is allergic to mold (urticaria) and tree pollens (nasal congestion). Her current medications are empagliflozin, glipizide, metformin, insulin degludec, lisinopril, gabapentin, oxycodone/acetaminophen, and simvastatin.

Her physical examination is remarkable for widely scattered papular lesions that are most prominent on her arms, shins, and trunk. There are also extensive excoriations in these areas. The appearance of the rash is shown (*see images*).

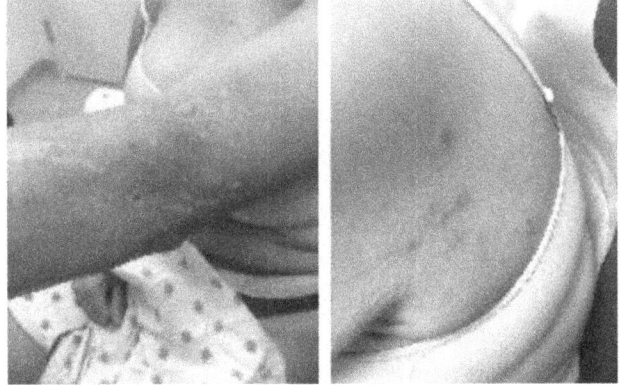

Laboratory test results:
   Her hemoglobin A_{1c} = 7.2% (4.0%-5.6%) (55 mmol/mol [20-38 mmol/mol])
   Estimated glomerular filtration rate = 81 mL/min per 1.73 m^2 (>60 mL/min per 1.73 m^2)
   AST, normal
   ALT, normal

Which of the following is the cause of the patient's pruritic skin condition?
   A. Hypersensitivity reaction to insect bites
   B. Necrobiosis lipoidica diabeticorum
   C. Perforating collagenosis
   D. Insulin allergy

Female Reproduction Board Review

Kathryn A. Martin, MD

1 A 53-year-old woman who had her final menstrual period 1 year ago seeks help for severe hot flashes. She would like to start menopausal hormone therapy. Her symptoms occur during the day, but they are worse at night and awaken her frequently. The lack of sleep is now affecting her ability to function well at work. She is otherwise in excellent health and has no history of hypertension, dyslipidemia, coronary heart disease, or venous thromboembolism. Menarche was at 14 years. She is G2, P2 (first pregnancy at age 24 years), and she has never had a breast biopsy. She has an intact uterus. Her father has type 2 diabetes mellitus, and there is no family history of breast cancer, stroke, venous thromboembolism, or coronary heart disease.

On physical examination, her blood pressure is 110/70 mm Hg and BMI is 21 kg/m^2.

You advise her that she is a good candidate for menopausal hormone therapy to treat her symptoms, as she is in her 50s, newly menopausal, and in good health. She is aware that prolonged use may be associated with an increased risk of breast cancer.

During treatment with menopausal hormone therapy (combined estrogen-progestin), she could expect a decreased risk of which of the following?
A. Stroke
B. Later dementia
C. Type 2 diabetes
D. Venous thromboembolism

2 A 28-year-old woman presents with a change in her intermenstrual interval. She had menarche at age 13 years and had regular menses during high school and college. She took an oral contraceptive pill from age 22 to 24 years. After stopping, she had 28- to 30-day cycles, but for the past 18 months, she has been having menses every 22 to 23 days. She has autoimmune hypothyroidism and takes a stable levothyroxine dosage. She exercises 3 times weekly for 1 hour each session. She has mild acne, no hot flashes, and no galactorrhea. Her BMI is 20 kg/m^2.

Laboratory test results from blood samples drawn on cycle day 3:
  FSH = 20.0 mIU/mL (2.0-12.0 mIU/mL [follicular]) (SI: 20.0 IU/L [2.0-12.0 IU/L])
  LH = 60.0 mIU/mL (1.0-18.0 mIU/mL [follicular]) (SI: 60.0 IU/L [1.0-18.0 IU/L])
  Estradiol = 28 pg/mL (10-180 pg/mL [follicular]) (SI: 102.8 pmol/L [36.7-660.8 pmol/L])
  Antimullerian hormone = 0.9 ng/mL (0.9-9.5 ng/mL) (SI: 6.4 pmol/L [6.4-67.9 pmol/L])
  TSH = 2.1 mIU/L (0.5-5.0 mIU/L)

In addition to karyotype analysis and genetic testing for the fragile X premutation, which of the following is most important to measure next?
A. Inhibin B
B. 21-Hydroxylase antibodies
C. IGF-1
D. Ovarian antibodies

3 A 46-year-old woman seeks advice for irregular menstrual cycles. She previously had 30- to 32-day cycles, but for the past 18 months, her menstrual periods have become unpredictable, occurring every 21 to 60 days. Her last menstrual period was 50 days ago. She has gained weight over the past 2 to 3 years. Current BMI is 31 kg/m^2. She wakes up often at night and feels tired during the day. She is very worried and would like an evaluation to determine the etiology of her symptoms.

Laboratory test results from blood samples drawn on cycle day 50:
  LH = 10.0 mIU/mL (1.0-18.0 mIU/mL [follicular]) (SI: 10.0 IU/L [1.0-18.0 IU/L])
  FSH = 18.0 mIU/mL (2.0-12.0 mIU/mL [follicular]) (SI: 18.0 IU/L [2.0-12.0 IU/L])

Estradiol = 450 pg/mL (10-180 pg/mL [follicular]) (SI: 1652.0 pmol/L [36.7-660.8 pmol/L])

Progesterone = 1.6 ng/mL (2.0-20.0 ng/mL [luteal]) (SI: 5.1 nmol/L [6.4-63.6 nmol/L])

Which of the following is the most likely cause of her clinical picture?

A. Menopausal transition (perimenopause)
B. Pregnancy
C. Obesity
D. Estradiol-secreting granulosa-cell tumor

4 A 26-year-old woman seeks evaluation for irregular menstrual cycles and potential infertility. She was on combined estrogen-progestin oral contraceptives from age 19 to 24 years for oligomenorrhea, acne, and excess facial hair. She has struggled with her weight since puberty. Two years ago, she stopped the pill to try and conceive. Her primary care physician suggested weight loss before pursuing fertility, and she lost 25 lb (11.4 kg) with diet and exercise. Her height is 65 in (165.1 cm) and her BMI decreased from 35 to 32 kg/m^2. Despite weight loss, she has menses every 60 days with no moliminal symptoms. One week ago, on cycle day 45, her primary care physician ordered laboratory tests. The patient comes to see you today to review her laboratory results and to discuss treatment plans.

Laboratory test results (sample drawn on cycle day 45):
LH = 100.0 mIU/mL (1.0-18.0 mIU/mL [follicular]) (SI: 100.0 IU/L [1.0-18.0 IU/L])
FSH = 12.0 mIU/mL (2.0-12.0 mIU/mL [follicular]) (SI: 12.0 IU/L [2.0-12.0 IU/L])
Estradiol = 275 pg/mL (10-180 pg/mL [follicular]) (SI: 1009.5 pmol/L [36.7-660.8 pmol/L])
Progesterone = 0.9 ng/mL (2.0-20.0 ng/mL [luteal]) (SI: 2.9 nmol/L [6.4-63.6 nmol/L])
TSH = 1.3 mIU/L (0.5-5.0 mIU/L)
Prolactin = 18 ng/mL (4-30 ng/mL) (SI: 0.78 nmol/L [0.17-1.30 nmol/L])

Which of the following conditions best explains her laboratory results?

A. Primary ovarian insufficiency
B. Midcycle LH surge
C. Polycystic ovary syndrome
D. Pregnancy

5 A 30-year-old transgender woman sees you for gender-affirming hormonal therapy (estrogen). She has a history of depression, but she is doing well on sertraline, 50 mg daily. She has no history of hypertension, dyslipidemia, type 2 diabetes mellitus, or venous thromboembolism. She is obese (BMI = 32 kg/m^2). You review treatment options with the patient.

Which of the following is the optimal hormonal therapy (route and dosage) for this patient?

A. Oral ethinyl estradiol, 50 to 100 mcg daily
B. Oral 17β-estradiol, 2 to 6 mg daily
C. Transdermal 17β-estradiol, 50 to 200 mcg once or twice weekly
D. Oral conjugated estrogens, 1.25 mg daily

6 A 32-year-old woman presents to your office to discuss fatigue. She has a history of polycystic ovary syndrome with menarche at age 11 years and hirsutism and acne since age 13 years. She has been on a combined estrogen-progestin contraceptive for the past 10 years. At work she has felt unusually tired, and she is struggling to achieve her productivity goals. Over the past 3 years, she has gained approximately 40 lb (18.2 kg) (from 160 to 200 lb [73 to 91 kg]). Two years ago, her hemoglobin A$_{1c}$ measurement was 6.0% (42 mmol/mol). She has a family history of hypertension and type 2 diabetes mellitus.

On physical examination, her blood pressure is 130/90 mm Hg and BMI is 34.3 kg/m^2. She has mild facial acne and terminal hair in the upper lip area.

Which of the following is the most likely diagnosis?

A. New-onset type 2 diabetes mellitus
B. Depression
C. Sleep apnea
D. Cushing syndrome

7 A 41-year-old woman with severe hot flashes and insomnia seeks advice regarding menopausal hormone therapy. She underwent normal menarche and had regular menses until age 40 years, when she noted some irregularity. Leiomyomata were diagnosed, and 6 months ago she underwent total abdominal hysterectomy and bilateral salpingo-oophorectomy. Since her surgery, she has had intractable hot flashes at night, as well as during the day. Her sleep is poor and she is having trouble functioning at work. She is otherwise in good health, takes no medications, and maintains a healthful diet and lifestyle. She has no family history of breast cancer, venous thromboembolism, coronary heart disease, or type 2 diabetes mellitus. Findings on physical examination are normal, and her BMI is 24 kg/m^2.

She has heard from many friends that taking estrogen is risky. You reassure her that estrogen replacement is important for young women who experience any type of early menopause (surgical [bilateral oophorectomy] or natural [primary ovarian insufficiency]). You recommend estrogen therapy until age 50 or 51 years (the average age of menopause) to manage her symptoms and to reduce the risk of premature development of coronary heart disease, stroke, and osteoporosis.

In this patient, estrogen therapy will also help reduce the risk of premature development of which of the following disorders?
  A. Dementia
  B. Migraine headaches
  C. Autoimmune disorders
  D. Osteoarthritis

8 A 30-year-old Hispanic woman seeks evaluation for irregular periods and possible infertility. She had early development of pubic hair at age 7 years. Menarche was at age 11 years. Her cycles have been irregular since then, and she has been treated intermittently with oral contraceptives but discontinued them 3 years ago. She and her husband have been trying to conceive for the past 2 years without success. Her menstrual periods occur every 2 to 3 months. She seeks advice on treatment options.

On physical examination, her BMI is 29 kg/m^2. She has hair on her chin, upper lip, neck, midsternum, and upper abdomen. Her Ferriman-Gallwey score is 10. She has no clitoromegaly, acne, or alopecia. Findings on pelvic examination are normal.

Laboratory test results (sample drawn on day 60 of her menstrual cycle):
  LH = 5.0 mIU/mL (1.0-18.0 mIU/mL)
    (SI: 5.0 IU/L [1.0-18.0 IU/L])
  FSH = 4.0 mIU/mL (2.0-12.0 mIU/mL)
    (SI: 4.0 IU/L [2.0-12.0 IU/L])
  Testosterone = 50 ng/dL (8-60 ng/dL)
    (SI: 1.7 nmol/L [0.3-2.1 nmol/L])
  17-Hydroxyprogesterone = 470 ng/dL (<80 ng/dL)
    (SI: 14.2 nmol/L [<2.42 nmol/L])

Prolactin = 18 ng/mL (4-30 ng/mL)
  (SI: 0.78 nmol/L [0.17-1.30 nmol/L])
TSH = 2.1 mIU/L (0.5-5.0 mIU/L)
Following a cosyntropin-stimulation test,
  17-hydroxyprogesterone = 1600 ng/dL
  (SI: 48.5 nmol/L)

Which of the following is the best initial therapy to restore ovulation?
  A. Dexamethasone
  B. Metformin
  C. Prednisone
  D. Letrozole

9 A 45-year-old woman seeks evaluation for night sweats and hot flashes during the day. Six months ago, she had a levonorgestrel-releasing intrauterine device inserted for contraception and has no periods. Her symptoms and lack of sleep are interfering with her ability to perform well at work. She is otherwise in good health. Her BMI is 32 kg/m^2.

Which of the following treatments would you suggest for this patient?
  A. Transdermal estradiol, 0.05 mg patch twice weekly
  B. Combined estrogen-progestin contraceptive (ethinyl estradiol, 20 mcg, with norethindrone acetate, 1 mg)
  C. Gabapentin, 300 mg orally at bedtime
  D. Conjugated estrogens, 0.3 mg orally daily

10 A 20-year-old woman with Turner syndrome sees you to transition her care from her pediatrician to an adult provider. She has a history of primary amenorrhea and short stature.

On physical examination, her blood pressure is 140/90 mm Hg. Her height is 56 in (142.2 cm) (BMI = 28 kg/m^2). She has absent breast development and scant pubic and axillary hair. She is on a combined estrogen-progestin regimen and has been seeing her pediatrician yearly. Last year, cardiac MRI showed no evidence of aortic dilatation and no significant cardiovascular anomalies.

Past laboratory test results:
    FSH = 35.0 mIU/mL (2.0-12.0 mIU/mL [follicular])
        (SI: 35.0 IU/L [2.0-12.0 IU/L])
    LH = 28.0 mIU/mL (1.0-18.0 mIU/mL [follicular])
        (SI: 28.0 IU/L [1.0-18.0 IU/L])
    Estradiol = <10 pg/mL (10-180 pg/mL [follicular])
        (SI: <36.7 pmol/L [36.7-660.8 pmol/L])
    Karyotype = 45,X

Which of the following tests should you do today (and at each yearly visit)?
    A. Hemoglobin A_{1c} measurement, renal ultrasonography, liver enzymes
    B. Thyroid function tests, hemoglobin A_{1c} measurement, liver enzymes
    C. Electrocardiography, celiac disease screening, hemoglobin A_{1c} measurement
    D. Complete blood cell count, thyroid function tests, echocardiography

11 A 28-year-old transgender man sees you to discuss testosterone therapy that he started last week (testosterone cypionate, 200 mg intramuscularly every 2 weeks). He wants to know whether he will experience an increase in muscle strength right away.

Which of the following effects is most likely to begin during the first few months of his new regimen?
    A. Deepening of the voice
    B. Increased oiliness of the skin and acne
    C. Increased body hair growth
    D. Alopecia

12 A 17-year-old girl presents with primary amenorrhea. She is otherwise healthy, and there is no family history of reproductive disorders. She has sparse axillary and pubic hair, but normal Tanner stage 5 breast development. Her pelvic examination reveals a blind vaginal vault, and no uterus is seen on transvaginal ultrasonography.

Initial laboratory test results:
    hCG = <3.0 mIU/L (<3.0 mIU/mL)
        (SI: <3.0 IU/L [<3.0 IU/L])
    FSH = 7.0 mIU/mL (2.0-12.0 mIU/mL [follicular])
        (SI: 7.0 IU/L [2.0-12.0 IU/L])
    LH = 18.0 mIU/mL (1.0-18.0 mIU/mL [follicular])
        (SI: 18.0 IU/L [1.0-18.0 IU/L])

Prolactin = 17 ng/mL (4-30 ng/mL)
    (SI: 0.7 nmol/L [0.17-1.30 nmol/L])

You order karyotype analysis. Which of the following is the most likely result?
    A. 45,X
    B. 46,XX
    C. 46,XY
    D. 47,XXY

13 A 44-year-old perimenopausal woman is referred to your office by her psychopharmacologist for consultation regarding perimenopausal symptoms. One year ago, she noted a change in her menstrual cycles (a decrease from a 28-day to 23-day intermenstrual interval), night sweats, and hot flashes that seem to be worse around the time of her period. She has also developed depression and is currently on citalopram, 30 mg daily. She still does not feel like herself and would like to modify her depression medication. She has a history of fairly severe premenstrual mood symptoms. They are now manageable, but not entirely gone on citalopram. She is otherwise in excellent health. She has no personal or family history of hypertension, coronary heart disease, or venous thromboembolism.

Laboratory test results (sample drawn on cycle day 3):
    FSH = 40.0 mIU/L (2.0-12.0 mIU/mL [follicular])
        (SI: 40.0 IU/L [2.0-12.0 IU/L])
    Prolactin = 15 ng/mL (4-30 ng/mL)
        (SI: 0.65 nmol/L [0.17-1.30 nmol/L])
    TSH = 2.0 mIU/L (0.5-5.0 mIU/L)
    hCG, negative

On physical examination, her blood pressure is 105/70 mm Hg and BMI is 21 kg/m^2.

Which of the following do you suggest next in this patient's management?
    A. Start oral estradiol, 2 mg daily, and micronized progesterone, 200 mg on days 1 to 12 of each calendar month
    B. Increase the citalopram dosage to 40 mg daily
    C. Start a low-dosage continuous estrogen-progestin oral contraceptive (20 mcg ethinyl estradiol; 1 mg norethindrone acetate)
    D. Refer for cognitive behavioral therapy

14 A 20-year-old woman presents to discuss treatment options for hirsutism. She had menarche at age 10 years and has always had irregular menses. Acne and abnormal hair growth began at puberty. Her BMI is 27 kg/m². Excess hair is observed on her upper lip, chin, and neck (modified Ferriman-Gallwey score = 7). No hair is present on her upper chest, upper back, or upper abdomen.

Laboratory test results:
Testosterone = 75 ng/dL (8-60 ng/dL)
(SI: 2.6 nmol/L [0.3-2.1 nmol/L])
DHEA-S = 330 µg/dL (44-332 µg/dL)
(SI: 8.9 µmol/L [1.19-9.00 µmol/L])

Which of the following is the best treatment option for improving hirsutism in this patient?
  A. Combined estrogen-progestin oral contraceptive: ethinyl estradiol, 20 mcg, and norethindrone, 1 mg
  B. Flutamide and ethinyl estradiol, 20 mcg, with levonorgestrel, 1 mg
  C. Spironolactone, 100 mg orally twice daily
  D. Photoepilation therapy (laser)

15 A 32-year-old woman is referred for infertility. She has a history of irregular periods, acne, hirsutism, and progressive weight gain. Polycystic ovary syndrome was diagnosed at age 16 years. Her current BMI is 33 kg/m². Her blood pressure is 130/80 mm Hg. She began metformin 3 months ago, and she has had 2 periods since then. Serum hCG is negative.

In this patient's case, which of the following treatments will most effectively induce ovulation and result in a live birth?
  A. Clomiphene citrate
  B. Progesterone suppositories
  C. Continue metformin
  D. Letrozole

16 A 32-year-old woman with polycystic ovary syndrome presents to your office to discuss the health risks associated with her diagnosis. She had early menarche at age 11 years, hirsutism and acne since age 13 years, and weight gain in her 20s (from 120 lb [54.5 kg] to 190 lb [86.4 kg]). She has a family history of hypertension and type 2 diabetes mellitus. She has been trying to lose weight on a low-carbohydrate diet, and she started an exercise program to improve her chance for fertility.

In addition to a cardiometabolic risk assessment (blood pressure, BMI, lipid profile, and oral glucose tolerance test), for which comorbidities should the patient be screened at her initial visit?
  A. Celiac disease
  B. Coronary heart disease
  C. Autoimmune thyroid disease
  D. Depression and anxiety

17 A 28-year-old woman presents to discuss options to treat severe premenstrual dysphoria. Menarche was at age 12 years, and she has regular menses every 28 days. Since her mid 20s, she has been experiencing mood symptoms the week before her menses. Recently, she has been unable to work 1 to 2 days per month because of her mood swings, irritability, and sense of hopelessness during this time. She feels better once her period starts. Her family history is notable for hypertension, diabetes mellitus, and depression.

On physical examination, her BMI is 28 kg/m², and the rest of the findings are normal.

Which of the following is the best option for treating her premenstrual syndrome?
  A. Refer her to a therapist
  B. Start a serotonin reuptake inhibitor
  C. Start a tricyclic antidepressant such as amitriptyline
  D. Start an estrogen-progestin oral contraceptive (cyclic regimen)

18 A 51-year-old woman seeks help for menopausal symptoms. She is having hot flashes 10 to 15 times during the day and is awakened 4 to 5 times at night with sweating. These symptoms are affecting her quality of life. She had menarche at age 10 years and has always had regular menses. Her last menses was 6 months ago. She engages in aerobic exercise 3 times weekly. Her family history is notable for osteoporosis and cardiovascular disease.

On physical examination, her BMI is 26 kg/m² and blood pressure is 110/70 mm Hg.

As you obtain further information from the patient's chart, which of the following is the most important laboratory finding that would help determine the optimal menopausal hormone regimen?

A. Estradiol = 26 pg/mL (SI: 95.4 pmol/L)
B. Serum LDL cholesterol = 110 mg/dL (SI: 2.85 mmol/L)
C. Hemoglobin A_{1c} = 5.9% (41 mmol/mol)
D. Serum triglycerides = 499 mg/dL (SI: 5.64 mmol/L)

19 A 24-year-old woman with Turner syndrome (gonadal dysgenesis) is pursuing pregnancy. She will be using donor oocytes and in vitro fertilization.

On physical examination, her height is 59 in (149.9 cm), BMI is 29 kg/m^2, and blood pressure is 130/80 mm Hg. She is healthy and takes no medications.

Which of the following would be the most common risk for this patient during pregnancy?

A. Placenta accreta
B. Adrenal insufficiency
C. Ruptured spleen
D. Preeclampsia

20 A 23-year-old woman presents with irregular menses followed by amenorrhea. Menarche was at age 14 years; her periods were irregular for 18 months, then regular every 28 days. About 2 years ago, her cycle length shortened to 25 days and then to 22 days. She has not had a period in 4 months. She is stressed in her new job. She runs 2 miles 3 times a week. Her BMI is 20 kg/m^2. She has no evidence of hirsutism or acne.

A pregnancy test is negative. Her TSH value is 2.1 mIU/L (0.5-5.0 mIU/L).

Which of the following are the best laboratory tests to order now?

A. FSH, LH, testosterone, and DHEA-S
B. FSH, estradiol, and prolactin
C. FSH, estradiol, and 17-hydroxyprogesterone
D. FSH, estradiol, and progesterone
E. FSH, ACTH, and cortisol

Male Reproduction Board Review

Frances J. Hayes, MB BCh, BAO

1 A 39-year-old man is found to have a low serum testosterone level during workup of decreased energy levels and libido. He is otherwise healthy and is taking no medications.

On physical examination, his BMI is 25 kg/m^2 and blood pressure is 120/80 mm Hg. He is well virilized and has no gynecomastia. He has no ecchymoses or striae. His testicular volume is 20 mL bilaterally. He has no difficulty rising from a squatting position.

Laboratory test results:
Total testosterone = 180 ng/dL (300-900 ng/dL)
(SI: 6.2 nmol/L [10.4-31.2 nmol/L])
Calculated free testosterone = 4.5 ng/dL
(9.0-30.0 ng/dL) (SI: 0.16 nmol/L
[0.31-1.04 nmol/L])
LH = 2.8 mIU/mL (1.0-9.0 mIU/mL) (SI: 2.8 IU/L
[1.0-9.0 IU/L])
FSH = 3.5 mIU/mL (1.0-13.0 mIU/mL)
(SI: 3.5 IU/L [1.0-13.0 IU/L])

Pituitary MRI findings are normal.

Which of the following is the most appropriate next test?
A. Late-night salivary cortisol measurement
B. Karyotype analysis
C. Testicular ultrasonography
D. Serum prolactin measurement

2 A 40-year-old man is referred for evaluation of fatigue, decreased sex drive, and lack of spontaneous erections. On review of systems, his only other complaint is pain in the small joints of his hands. He takes no medications. His mother has psoriatic arthropathy.

On physical examination, his BMI is 26 kg/m^2 and blood pressure is 130/80 mm Hg. He has normal secondary sexual characteristics and no gynecomastia. He has no striae, bruises, joint swelling or evidence of psoriasis and has no difficulty rising from a squatting position. Testicular volume is 20 mL bilaterally.

Laboratory test results:
Total testosterone = 195 ng/dL (300-900 ng/dL)
(SI: 6.8 nmol/L [10.4-31.2 nmol/L])
Serum prolactin = 20 ng/mL (4-18 ng/mL)
(SI: 0.87 nmol [0.17-1.00 nmol/L])
FSH = 3.0 mIU/mL (1.0-13.0 mIU/mL)
(SI: 3.0 IU/L [1.0-13.0 IU/L])
LH = 3.0 mIU/mL (1.0-9.0 mIU/mL) (SI: 3.0 IU/L
[1.0-9.0 IU/L])

Pituitary MRI shows a 5-mm hypoenhancing lesion.

Which of the following conditions most likely explains this patient's presentation?
A. Hereditary hemochromatosis
B. Opioid abuse
C. Cushing disease
D. Hyperprolactinemia with hook effect

3 An 18-year-old high school senior is referred because of absent pubertal development. He grew normally in childhood but never experienced a growth spurt. He has a normal sense of smell. He does not take any medications but admits to occasional marijuana use. His two older brothers and his father went through puberty at a normal age.

On physical examination, his height is 67 in (170 cm), arm span is 70 in (177.8 cm), and BMI is 22 kg/m^2. He has slight axillary hair and Tanner stage 2 pubic hair but no facial or chest hair. He has no gynecomastia. His testes measure 2 mL bilaterally. His visual fields are full to confrontation.

Laboratory test results (sample drawn at 8 AM):
Total testosterone = 40 ng/dL (300-900 ng/dL)
(SI: 1.4 nmol/L [10.4-31.2 nmol/L])

Free T$_4$ = 1.3 ng/dL (0.8-1.8 ng/dL) (SI: 16.7 pmol/L [10.30-23.17 pmol/L])

TSH = 1.41 mIU/L (0.5-5.0 mIU/L)

LH = <0.2 mIU/mL (1.0-9.0 mIU/mL) (SI: <0.2 IU/L [1.0-9.0 IU/L])

FSH = 0.3 mIU/mL (1.0-13.0 mIU/mL) (SI: 0.3 IU/L [1.0-13.0 IU/L])

Prolactin = 10 ng/mL (4-23 ng/mL) (SI: 0.43 nmol/L [0.17-1.00 nmol/L])

Cortisol (8 AM) = 20.0 µg/dL (5-25 µg/dL) (SI: 551.8 nmol/L [137.9-689.7 nmol/L])

IGF-1, low-normal for age and sex

Which of the following is the most likely diagnosis?
   A. Constitutional delay of growth and puberty
   B. Congenital hypogonadotropic hypogonadism
   C. Pathogenic variant in the *PROP1* gene
   D. Pathogenic variant in the *LEPR* gene (leptin receptor)

A 19-year-old man is referred for evaluation of small testes noted on his first physical examination by an adult provider. He reports normal sexual function. He has a history of attention-deficit/hyperactivity disorder, for which he is being treated with amphetamine-dextroamphetamine. He has no history of testicular pain, swelling, or trauma. He takes no prescribed medications but recently started taking biotin, 5000 mcg daily, for hair loss. He has a normal sense of smell.

On physical examination, his height is 72 in (182.9 cm), arm span is 71 in (180.3 cm), and BMI is 23 kg/m^2. His blood pressure is 110/70 mm Hg. He is well virilized. He has mild gynecomastia. He has a normal phallus with no hypospadias. His testes are small and firm, measuring 6 mL bilaterally.

Laboratory test results:
   Total testosterone = 325 ng/dL (300-900 ng/dL) (SI: 11.3 nmol/L [10.4-31.2 nmol/L])
   Free testosterone = 5.0 (9.0-30.0 ng/dL) (SI: 1.17 nmol/L [0.31-1.04 nmol/L])
   Estradiol = 30 pg/mL (10-40 pg/mL) (SI: 110.1 pmol/L [36.7-146.8 pmol/L])
   FSH = 38.0 mIU/mL (1.0-13.0 mIU/mL) (SI: 38.0 IU/L [1.0-13.0 IU/L])
   LH = 18.0 mIU/mL (1.0-9.0 mIU/mL) (SI: 18.0 IU/L [1.0-9.0 IU/L])

Which of the following is the most likely cause of this patient's presentation?
   A. Inactivating pathogenic variant in the gene encoding the FSH receptor
   B. Klinefelter syndrome
   C. Interference with FSH assay due to biotin
   D. Mumps orchitis

A 47-year-old man presents with a 2-year history of increasing fatigue, loss of libido, and erectile dysfunction. He underwent normal puberty. HIV infection was diagnosed 3 years ago, and his CD$_4$ cell count is currently stable on treatment. He states that he does not use androgens or recreational drugs.

On physical examination, the patient is normally virilized. His BMI is 24.5 kg/m^2. He has bilateral, nontender gynecomastia. Testes are 15 mL bilaterally.

Laboratory test results:
   Total testosterone (8 AM) (by liquid chromatography tandem mass spectrometry) = 865 ng/dL (300-900 ng/dL) (SI: 30 nmol/L [10.4-31.2 nmol/L]) (repeated measurement = 808 ng/dL [SI: 28.0 nmol/L])
   LH = 5.6 mIU/mL (1.0-13.0 mIU/mL) (SI: 5.6 IU/L [1.0-13.0 IU/L])
   FSH = 6.1 mIU/mL (1.0-9.0 mIU/mL) (SI: 6.1 IU/L [1.0-9.0 IU/L])
   TSH = 2.2 mIU/L (0.5-5.0 mIU/L)

Which of the following is the best next diagnostic step in this patient's evaluation?
   A. Measure free testosterone by equilibrium dialysis
   B. Determine the urinary testosterone-to-epitestosterone ratio
   C. Screen for pathogenic variants in the androgen receptor gene
   D. Measure estradiol

A 20-year-old man is seeing you for the first time after transitioning from pediatric care. Adrenal insufficiency was diagnosed at age 3 years, and he has since been treated with hydrocortisone and fludrocortisone. At age 18 years, hypogonadotropic hypogonadism was diagnosed when he showed no signs of puberty and was found to have a serum testosterone level of 45 ng/dL (1.6 nmol/L) and undetectable gonadotropins. His free T$_4$ and prolactin levels were normal, as was sellar imaging. He has been treated with testosterone since age 18 years, and his total testosterone levels are normal on treatment. He has a normal sense of smell.

On physical examination, his blood pressure is 95/60 mm Hg with no postural drop. He is well virilized and has no gynecomastia. He has slight pigmentation of the buccal mucosa and palmar creases. Testes are 4 mL bilaterally.

You obtain a copy of his original cosyntropin-stimulation test:

Baseline cortisol = 1.8 μg/dL (5-25 μg/dL)
   (SI: 49.7 nmol/L [137.9-689.7 nmol/L])
Baseline ACTH = 250 pg/mL (10-60 pg/mL)
   (SI: 55.0 pmol/L [2.2-13.2 pmol/L])
Cortisol 1 hour after administration of 250 mcg
   intravenous cosyntropin = 3.5 μg/dL
   (SI: 96.6 nmol/L)

A pathogenic variant in which of the following genes is the most likely explanation for this patient's presentation?
   A. *PROP1* (PROP paired-like homeobox 1)
   B. *AIRE* (autoimmune regulator)
   C. *NR0B1* (formerly *DAX1*) (nuclear receptor subfamily 0 group B member 1)
   D. *ANOS1* (formerly *KAL1*) (anosmin 1)

7 A 45-year-old white man is referred by his primary care physician to discuss testosterone replacement therapy. During workup for fatigue, decreased libido, and erectile dysfunction, hypogonadism was diagnosed and he is eager to start therapy. He has no lower urinary tract symptoms. His family history is negative for prostate cancer.

On physical examination, he has a BMI of 31 kg/m^2. He appears healthy, is well virilized, and has normal testes. His prostate feels normal in size on rectal examination.

Laboratory test results:
   Total testosterone (8 AM) = 160 ng/dL
      (300-900 ng/dL) (SI: 5.5 nmol/L
      [10.4-31.2 nmol/L]) (repeated value = 180 ng/dL
      [SI: 6.2 nmol/L])
   Free testosterone = 5.0 ng/dL (9.0-30.0 ng/dL)
      (SI: 0.17 nmol/L [0.31-1.04 nmol/L])
   LH = 5.9 mIU/mL (1.0-9.0 mIU/mL) (SI: 5.9 IU/L
      [1.0-9.0 IU/L])

FSH = 6.2 mIU/mL (1.0-13.0 mIU/mL)
   (SI: 6.2 IU/L [1.0-13.0 IU/L])
Prolactin = 8.9 ng/mL (4-18 ng/mL)
   (SI: 0.39 nmol/L [0.17-0.78 nmol/L])
Hematocrit = 45% (41%-50%) (SI: 0.45 [0.41-0.50])

Which of the following is the best next step in this patient's management?
   A. Start testosterone replacement therapy
   B. Start a phosphodiesterase inhibitor
   C. Measure PSA
   D. Order karyotype analysis

8 A 67-year-old man returns to clinic for follow-up of hypogonadism 12 months after starting testosterone therapy. At the time of diagnosis, his prostate examination was normal and his PSA level was 1.5 ng/mL (1.5 μg/L). Following treatment with a 1.62% testosterone gel, 40.5 mg daily, his testosterone level has been restored to the mid-normal range. The patient reports a significant improvement in energy levels, mood, and libido since starting treatment, and he has no lower urinary tract symptoms.

On physical examination, his prostate examination findings are unchanged.

His current PSA level is 3.5 ng/mL (<5.3 ng/mL) (SI: 3.5 μg/L [<5.3 μg/L]).

Which of the following is the best next step in this patient's management?
   A. Discontinue testosterone therapy
   B. Refer for prostate biopsy
   C. Recheck his PSA level
   D. Start a 5α-reductase inhibitor

9 A 65-year-old man was prescribed testosterone therapy by his primary care physician to treat hypogonadism. However, he was reluctant to start it due to concerns about its impact on prostate health, and he requested a specialist referral to discuss further. He is generally healthy apart from being overweight. He reports nocturia once nightly but no other lower urinary tract symptoms, and he has a mildly enlarged, smooth prostate without nodules on examination. His pretreatment PSA level was 1.9 ng/mL (<5.3 ng/mL) (SI: 1.9 μg/L [<5.3 μg/L]).

If this patient were to start testosterone therapy, which of the following prostate outcomes would be most likely?

A. Increased risk of detecting subclinical prostate cancer
B. Aggravation of his lower urinary tract symptoms
C. Significant increase in his PSA levels
D. Increased risk of developing prostatitis

10 A 56-year-old man returns for monitoring of testosterone therapy for opioid-induced hypogonadism. Following an initial discussion of the different formulations available to treat his condition, he opted for a gel delivery system and has been applying 40.5 mg of a 1.62% testosterone gel every morning. At his last evaluation on this testosterone dosage 6 months ago, his total testosterone concentration was 475 ng/dL (16.5 nmol/L) and hematocrit was 47% (0.47). He currently reports normal energy levels, libido, and sexual function.

Current laboratory test results (sample drawn at 7 AM yesterday):
Total testosterone = 1100 ng/dL (300-900 ng/dL) (SI: 38.2 nmol/L [10.4-31.2 nmol/L])
Hematocrit = 47.2% (41%-50%) (SI: 0.472 [0.41-0.50])
PSA = 1.3 ng/mL (<3.8 ng/mL) (SI: 1.3 µg/L [<3.8 µg/L])

Which of the following is the best next step?

A. Discontinue testosterone therapy due to evidence of androgen abuse
B. Reduce the dosage of his 1.62% testosterone gel to 20.25 mg daily
C. Measure testosterone 2 to 8 hours after the gel has been applied
D. Switch to intramuscular injections of testosterone enanthate

11 A 68-year-old man is referred to discuss treatment options for hypogonadism. He is not keen on the idea of having to apply a testosterone gel or patch daily and expresses a preference for injections. He has read about the long-acting depot formulation of testosterone undecanoate. He likes the fact that the injection must only be administered every 10 weeks and asks for additional information about its safety profile.

Which of the following is a potential adverse effect that this patient might experience as a result of this regimen?

A. Marked fluctuations in energy levels and mood
B. Abnormal liver function test results
C. Cough and shortness of breath following the injection
D. Skin irritation

12 A 55-year-old man is referred by his primary care physician for management of hypogonadism. At the time of diagnosis, he described decreased energy and libido and was found to have 2 morning testosterone values in the hypogonadal range (190 and 215 ng/dL [6.6 and 7.5 nmol/L]). For the past 6 months, he has been treated with intramuscular injections of testosterone enanthate, 150 mg every 2 weeks. Although he feels better overall on this regimen, he reports feeling depressed and tired in the few days before each injection.

His testosterone level drawn 5 days after his last injection was 405 ng/dL (14.1 nmol/L).

Which of the following is the best next step in this patient's management?

A. Recommend that he talk to his primary care physician about starting an antidepressant
B. Switch from testosterone enanthate to cypionate at the current dosage
C. Discontinue testosterone therapy due to lack of efficacy
D. Measure a trough testosterone level

13 A 30-year-old man is referred by his oncologist for a fertility consultation. He has completed chemotherapy with cyclophosphamide for Hodgkin lymphoma. He feels well and is now in complete remission from his cancer. A semen analysis shows azoospermia.

Which of the following hormone profiles is most likely in this patient?

Answer	Testosterone	LH	FSH
A.	Normal	Normal	Normal
B.	Normal	Normal	High
C.	Low	Low	Low
D.	Low	Low	High

14 A 35-year-old man is referred for evaluation of azoospermia noted during workup for primary infertility. He and his wife have been having unprotected intercourse for the past 2 years without a confirmed pregnancy. The patient underwent normal puberty and reports normal libido and erections. His wife is 32 years old and her infertility workup is normal.

On physical examination, his BMI is 25.5 kg/m². He is well virilized and has no gynecomastia. His testes are 15 mL bilaterally.

Laboratory test results:
Total testosterone = 625 ng/dL (300-900 ng/dL)
(SI: 21.7 nmol/L [10.4-31.2 nmol/L])
FSH = 21.5 mIU/mL (1.0-13.0 mIU/mL)
(SI: 21.5 IU/L [1.0-13.0 IU/L])
LH = 5.0 mIU/mL (1.0-9.0 mIU/mL) (SI: 5.0 IU/L
[1.0-9.0 IU/L])
Karyotype = 46,XY

A second semen analysis documents a pH of 7.5 and volume of 3 mL and confirms azoospermia.

Which of the following genetic conditions does this patient most likely have?
A. Y-Chromosome microdeletion
B. Kallmann syndrome
C. Mosaic Klinefelter syndrome
D. Congenital bilateral absence of the vas deferens

15 A 30-year-old man seeks a second opinion for management of infertility after being diagnosed with adult-onset hypogonadotropic hypogonadism. He and his wife have had regular unprotected intercourse for 18 months without a documented pregnancy. His wife's workup is normal. Previously ordered laboratory tests document the following:
Total testosterone (8 AM) = 225 ng/dL
(300-900 ng/dL) (SI: 7.8 nmol/L
[10.4-31.2 nmol/L])
Free testosterone = 5.2 ng/dL (9.0-30.0 ng/dL)
(SI: 1.18 nmol/L [0.31-1.04 nmol/L])
LH = 5.5 mIU/mL (1.0-9.0 mIU/mL) (SI: 5.5 IU/L
[1.0-9.0 IU/L])
FSH = 4.0 mIU/mL (1.0-13.0 mIU/mL)
(SI: 4.0 IU/L [1.0-13.0 IU/L])
Prolactin = 12 ng/mL (4-18 ng/mL)
(SI: 0.52 nmol/L [0.17-0.78 nmol/L])
Transferrin saturation = 38% (14%-50%)

Previously ordered semen analysis documented azoospermia. He was started on hCG, 1500 units 3 times weekly.

On physical examination, he is an obese, otherwise healthy man who is well virilized. His testes are 20 mL bilaterally, but you have difficulty palpating his vas deferens.

His testosterone level measured on the day his hCG injection is due is 490 ng/dL (17.0 nmol/L), but he remains azoospermic.

Which of the following is the most appropriate next step?
A. Add recombinant FSH injections
B. Arrange for transrectal ultrasonography
C. Increase the hCG dosage to 2000 units 3 times weekly
D. Encourage the patient to consider use of donor sperm

16 A 35-year-old man presents for evaluation of secondary infertility. His wife is 32 years old and they have a 5-year-old daughter. They have been having regular unprotected intercourse for the past year without success. He has a history of a hypophysectomy for a nonsecreting pituitary macroadenoma 3 years ago, following which he developed secondary hypogonadism. He is currently being treated with testosterone gel, and he has normal libido and erections.

On physical examination, he has normal secondary sexual characteristics and a testicular volume of 20 mL bilaterally.

Laboratory test results 2 weeks after discontinuing testosterone therapy:
Total testosterone = 52 ng/dL (300-900 ng/dL)
(SI: 1.8 nmol/L [10.4-31.2 nmol/L])
LH = 1.0 mIU/mL (1.0-13.0 mIU/mL) (SI: 1.0 IU/L
[1.0-13.0 IU/L])
FSH = 1.8 mIU/mL (1.0-9.0 mIU/mL) (SI: 1.8 IU/L
[1.0-9.0 IU/L])

Semen analyses show normal semen volume with azoospermia.

Which of the following is the best initial treatment option to restore fertility in this patient?
- A. Clomiphene
- B. hCG and FSH injections
- C. Pulsatile GnRH therapy
- D. hCG injections

17 A 32-year-old man presents for evaluation of a 6-month history of tender gynecomastia. On questioning, he also endorses recent onset of fatigue and decreased libido, although he can still get and sustain an erection. He has been taking finasteride for male-pattern balding.

On physical examination, his BMI is 22 kg/m^2 and pulse rate is 68 beats/min. His thyroid gland is normal in size with no palpable nodules. He has normal facial, axillary, and pubic hair. He has bilateral gynecomastia, right greater than left, which is tender to palpation. His phallus is normal, and testes are 15 mL bilaterally with no palpable masses.

Laboratory test results:
Total testosterone = 150 ng/dL (300-900 ng/dL)
(SI: 5.2 nmol/L [10.4-31.2 nmol/L])
Estradiol = 160 pg/mL (10-40 pg/mL)
(SI: 587.4 pmol/L [36.7-146.8 pmol/L])
FSH = 1.0 mIU/mL (1.0-13.0 mIU/mL)
(SI: 1.0 IU/L [1.0-13.0 IU/L])
LH = 0.5 mIU/mL (1.0-9.0 mIU/mL) (SI: 0.5 IU/L
[1.0-9.0 IU/L])
β–hCG, negative

Which of the following most likely explains his hormone profile?
- A. Anabolic steroid use
- B. Decreased 5α-reductase activity due to finasteride
- C. Estrogen-secreting testicular tumor
- D. Hyperthyroidism

18 An 18-year-old man presents for evaluation of bilateral breast enlargement, which has been present for 4 years. The breast tissue is no longer growing and the tenderness that he initially experienced has now resolved. However, he has started dating and is embarrassed by the cosmetic appearance. He takes no medications or herbal products and does not use illicit drugs.

On physical examination, the patient is well virilized and has facial acne. Palpation of the breasts reveals rubbery, mobile subareolar tissue. There is no nipple discharge or retraction. Findings on genital examination are age appropriate, with a normal phallus, testes of 15 mL bilaterally, and Tanner stage 5 pubic hair.

Laboratory test results:
Total testosterone = 400 ng/dL (300-900 ng/dL)
(SI: 13.9 nmol/L [10.4-31.2 nmol/L])
Estradiol = 25 pg/mL (10-40 pg/mL)
(SI: 91.8 pmol/L [36.7-146.8 pmol/L])
LH = 4.5 mIU/mL (1.0-13.0 mIU/mL) (SI: 4.5 IU/L
[1.0-13.0 IU/L])
FSH = 3.0 mIU/mL (1.0-9.0 mIU/mL) (SI: 3.0 IU/L
[1.0-9.0 IU/L])
TSH = 1.5 mIU/mL (0.5-5.0 mIU/mL)

Which of the following is the most likely diagnosis?
- A. Mosaic Klinefelter syndrome
- B. Persistent postpubertal gynecomastia
- C. Leydig-cell tumor
- D. Inadvertent estrogen exposure

19 A 35-year-old transgender woman is self-referred for ongoing management of hormone therapy. She has a strong family history of hyperlipidemia, and hypertriglyceridemia was diagnosed when she was in her late teens. She was prescribed rosuvastatin and fenofibrate, but she has not taken her medications consistently. She has been treated with conjugated equine estrogens, 1.25 mg daily, and spironolactone, 100 mg twice daily, since age 18 years when she started living as a woman. In her late 20s, she had breast augmentation and facial feminization surgery. She consumes 1 to 2 glasses of wine per week and does not smoke cigarettes.

Laboratory test results (sample drawn while fasting):
Total testosterone = 125 ng/dL (8-60 ng/dL)
(SI: 4.3 nmol/L [0.3-2.1 nmol/L])
Estradiol = 25 pg/mL (SI: 91.8 pmol/L)
Triglycerides = 1050 mg/dL (<150 mg/dL
[optimal]) (SI: 11.87 mmol/L [<1.70 mmol/L])
Glucose = 90 mg/dL (70-99 mg/dL) (SI: 5.0 mmol/L
[3.9-5.5 mmol/L])

Following discontinuation of hormone therapy, her triglyceride level decreased to 380 mg/dL (4.29 mmol/L).

Which of the following is the most appropriate management option for this patient?

    A. Resume spironolactone but remain off conjugated equine estrogen

    B. Switch her regimen to a GnRH agonist with a 0.05-mg estradiol patch

    C. Tell the patient that she is not a candidate for any further hormone therapy

    D. Resume spironolactone and switch her estrogen regimen to ethinyl estradiol

20 You are asked to consult on a 61-year old man with gynecomastia who was admitted to the medicine service with pneumonia. His medical history is notable for surgery for right-sided cryptorchidism as a child, as well as hypothyroidism treated with levothyroxine, 112 mcg daily.

On physical examination, he has diminished facial and axillary hair, bilateral nontender breast enlargement, microphallus, hypospadias, and testes measuring 3 mL bilaterally.

Laboratory test results:

    Total testosterone = 760 ng/dL (300-900 ng/dL)
      (SI: 26.4 nmol/L [10.4-31.2 nmol/L])

    LH = 24.0 mIU/mL (1.0-13.0 mIU/mL)
      (SI: 24.0 IU/L [1.0-13.0 IU/L])

    FSH = 18.0 mIU/mL (1.0-9.0 mIU/mL)
      (SI: 18.0 IU/L [1.0-9.0 IU/L])

    TSH = 3.8 mIU/L (0.5-5.0 mIU/L)

Which of the following is the most likely diagnosis?

    A. Klinefelter syndrome with concomitant testosterone therapy

    B. 5α-Reductase deficiency

    C. Polyglandular autoimmune syndrome type 2

    D. Partial androgen insensitivity syndrome

Obesity & Lipids Board Review
Andrea D. Coviello, MD

1 A 38-year-old woman is referred to you for weight loss. She has features of the metabolic syndrome, including impaired fasting glucose and dyslipidemia. Her height is 66 in (167.6 cm), and weight is 178 lb (80.9 kg) (BMI = 28.7 kg/m^2). She has had slow, steady weight gain since puberty. Menarche was at age 13 years, and she has always had normal menses. She has never been pregnant. She has a strong family history of obesity. Her mother underwent gastric bypass surgery at age 52 years and lost approximately 60 lb (27.3 kg). Her father was recently diagnosed with steatohepatitis and both of her brothers are obese. She currently takes metformin but no other medications.

Physical examination is notable for generalized adiposity but findings are otherwise normal.

A predisposing variant in which of the following genes is most likely to be present in this family?
  A. *MC4R* (melanocortin 4 receptor)
  B. *LEP* (leptin)
  C. *LEPR* (leptin receptor)
  D. *FTO* (fat mass and obesity associated)

2 You have been working with a 36-year-old woman to lose weight and improve her health. Her height is 67 in (170.2 cm), and weight is 245 lb (111.4 kg) (BMI = 38.4 kg/m^2). She has type 2 diabetes mellitus and dyslipidemia. You recommended a low–glycemic index, reduced-calorie diet (–500 kcal daily) in addition to an exercise regimen of aerobic exercise (walking on a treadmill for an hour) 5 days a week and resistance training 3 days a week. She keeps a daily food diary with an app on her phone. She has lost 40 lb (18.2 kg) over 2 years, but over the last 3 months, she regained 8 lb (3.6 kg). You review her food diary (on the phone app), and it shows that she is consuming 1200 to 1400 kcal daily. She states she has maintained her exercise regimen, which is confirmed by her pedometer. She is frustrated and very concerned about the weight regain.

Which of the following is the main cause of her weight regain?
  A. Increased energy expenditure
  B. Decreased satiety
  C. Decreased energy expenditure
  D. Increased appetite

3 A 46-year-old women presents to your clinic for medically supervised weight loss with a meal replacement program. She has migraines, hypertension, type 2 diabetes mellitus, hyperlipidemia, depression, and kidney stones. She has had a cholecystectomy for cholelithiasis. Current medications are lisinopril, metformin, glipizide, atorvastatin, escitalopram, and norethindrone.

On physical examination, her height is 65 in (165.1 cm) and weight is 205 lb (93.2 kg) (BMI = 34.1 kg/m^2). Her blood pressure is 162/88 mm Hg, and pulse rate is 76 beats/min. Waist circumference is 40 in (101.5 cm).

Of the patient's medications, which of the following is considered weight promoting?
  A. Lisinopril
  B. Metformin
  C. Glipizide
  D. Atorvastatin
  E. Escitalopram

4 A 46-year-old woman presents to your clinic for medically supervised weight loss with a meal replacement program. She has migraines, hypertension, type 2 diabetes mellitus, hyperlipidemia, depression, and kidney stones. She has had a cholecystectomy for cholelithiasis.

On physical examination, her height is 65 in (165.1 cm) and weight is 205 lb (93.2 kg) (BMI = 34.1 kg/m^2).

You stop glipizide and start canagliflozin. You recommend a 500 kcal-reduced, low-fat, high-fiber diet and walking (10,000 steps daily). She loses 12 lb (5.5 kg) in 3 months, 6 lb (2.7 kg) in the following 3 months, and then plateaus at 190 lb (86.4 kg).

Current medications are lisinopril, metformin, canagliflozin, atorvastatin, escitalopram, and norethindrone.

On physical examination, her current weight is 187 lb (85 kg) (BMI = 31.1 kg/m^2) and waist circumference is 38 in (96.5 cm). Her blood pressure is 160/84 mm Hg, and pulse rate is 72 beats/min.

Given her medical problems and current medications, which of the following weight-loss medications would you recommend?
- A. Lorcaserin
- B. Liraglutide
- C. Phentermine/topiramate
- D. Topiramate
- E. Naltrexone/bupropion

5 A 68-year-old man with osteoarthritis of the knees seeks assistance with weight loss. His height is 70 in (177.8 cm) and weight is 315 lb (143.2 kg) (BMI = 45.2 kg/m^2). He has debilitating joint pain and increasing difficulty with mobility, which he notes is contributing to his weight gain. He wants to pursue knee replacement, but his orthopedic surgeon told him he must lose approximately 45 lb (20.5 kg) (BMI = 39 kg/m^2). He also has type 2 diabetes mellitus, stage 3 chronic kidney disease, hypertension, fatty liver, dyslipidemia, and cholelithiasis. His current medications are metformin, sitagliptin, lisinopril, and atorvastatin. His hemoglobin A$_{1c}$ level is 8.2% (66 mmol/mol).

Given his overall clinical picture, you are hesitant to prescribe a very low-calorie diet due to which of the following?
- A. Fatty liver disease
- B. Dyslipidemia
- C. Cholelithiasis
- D. Hypertension
- E. Type 2 diabetes mellitus

6 A 57-year-old woman had a laparoscopic gastric banding procedure done in another state 4 years ago. One year after surgery, she had lost 71 lb (32.3 kg) (from a peak lifetime weight of 290 lb [131.8 kg] to a weight nadir of 219 lb [99.5 kg]). She initially did well, but over the last 6 months, she has gained weight and currently weighs 282 lb (128.2 kg). Over the last

10 days, she has noted increasing abdominal pain and bloating associated with redness and tenderness over her injection port.

On physical examination, she has moderate abdominal tenderness and decreased bowel sounds.

Which of the following is the most likely diagnosis?
- A. Surreptitious manipulation of the injection port
- B. Staple line dehiscence
- C. Anastomotic leak
- D. Gastric band erosion
- E. Food impaction in the band

7 An 18-year-old man is brought to clinic by his family for help losing weight. At birth he was hypotonic and had trouble feeding. He received tube feedings shortly after birth. As he got older, he developed a ravenous appetite and became overweight and then markedly obese. He had cryptorchidism, which was treated surgically at age 5 years. He had developmental delay and the family was told that he had mild cognitive impairment.

On physical examination, his height is 61 in (154.9 cm) and weight is 290 lb (131.8 kg) (BMI = 54.8 kg/m^2). He has almond-shaped eyes, small hands and feet, and underdeveloped genitalia.

Which of the following is the most likely genetic defect in this patient?
- A. Deletion in the 15q11.2-q13 chromosomal region (Prader-Willi syndrome)
- B. Pathogenic variant in the *MC4R* gene (associated with early-onset obesity)
- C. Pathogenic variant in the *LEPR* gene (leptin receptor deficiency)
- D. Pathogenic variant in the *ALMS1* gene (Alstrom syndrome)
- E. Pathogenic variant in the *BBS1* gene (Bardet-Biedl syndrome)

8 A 64-year-old man with type 2 diabetes mellitus asks your advice on weight-loss surgery, which he has been considering due to his severe obesity. He has hypertension and hyperlipidemia, and he has had 2 stents placed for coronary artery disease. He also has osteoarthritis in his knees and has been told that he needs bilateral knee replacements, but his surgeon has said that his weight must be under 300 lb (<136.4 kg) (>20% weight loss) before considering surgery.

On physical examination, his height is 70 in (177.8 cm) and weight is 365 lb (165.9 kg) (BMI = 52.4 kg/m^2) (class 3 obesity).

Which of the following bariatric procedures will most likely result in the greatest weight loss for this patient?
  A. Sleeve gastrectomy
  B. Roux-en-Y gastric bypass
  C. Laparoscopic banding procedure
  D. Biliopancreatic diversion
  E. Endoscopically placed duodenal sleeve

9 A 54-year-old woman with class 3 obesity (weight 267 lb [121.4 kg]; BMI = 43 kg/m^2) and type 2 diabetes mellitus had Roux-en-Y gastric bypass 3 years ago. She lost 110 lb (50 kg) (current weight = 157 lb [71.4 kg]; BMI = 25 kg/m^2) and diabetes resolved. In the last few months, she has developed recurrent episodes when she felt shaky, sweaty, and irritable. The episodes almost always occur after lunch or dinner. Last week, her daughter found her unarousable, and emergency medical technicians documented a blood glucose value of 29 mg/dL (1.6 mmol/L).

Laboratory test results:
  Hemoglobin A$_{1c}$ = 4.9% (4.0%-5.6%)
    (20-38 mmol/mol)
  Fasting glucose = 87 mg/dL (70-99 mg/dL)
    (SI: 4.8 mmol/L [3.9-5.5 mmol/L])
  C-peptide = 4.0 ng/mL (0.9-4.3 ng/mL)
    (SI: 1.3 nmol/L [0.30-1.42 nmol/L])
  72-hour fast, normal response

You recommend she adjust her diet by reducing simple carbohydrates and eating small mixed meals (low–glycemic index carbohydrates with protein and fat) during the day. She makes these changes and returns in a few months with some improvement. However, she still has 1 severe episode each week.

Which of the following is the most appropriate next treatment?
  A. GLP-1 receptor agonist
  B. Partial pancreatectomy
  C. Octreotide
  D. Acarbose

10 A 27-year-old woman seeks advice on weight loss. She is a student and has been writing her dissertation, which has changed her lifestyle considerably. She sits at her computer most of the day, gets little exercise, and has been craving junk food. She has gained 25 lb (11.4 kg) in the last year. Her current BMI is 30.5 kg/m^2. She wants to lose weight but does not want to start medication. She would like to begin a diet, but she is unsure which one would have the best results. She asks about the evidence supporting various diets.

You tell her that in comparison to a traditional daily caloric restriction diet (500 kcal reduced daily calorie diet), an alternate day fasting diet results in which of the following?
  A. Same amount of weight loss
  B. More weight loss
  C. Less weight loss
  D. Weight gain

11 A 42-year-old man with a peak lifetime BMI of 48 kg/m^2 had a laparoscopic gastric bypass in another state 2 years ago, after which he lost 60 lb (27.3 kg). Eight months after his surgery, his employer transferred him to Mumbai, so he was unable to follow-up with his bariatric surgeon over the last year. He is home on vacation, and he comes to see you for a checkup. He takes no medications and relates that he was taking his vitamin supplements postoperatively, but ran out more than 6 months ago. He has developed numbness and tingling in his feet and hands. He also thinks he has a middle ear problem after the long flight home because he feels off-balance. Routine bloodwork indicates mild anemia.

This patient most likely has a deficiency of which of the following?
  A. Vitamin B$_{12}$
  B. Folate
  C. Thiamine
  D. Zinc

12 After diagnosing the above patient, you recommend a daily multivitamin, a B complex supplement, and a vitamin D supplement. You discuss appropriate follow-up after bariatric surgery and outline a treatment plan.

Which of the following should be done as part of this patient's routine monitoring?
- A. Cardiac stress test
- B. Right upper-quadrant ultrasonography for gallstones
- C. Single-view abdominal film to screen for kidney stones
- D. DXA scan for bone mineral density
- E. 24-Hour urine collection for measurement of calcium and creatinine

13 A 36-year-old woman with polycystic ovary syndrome presents for weight management. She gained a significant amount of weight after the birth of her second child, and she has been not been able to lose this weight. Her first pregnancy was complicated by gestational diabetes mellitus that was controlled with diet. Diabetes resolved after delivery. She had gestational diabetes with her second pregnancy, but hyperglycemia persisted after delivery. Prediabetes was diagnosed, and metformin was initiated. She would like to lose weight in hopes that her prediabetes will reverse. She is finished child bearing and has an intrauterine device.

Which of the following is the best choice for medical therapy in this patient?
- A. Phentermine
- B. Phentermine/topiramate ER
- C. Naltrexone/bupropion ER
- D. Lorcaserin

14 You refer one of your patients, a 36-year old obese man (BMI = 38 kg/m^2) with dyslipidemia and type 2 diabetes mellitus (hemoglobin A_{1c} = 7.4% [57 mmol/mol]), to a hepatologist because of chronically elevated liver function tests (ALT = 120 U/L [2.00 µkat/L], AST = 90 U/L [1.50 µkat/L]). He comes to see you after having a liver biopsy and being diagnosed with nonalcoholic steatohepatitis (NASH) with stage 3 fibrosis. He was informed that he is at high risk for cirrhosis and is very distressed. He wants to know what he should do to avoid liver cirrhosis. His hepatologist prescribed pioglitazone.

Which of the following treatments has the greatest chance of NASH regression over the next year?
- A. Lifestyle modification to achieve 5% to 10% weight loss
- B. Liraglutide, 1.8 mg daily
- C. Canagliflozin, 100 mg daily
- D. Metformin, 500 mg twice daily

15 A 67-year-old woman presents for help with weight loss. After retiring last year, she focused on improving her health. Her medical history is notable for prediabetes, nonalcoholic fatty liver disease, migraines, and glaucoma. Her peak weight was 270 lb (122.7 kg) (BMI = 43 kg/m^2). She lost 25 lb (11.4 kg) by increasing physical activity (30 minutes walking daily) and participating in an app-based weight-loss program. She was able to lower her BMI to 39.5 kg/m^2. She then regained 10 lb (4.5 kg), which prompted her primary care physician to prescribe phentermine; she then lost 15 lb (6.8 kg) over 6 months. She is interested in combination therapy with topiramate, which she has heard is even more effective when used with phentermine.

Which of her current medications would preclude her from starting combination therapy with topiramate?
- A. Metoprolol
- B. Travoprost ophthalmic solution
- C. Pioglitazone
- D. Metformin

16 A 37-year-old man comes to see you for hyperlipidemia. A cholesterol panel was done 1 year ago, and a repeated panel was done last week.

Measurement	1 Year Ago	Current
Total cholesterol	190 mg/dL (SI: 4.92 mmol/L)	220 mg/dL (SI: 5.70 mmol/L)
Triglycerides	115 mg/dL (SI: 1.30 mmol/L)	130 mg/dL (SI: 1.47 mmol/L)
LDL cholesterol	123 mg/dL (SI: 3.19 mmol/L)	150 mg/dL (SI: 3.89 mmol/L)
HDL cholesterol	43 mg/dL (SI: 1.11 mmol/L)	44 mg/dL (SI: 1.14 mmol/L)

He is concerned about the increase in his cholesterol. Since his cholesterol was checked 1 year ago, he has gained 12 lb (5.5 kg) (BMI 28 kg/m^2). He reports he has been working longer hours (sedentary desk job), sleeping less, and feeling quite fatigued. He has changed his diet and eliminated fried foods and sweets. He has been exercising regularly to lose weight. His wife states that he has been snoring a lot lately. He has a family history of type 2 diabetes, but his hemoglobin A_{1c} level last year was 5.2% (33 mmol/mol).

Which of the following is the most likely cause of the increase in his cholesterol?

A. Sleep apnea
B. Hypothyroidism
C. Weight gain
D. Undiagnosed diabetes mellitus

17 A 20-year-old woman with a family history of premature coronary artery disease comes to see you for evaluation of an increased cholesterol level.

On physical examination, she has bilateral Achilles tendon thickening. The rest of her examination findings are normal.

Fasting lipid profile:
Total cholesterol = 301 mg/dL (<200 mg/dL [optimal]) (SI: 7.80 mmol/L [<5.18 mmol/L])
Triglycerides = 130 mg/dL (<150 mg/dL [optimal]) (SI: 1.47 mmol/L [<1.70 mmol/L])
HDL cholesterol = 51 mg/dL (>60 mg/dL [optimal]) (SI: 1.32 mmol/L [>1.55 mmol/L])
LDL cholesterol = 130 mg/dL (<100 mg/dL [optimal]) (SI: 3.37 mmol/L [<2.59 mmol/L])
Hematocrit = 32% (35%-45%) (SI: 0.32 [0.35-0.45])

Which of the following is the most likely cause of her lipid profile?

A. Cerebrotendinous xanthomatosis
B. Familial combined hyperlipidemia
C. Familial defective apolipoprotein B_{100}
D. Familial hypercholesterolemia
E. Sitosterolemia

18 A 59-year-old man had a non–q-wave myocardial infarction 8 months ago. His LDL-cholesterol level decreased dramatically after atorvastatin, 80 mg daily, was prescribed. However, he developed pain in his lower extremities and a rise in his creatine kinase level twice the upper normal limit. He stopped the atorvastatin and the pain resolved. His TSH level is normal. His triglyceride level has been in the range of 220 to 270 mg/dL (2.49-3.05 mmol/L) each time it has been checked since his myocardial infarction.

Which of the following is the best next step?

A. Start rosuvastatin, 10 mg daily
B. Start fenofibrate, 145 mg daily
C. Start ezetimibe, 10 mg daily
D. Restart atorvastatin, 80 mg daily
E. Start alirocumab, 75 mg every 2 weeks

19 A 54-year-old man comes to see you for follow-up of type 2 diabetes mellitus. His BMI is 34 kg/m^2, and his hemoglobin A_{1c} level is 7.5% (58 mmol/mol) on metformin and canagliflozin. He is taking rosuvastatin, 40 mg daily, and tolerating it well. His fasting lipid panel reveals the following:
LDL cholesterol = 88 mg/dL (<100 mg/dL [optimal]) (SI: 2.28 mmol/L [<2.59 mmol/L])
HDL cholesterol = 38 mg/dL (>60 mg/dL [optimal]) (SI: 0.98 mmol/L [>1.55 mmol/L])
Triglycerides = 274 mg/dL (<150 mg/dL [optimal]) (SI: 3.10 mmol/L [<1.70 mmol/L])

Which of the following would be the most appropriate medication to start?

A. Gemfibrozil
B. Fenofibrate
C. Liraglutide
D. Niacin
E. Omega-3 fatty acid supplement

20 You are referred a 36-year-old man for hyperlipidemia. He has no known coronary disease, but he does have a strong family history of early-onset cardiovascular disease with multiple first-degree male relatives having a myocardial infarction in their 40s. He does not have diabetes and there is no family history of diabetes. His son, age 12 years, also has a high cholesterol level for his age, but his daughter, age 10 years, does not. The patient's primary care physician has recommended a statin, but he is not sure if he should start one now.

Total cholesterol = 326 mg/dL (<200 mg/dL [optimal]) (SI: 8.44 mmol/L [<5.18 mmol/L])
LDL cholesterol = 251 mg/dL (<100 mg/dL [optimal]) (SI: 6.50 mmol/L [<2.59 mmol/L])
HDL cholesterol = 45 mg/dL (>60 mg/dL [optimal]) (SI: 1.17 mmol/L [>1.55 mmol/L])
Triglycerides = 148 mg/dL (<150 mg/dL [optimal]) (SI: 1.67 mmol/L [<1.70 mmol/L])

On physical examination, you note arcus corneal arcus bilaterally and look specifically for which of the following?

    A. Lipemia retinalis

    B. Achilles tendon xanthomas

    C. Eruptive xanthomas

    D. Palmar xanthoma

    E. Orange tonsils

21 A 38-year-old man comes to see you for ongoing care of type 2 diabetes mellitus complicated by nephropathy. He developed diabetes at the age of 25 years.

Laboratory test results:

    Hemoglobin A_{1c} = 7.8% (4.0%-5.6%)

       (62 mmol/mol [20-38 mmol/mol])

    Urinary albumin-to-creatinine ratio = >30 mg/g

       creat (<30 mg/g creat)

His medications include metformin, once-weekly dulaglutide, and lisinopril. You use the American Heart Association risk calculator to assess his cardiovascular disease risk; his 10-year risk is 5.2% and his lifetime risk is 42%.

Which of the following is the best treatment recommendation?

    A. Do not recommend statin therapy given that he is younger than 40 years

    B. Do not recommend statin therapy because his 10-year cardiovascular disease risk is <7.5%

    C. Recommend statin therapy because his lifetime cardiovascular disease risk is >20%

    D. Recommend statin therapy because he has had type 2 diabetes for more than 10 years and he has nephropathy

22 A 24-year-old man is referred to you for management of high triglycerides. Two weeks ago, he was hospitalized with acute pancreatitis after attending a party. He notes that he had only "a few beers" and normally does not drink alcohol at all. His peak triglyceride level was 4800 mg/dL (54.24 mmol/L).

On physical examination, he has a rash of small eruptive xanthomas (*see image*) and lipemia retinalis on fundoscopic exam. He relates that as a teenager and in college he had episodes of severe abdominal pain after eating too many cheeseburgers and fries.

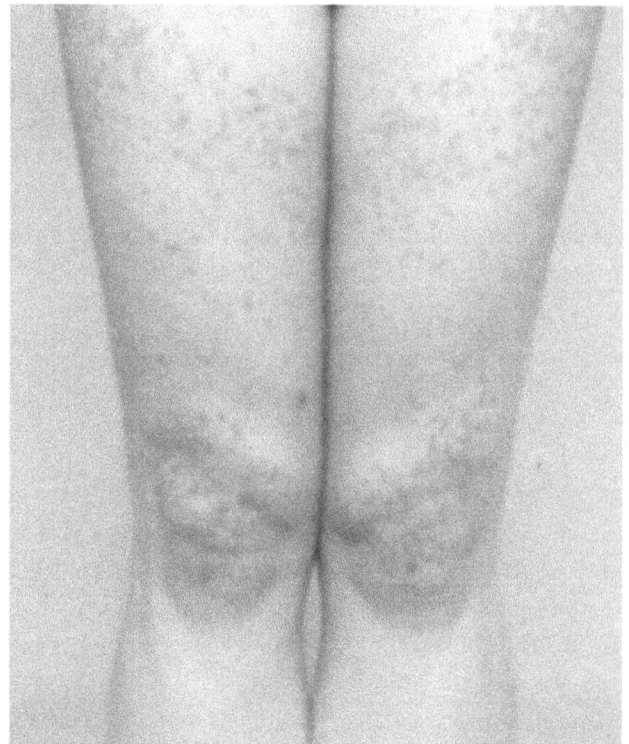

Which of the following is the most likely etiology of his hypertriglyceridemia?

    A. Apolipoprotein B elevation

    B. Adipose triglyceride lipase deficiency

    C. Hepatic lipase deficiency

    D. Lipoprotein lipase deficiency

    E. Pancreatic lipase deficiency

23 A 39-year-old man seeks help treating elevated cholesterol. His father died of a myocardial infarction at age 29 years and his brother developed angina at age 32 years. He has intermittent chest pain that is consistent with angina, but he has not had any diagnostic testing. He takes atorvastatin, 80 mg daily, and on this medication his fasting LDL-cholesterol level is 245 mg/dL (6.35 mmol/L).

On physical examination, he has thickened Achilles tendons and nodules on the extensor tendons of his hands and corneal arcus.

Which of the following medications should be added to his regimen as the best next step?

    A. Ezetimibe

    B. Fenofibrate

    C. Evolocumab

    D. Niacin

24 A 24-year-old graduate student from Japan comes to see you for a high cholesterol level identified by screening at the student health clinic. He is healthy and takes a multivitamin but no other medications. He drinks a couple beers 2 or 3 times a week but does not binge drink.

Fasting lipid levels:
Total cholesterol = 220 mg/dL (<200 mg/dL [optimal]) (SI: 5.70 mmol/L [<5.18 mmol/L])
HDL cholesterol = 115 mg/dL (>60 mg/dL [optimal]) (SI: 2.98 mmol/L [>1.55 mmol/L])
Triglycerides = 78 mg/dL(<150 mg/dL [optimal]) (SI: 0.88 mmol/L [<1.70 mmol/L])
LDL cholesterol = 89 mg/dL (<100 mg/dL [optimal]) (SI: 2.31 mmol/L [<2.59 mmol/L])

Which of the following is the most likely explanation for his lipid levels?
A. Alcohol use
B. Cholesteryl ester transfer protein deficiency
C. Interference with lipid assays
D. Apolipoprotein A1 deficiency
E. Lipoprotein lipase deficiency

25 A 32-year-old woman with hypertriglyceridemia is planning to have a second child. She has a history of gestational diabetes mellitus with her first pregnancy that progressed to type 2 diabetes after delivery. She has been on metformin, sitagliptin, and gemfibrozil, which has maintained her triglycerides around 300 mg/dL (3.39 mmol/L). She is seeking guidance regarding her lipid medication.

Laboratory test results (drawn while patient is off medications):
Total cholesterol = 300 mg/dL (<200 mg/dL [optimal]) (SI: 7.77 mmol/L [<5.18 mmol/L])
Triglycerides = 815 mg/dL (<150 mg/dL [optimal]) (SI: 9.21 mmol/L [<1.70 mmol/L])
HDL cholesterol = 31 mg/dL (>60 mg/dL [optimal]) (SI: 0.80 mmol/L [>1.55 mmol/L])
Fasting glucose = 105 mg/dL (70-99 mg/dL) (SI: 5.8 mmol/L [3.9-5.5 mmol/L])
Hemoglobin A_{1c} = 7.0% (4.0%-5.6%) (53 mmol/mol [20-38 mmol/mol])

Which of the following is the most reasonable strategy now?
A. Continue gemfibrozil
B. Change gemfibrozil to fenofibrate
C. Stop gemfibrozil
D. Change gemfibrozil to a statin

26 You are referred a 53-year-old woman for high cholesterol, which her physician checked after menopause. She has been in good health and has no personal or family history of vascular disease. After menopause, she gained 20 lb (9.1 kg), and during the past year she has attempted to reduce her weight with a high-fat, low-carbohydrate diet. On this diet, her BMI has decreased from 35 to 29 kg/m^2. Moreover, she is unaware that she had a cholesterol problem. Her total cholesterol concentration is greater than 600 mg/dL (>15.54 mmol/L) with an equal increase in triglycerides. Thyroid function is normal.

Which of the following should you order to diagnose this patient's disorder?
A. Apolipoprotein A1 measurement
B. Assessment of LDL particle size
C. Apolipoprotein E genotyping
D. Lipoprotein (a) genotyping

27 A 52-year-old man presents with class 3 obesity, BMI of 48 kg/m^2, type 2 diabetes mellitus (hemoglobin A_{1c} = 8.2% [66 mmol/mol]), and nonalcoholic fatty liver disease. His American Heart Association 10-year risk of cardiovascular disease is 16%. His primary care physician recommended starting atorvastatin, 40 mg daily. Due to his fatty liver disease, his liver transaminases (ALT, AST) are chronically elevated. He is concerned about taking atorvastatin, as he has read that statins can cause liver injury.

Laboratory test results (sample drawn while fasting):
LDL cholesterol = 164 mg/dL (<100 mg/dL [optimal]) (SI: 4.25 mmol/L [<2.59 mmol/L])
Triglycerides = 242 mg/dL (<150 mg/dL [optimal]) (SI: 2.73 mmol/L [<1.70 mmol/L])
ALT = 88 U/L (10-40 U/L) (SI: 1.47 µkat/L [0.17-0.67 µkat/L])
AST = 76 U/L (20-48 U/L) (SI: 1.27 µkat/L [0.33-0.80 µkat/L])

In addition to dietary counseling, which of the following treatments is the best approach to this patient's management?

A. Atorvastatin

B. Omega-3 fatty acids

C. Fenofibrate

D. Ezetimibe

E. Niacin

28 A 52 year-old man presents for aggressive treatment of his dyslipidemia. There is a strong history of cardiovascular disease in male family members (in their 50s). His brother had a myocardial infarction at age 56 years, and his father had a fatal myocardial infarction at age 52 years. The patient has had type 2 diabetes for 15 years and takes metformin, once-daily insulin glargine, and once-weekly semaglutide. He also has hypertension, but his blood pressure is well controlled on lisinopril. His BMI is 38 kg/m^2.

He has been on atorvastatin, 80 mg daily, for the last 7 years and added ezetimibe, 10 mg daily, 3 years ago.

Current laboratory test results:

Hemoglobin A$_{1c}$ = 7.4% (4.0%-5.6%)
(53 mmol/mol [20-38 mmol/mol])

Total cholesterol = 179 mg/dL (<200 mg/dL
[optimal]) (SI: 4.64 mmol/L [<5.18 mmol/L])

LDL cholesterol = 86 mg/dL (<100 mg/dL
[optimal]) (SI: 2.23 mmol/L [<2.59 mmol/L])

HDL cholesterol = 39 mg/dL (>60 mg/dL
[optimal]) (SI: 1.01 mmol/L [>1.55 mmol/L])

Triglycerides = 270 mg/dL (<150 mg/dL [optimal])
(SI: 3.05 mmol/L [<1.70 mmol/L])

ALT = 52 U/L (10-40 U/L) (SI: 0.87 µkat/L
[0.17-0.67 µkat/L])

Which of the following is the best next step to further reduce this patient's risk of cardiovascular disease?

A. No change in current therapy

B. Gemfibrozil, 600 mg twice daily

C. Icosapent ethyl, 2 g twice daily

D. Fenofibrate, 160 mg daily

E. Niacin ER, 3 g daily

29 A 45-year-old man with hyperlipidemia seeks advice for secondary prevention of cardiovascular disease. He had a myocardial infarction 6 months ago complicated by a stroke. He does not smoke cigarettes. He started exercising, and started a high-intensity statin (atorvastatin, 80 mg daily). His LDL-cholesterol level decreased from 174 to less than 100 mg/dL (<2.59 mmol/L). Despite aggressive risk factor modification, he had a second heart attack 3 months ago. He had a twin brother who died suddenly of a myocardial infarction last year at age 44 years.

On physical examination, his blood pressure is 126/74 mm Hg and pulse rate is 72 beats/min. BMI is 27 kg/m^2, and waist circumference is 36 in (91.4 cm).

Laboratory test results:

Total cholesterol = 155 mg/dL (<200 mg/dL
[optimal]) (SI: 4.01 mmol/L [<5.18 mmol/L])

LDL cholesterol = 85 mg/dL (<100 mg/dL
[optimal]) (SI: 2.20 mmol/L [<2.59 mmol/L])

HDL cholesterol = 44 mg/dL (>60 mg/dL
[optimal]) (SI: 1.14 mmol/L [>1.55 mmol/L])

Triglycerides = 128 mg/dL (<150 mg/dL [optimal])
(SI: 1.45 mmol/L [<1.70 mmol/L])

Hemoglobin A$_{1c}$ = 5.3% (4.0%-5.6%)
(34 mmol/mol [20-38 mmol/mol])

TSH = 2.24 mIU/L (0.5-5.0 mIU/L)

ALT = 24 U/L (10-40 U/L) (SI: 0.40 µkat/L
[0.17-0.67 µkat/L])

Which of the following most likely explains his high cardiovascular disease risk despite good response to statin therapy?

A. Apolipoprotein A1 deficiency

B. Elevated lipoprotein (a)

C. ABCA1 deficiency

D. Elevated apolipoprotein B

30 A 58-year-old man consults with you for primary prevention of cardiovascular disease. He has had elevated LDL cholesterol that decreased from 172 mg/dL (4.45 mmol/L) to 150 mg/dL (3.89 mmol/L) over the last few years while he has been adhering to a low-cholesterol, low-fat diet. He exercises regularly, and his blood pressure is in the target range at 118/76 mm Hg. He does not currently take a statin or aspirin. He does not have diabetes and is a lifelong nonsmoker. You calculate his American Heart

Association/American College of Cardiology 10-year risk of cardiovascular disease to be 7.6% (American Heart Association Group 4 for statin benefit) with a lifetime risk of 46%. His optimal 10-year cardiovascular disease risk would be 4.1%. He is hesitant to start statin therapy. He has no family history of cardiovascular disease.

Laboratory test results:

Total cholesterol = 224 mg/dL (<200 mg/dL [optimal]) (SI: 5.80 mmol/L [<5.18 mmol/L])

LDL cholesterol = 152 mg/dL (<100 mg/dL [optimal]) (SI: 3.94 mmol/L [<2.59 mmol/L])

HDL cholesterol = 46 mg/dL (>60 mg/dL [optimal]) (SI: 1.19 mmol/L [>1.55 mmol/L])

Triglycerides = 130 mg/dL (<150 mg/dL [optimal]) (SI: 1.47 mmol/L [<1.70 mmol/L])

Non-HDL cholesterol = 168 mg/dL (<130 mg/dL [optimal]) (SI: 4.35 mmol/L [<3.37 mmol/L])

Hemoglobin A_{1c} = 5.3% (4.0%-5.6%) (34 mmol/mol [20-38 mmol/mol])

ALT = 21 U/L (10-40 U/L) (SI: 0.35 μkat/L [0.17-0.67 μkat/L])

Which of the following is the best next step?

A. Nuclear magnetic resonance spectroscopy for LDL-particle size

B. Assessment of the coronary artery calcium score

C. Apolipoprotein B measurement

D. Antioxidant profile

Pituitary Board Review

Laurence Katznelson, MD

1 Following transsphenoidal surgery, a 56-year-old woman with acromegaly has residual tumor in the cavernous sinus. Her postoperative GH level is 9.0 ng/mL (9.0 µg/L) and her IGF-1 level 12 weeks after surgery is 690 ng/mL (78-220 ng/mL) (SI: 90.4 nmol/L [10.2-28.8 nmol/L]). She has significant headaches, which are bothersome. She has diet-controlled diabetes mellitus. Her physical examination reveals coarse facial features.

Which of the following treatment options would you recommend now?
  A. Cabergoline
  B. Lanreotide depot monthly
  C. Another transsphenoidal surgery
  D. Pegvisomant weekly

2 A 29-year-old man is referred to restart GH replacement therapy. He states that he received GH injections for many years as a child and stopped when he completed growth at age 18 years. He has also taken thyroid hormone replacement since age 12 years. During his 20s, he has noted persistent fatigue, and he has had difficulty losing weight. He had a concussion at age 16 years while playing football.

On physical examination, he has increased abdominal girth, normal virilization, and 25-mL testes bilaterally.

Laboratory testing reveals a serum IGF-1 concentration of 60 ng/mL (117-321 ng/mL) (SI: 7.9 nmol/L [15.3-42.1 nmol/L]). Following a glucagon-stimulation test, the peak GH value is 0.8 ng/mL (0.8 µg/L).

MRI is shown (*see image*).

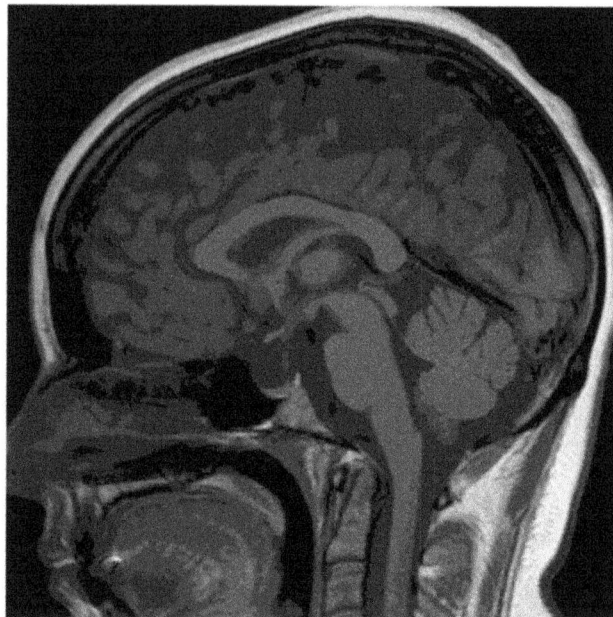

Which of the following is the most likely cause of these biochemical findings?
  A. Pathogenic variant in the *PROP1* gene
  B. Trauma-induced pituitary infarction
  C. Burnt-out hypothalamic/pituitary sarcoidosis
  D. Langerhans cell histiocytosis
  E. Hemochromatosis

3 A 19-year-old man is evaluated because of headaches, decreased libido, and progressive fatigue and is found to have what appears to be an 11-mm Rathke cleft cyst on MRI. He recalls having some problems with increased urinary frequency and thirst several years ago, but he no longer has these symptoms.

On physical examination, he has a sallow complexion, a normal-sized phallus and testes, and a sparse beard.

Laboratory test results (8 AM):
  Serum sodium = 144 mEq/L (136-142 mEq/L)
  (SI: 144 mmol/L [136-142 mmol/L])
  Urine specific gravity = 1.004

Serum cortisol (8 AM) = 7.0 µg/dL (5-25 µg/dL)
(SI: 193.1 nmol/L [137-39-689.7 nmol/L])
Free T$_4$ = 0.5 ng/dL (0.8-1.8 ng/dL) (SI: 6.4 pmol/L
[10.3-23.2 pmol/L])
TSH = 1.4 mIU/L (0.5-5.0 mIU/L)
Testosterone = 293 ng/dL (300-900 ng/dL)
(SI: 10.2 nmol/L [10.4-31.2 nmol/L])

Which of the following might be expected with initiation of hydrocortisone and levothyroxine?
A. Rapid development of hyponatremia
B. Increase in polyuria and polydipsia
C. Marked decrease in libido
D. Orthostatic hypotension

4 A 53-year-old woman has a classic history and examination findings of Cushing syndrome. Her urinary free cortisol excretion is 3-fold above the reference range, and her ACTH level and morning cortisol level are 2-fold above their respective reference ranges. On MRI, her pituitary is modestly increased to a height of about 12 mm, and there is global pituitary gland enhancement but no focal lesion. Inferior petrosal sinus sampling using corticotropin-releasing hormone stimulation shows a central step-up of ACTH levels (about 5-fold compared with peripheral levels), but no clear lateralization.

Which of the following should be performed as the next management step?
A. Corticotropin-releasing hormone test
B. Dexamethasone corticotropin-releasing hormone test
C. ^{68}Ga DOTATATE scan
D. Inferior petrosal sinus sampling again
E. High-dose dexamethasone suppression test

5 A 23-year-old woman was previously well and had regular menses. After discontinuing barrier contraception, she became pregnant within 2 months. Her pregnancy went well, but during her third trimester she developed headaches and mild weakness.

On physical examination, she is an ill-appearing woman. Her blood pressure is 96/68 mm Hg, and pulse rate is 74 beats/min. She uterus is appropriately sized for 36 weeks' gestation.

Laboratory test results:
Free T$_4$ = 0.9 ng/dL (0.8-1.8 ng/dL) (SI: 11.6 pmol/L
[10.3-23.2 pmol/L])
TSH = 1.3 mIU/L (0.5-5.0 mIU/L)
Prolactin = 198 ng/mL (4-30 ng/mL)
(SI: 8.61 nmol/L [0.17-1.30 nmol/L])

MRI shows a 1.5-cm, diffusely enhancing, symmetric, sellar lesion extending above the sella and impinging the optic chiasm (*see images*). A Goldmann visual field examination shows a small degree of bilateral superior and temporal visual field defects.

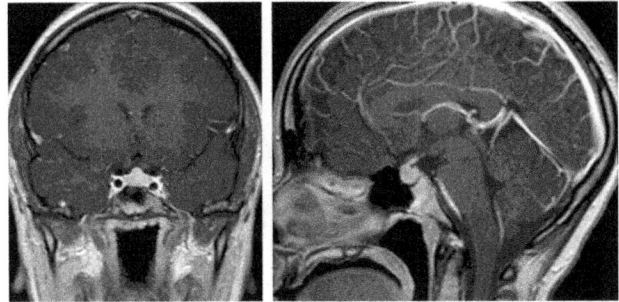

Which of the following is the most likely diagnosis?
A. Prolactinoma
B. Clinically nonfunctioning pituitary adenoma
C. Craniopharyngioma
D. Lymphocytic hypophysitis
E. Pituitary apoplexy

6 A 31-year-old woman with a history of prolactinoma is now in her 34th week of pregnancy. Two years ago, a 14-mm prolactinoma was identified. Her initial prolactin level was 320 ng/mL (4-30 ng/mL) (SI: 13.9 nmol/L [0.17-1.30 nmol/L]), and there was minimal suprasellar extension on MRI, without chiasmal compression. With bromocriptine, 2.5 mg nightly, her prolactin normalized, galactorrhea and amenorrhea resolved, and the tumor decreased in size to 5 mm. She stopped bromocriptine when she learned she was pregnant. She now reports minimal headaches. The serum prolactin concentration is now 427 ng/mL (18.6 nmol/L). Findings on Goldmann visual field testing are normal.

Which of the following is the best next step in this patient's management?
  A. Restart bromocriptine now
  B. Deliver the baby
  C. Start cabergoline
  D. Perform a pituitary-directed MRI
  E. Continue to monitor clinical progress

7 A 33-year-old woman has developed Cushing syndrome during her second month of pregnancy. She has hypertension, diabetes mellitus, hirsutism, and wide, purple striae on her abdomen.

Laboratory test results:
  Serum cortisol (8 AM) = 37 µg/dL (5-25 µg/dL)
    (SI: 1020.8 nmol/L [137-39-689.7 nmol/L])
  ACTH = 129 pg/mL (10-60 pg/mL)
    (SI: 28.4 pmol/L [2.2-13.2 pmol/L])
  Urinary free cortisol = 475 µg/24 h (4-50 µg/24 h)
    (SI: 1311 nmol/d [11-138 nmol/d])

MRI shows a 6-mm pituitary adenoma.

Which of the following treatment options is absolutely contraindicated?
  A. Mifepristone
  B. Metyrapone
  C. Transsphenoidal surgery in the second trimester
  D. Pasireotide
  E. Cabergoline

8 An 18-year-old girl had a craniopharyngioma resected at age 15 years with resultant pan-hypopituitarism. She has been treated with levothyroxine, hydrocortisone, and GH. An oral contraceptive for estrogen and progesterone replacement was recently started. Over the past year, she has only grown 1 cm and her height is now 64 in (162.6 cm). A recent hand and wrist film shows almost complete epiphyseal closure. After 1 month off GH therapy, her IGF-1 concentration is –2.7 standard deviations.

If she does not continue GH treatment, which of the following is most likely?
  A. Significant weight gain
  B. Glucose intolerance
  C. Reduced mortality rate
  D. Markedly decreased energy levels
  E. Decreased peak bone mass

9 A 48-year-old man is referred after a head MRI performed for evaluation of headache showed a pituitary mass—a 0.9-cm right-sided pituitary adenoma without parasellar extension (*see image*). He has been feeling well. He has no vision symptoms.

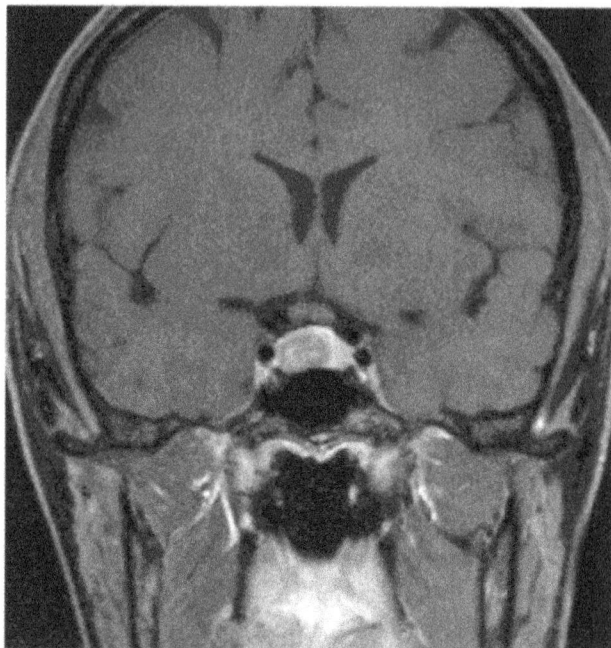

On physical examination, his blood pressure is 136/70 mm Hg and pulse rate is 74 beats/min. His skin has normal texture, and his reflexes are normal. He saw a local neurosurgeon who recommended surgery.

Laboratory test results (8 AM):
  Testosterone = 325 ng/dL (300-900 ng/dL)
    (SI: 11.3 nmol/L [10.4-31.2 nmol/L])
  LH = 2.3 mIU/mL (1.0-9.0 mIU/mL) (SI: 2.3 IU/L
    [1.0-9.0 IU/L])
  FSH = 1.4 mIU/mL (1.0-13.0 mIU/mL) (SI: 1.4 IU/L
    [1.0-13.0 IU/L])
  Cortisol (8 AM) = 15.7 µg/dL (5-25 µg/dL)
    (SI: 433.1 nmol/L [137-39-689.7 nmol/L])
  Prolactin = 5.7 ng/mL (4-23 ng/mL) (SI: 0.2 nmol/L
    [0.17-1.00 nmol/L])
  Free T$_4$ = 1.2 ng/dL (0.8-1.8 ng/dL) (SI: 15.4 pmol/L
    [10.3-23.2 pmol/L])
  Serum sodium = 143 mEq/L (136-142 mEq/L)
    (SI: 143 mmol/L [136-142 mmol/L])

Which of the following is the best next step in this patient's management?

   A. Visual field testing

   B. Transsphenoidal surgery

   C. Another MRI in 12 months

   D. Radiotherapy

10 A 30-year-old woman develops progressive, severe headaches, nausea, vomiting, and fatigue during her 33rd week of pregnancy. She has no notable medical history and was able to become pregnant within 2 months of trying. Her pregnancy course had been smooth until now.

Physical examination findings are normal for 33 weeks' gestation. Her obstetrician persuades the radiologist to perform a noncontrast MRI of her head, and the patient is found to have a diffusely enlarged pituitary, measuring 16 mm in height, without abutment of the optic chiasm.

Laboratory test results:
   Total T$_4$ = 13.0 μg/dL (5.5-12.5 μg/dL)
     (SI: 167.3 nmol/L [70.8-160.9 nmol/L])
   TSH = 1.3 mIU/L (0.5-5.0 mIU/L)
   Cortisol (8 AM) = 9.0 μg/dL (5-25 μg/dL)
     (SI: 248.3 nmol/L [137.9-689.7 nmol/L])
   Prolactin = 137 ng/mL (4-30 ng/mL)
     (SI: 6.0 nmol/L [0.17-1.30 nmol/L])

Which of the following is the best next step in this patient's management?

   A. Start dexamethasone

   B. Arrange for urgent cesarean delivery

   C. Start bromocriptine

   D. Start hydrocortisone

11 A 53-year-old woman has a medical history of stage 2 breast cancer diagnosed 4 years ago, status post mastectomy, local radiation therapy, and adjuvant chemotherapy. She is currently in remission. She recently slipped and struck her head, without loss of consciousness. However, given persistent headaches, she underwent head CT, which revealed a 1.5-cm sellar mass with suprasellar extension. In retrospect, she noted abrupt onset of frequent urination and increased thirst in the previous 3 weeks. MRI is performed 4 weeks later and shows that the mass is now 2 cm.

On physical examination, she is a tired-appearing woman with a blood pressure of 98/66 mm Hg, pulse rate of 92 beats/min, and BMI of 21.1 kg/m^2.

Laboratory test results:
   Serum sodium = 152 mEq/L (136-142 mEq/L)
     (SI: 152 mmol/L [136-142 mmol/L])
   Prolactin = 122 ng/mL (4-30 ng/mL)
     (SI: 5.30 nmol/L [0.17-1.30 nmol/L])
   FSH = 65.0 mIU/mL (>30 mIU/mL
     [postmenopausal]) (SI: 65.0 IU/L [>30 IU/L])
   LH = 95.0 mIU/mL (>30 mIU/mL
     [postmenopausal]) (SI: 95.0 IU/L [>30 IU/L])
   Plasma glucose = 89 mg/dL (70-99 mg/dL)
     (SI: 4.9 mmol/L [3.9-5.5 mmol/L])

Which of the following is the most likely diagnosis?

   A. Clinically nonfunctioning pituitary adenoma

   B. Prolactinoma

   C. Craniopharyngioma

   D. Metastasis

12 A 37-year-old woman is being evaluated for persistent fatigue and forgetfulness. Ten years ago, she had partial resection of a TSH-secreting pituitary tumor with subsequent radiotherapy for the residual tumor. Her current medications include levothyroxine, 137 mcg daily; hydrocortisone, 10 mg in the morning and 5 mg in the afternoon; and a low-dosage oral contraceptive. She read on the Internet that GH treatment might improve her energy levels.

On physical examination, she is a well-appearing woman. Her blood pressure is 124/78 mm Hg, pulse rate is 76 beats/min, and BMI is 24.1 kg/m^2.

Laboratory test results:
   Free T$_4$ = 1.6 ng/dL (0.8-1.8 ng/dL)
     (SI: 20.59 pmol/L [10.30-23.17 pmol/L])
   Prolactin = 7.6 ng/mL (4-30 ng/mL)
     (SI: 0.33 nmol/L [0.17-1.30 nmol/L])
   IGF-1 = 115 ng/dL (106-277 ng/dL)
     (SI: 15.1 nmol/L [13.9-36.3 nmol/L])
   Comprehensive chemistry panel, normal
   Complete blood cell count, normal

Which of the following is the best next step in evaluating for GH deficiency in this patient?

A. Measure a random GH level

B. Perform a glucagon-stimulation test to assess GH levels

C. Measure IGF-1 again

D. No assessment for GH deficiency is indicated

13 A 71-year-old woman with metastatic melanoma is being treated with chemotherapy. Approximately 6 weeks after starting chemotherapy, she develops fatigue, weight loss, confusion, and weakness. On hospital admission, she has lethargy and orthostatic hypotension.

Laboratory test results:

Serum sodium = 123 mEq/L (136-142 mEq/L) (SI: 123 mmol/L [136-142 mmol/L])

Random cortisol = 1.5 µg/dL (2-14 µg/dL) (SI: 41.4 nmol/L [55.2-386.2 nmol/L])

ACTH = <5 pg/mL (10-60 pg/mL) (SI: <1.1 pmol/L [2.2-13.2 pmol/L])

LH = 0.3 mIU/mL (>30 mIU/mL [postmenopausal]) (SI: 0.3 IU/L [>30 IU/L])

FSH = 2.0 mIU/mL (>30 mIU/mL [postmenopausal]) (SI: 2.0 IU/L [>30 IU/L])

Prolactin = 1.8 ng/mL (4-30 ng/mL) (SI: 0.08 nmol/L [0.17-1.30 nmol/L])

TSH = 0.2 mIU/L (0.5-5.0 mIU/L)

Free T_4 = 0.5 ng/dL (0.8-1.8 ng/dL) (SI: 6.44 pmol/L [10.30-23.17 pmol/L])

MRI shows mildly homogeneous enlargement of the pituitary and stalk.

Which of the following medications is the most likely cause of these pituitary abnormalities?

A. Ipilimumab

B. Bevacizumab

C. Temozolomide

D. Sunitinib

14 A 46-year-old man presents with loss of libido and erectile dysfunction. His primary care physician documented his testosterone level to be 180 ng/dL (6.2 nmol/L) and referred him for further evaluation.

Laboratory test results (sample drawn at 8 AM):

Repeated testosterone = 171 ng/dL (300-900 ng/dL) (SI: 5.9 nmol/L [10.4-31.2 nmol/L])

LH = 0.9 mIU/mL (1.0-9.0 mIU/L) (SI: 0.9 IU/L [1.0-9.0 IU/L])

FSH = 1.1 mIU/mL (1.0-13.0 mIU/L) (SI: 1.1 IU/L [1.0-13.0 IU/L])

Prolactin = 2513 ng/mL (4-23 ng/mL) (SI: 109.3 nmol/L [0.17-1.00 nmol/L])

TSH, normal

Cortisol, normal

MRI shows a 1.7-cm adenoma with substantial extension into the left cavernous sinus.

At a cabergoline dosage of 1.0 mg twice weekly, his prolactin level normalizes, his tumor is greatly reduced in size, his testosterone level increases to 602 ng/dL (20.9 nmol/L), and his erectile function returns. However, his wife complains that he has recently become obsessed with sexuality, to the point that it is hindering their relationship.

Which of the following is the most likely explanation for his current behavior?

A. Restoring testosterone to normal has unmasked previously suppressed obsessive behavior

B. Hypothalamic damage from the tumor

C. An adverse effect of cabergoline

D. Behavior change unrelated to his tumor or treatment

15 A 43-year-old woman presents with weight loss, tremor, palpitations, and sweating. She has had mild frontal headaches, and her menses are irregular. She is found to have atrial fibrillation.

Laboratory test results:

Free T_4 = 2.8 ng/dL (0.8-1.8 ng/dL) (SI: 36.0 pmol/L [10.30-23.17 pmol/L])

Total T_3 = 413 ng/dL (70-200 ng/dL) (SI: 6.36 nmol/L [1.08-3.08 nmol/L])

TSH = 1.9 mIU/L (0.5-5.0 mIU/L)

Prolactin = 28 ng/mL (4-30 ng/mL) (SI: 1.21 nmol/L [0.17-1.30 nmol/L])

A radioiodine scan reveals 50% uptake in a heterogeneous pattern in the thyroid gland. Brain MRI reveals a 2.1-cm pituitary adenoma invading the cavernous sinus. She is caring for her elderly parent and cannot take time off for surgery.

Which of the following is the best next step for managing both the hyperthyroidism and the adenoma?

A. Cabergoline
B. Methimazole
C. Radioactive iodine
D. Octreotide long-acting release

16 A 52-year-old woman has had hypopituitarism for 10 years after resection of a nonfunctioning pituitary adenoma. She has been treated with levothyroxine, hydrocortisone, a low-dosage oral contraceptive pill, and daily GH injections. Because her sister recently developed breast cancer, the patient has decided to stop her oral contraceptive. During the next month, she notices progressive joint aches and sweating.

Which of the following is the next step for endocrine management to relieve these new symptoms?

A. Increase the levothyroxine dosage
B. Decrease the GH dosage
C. Increase the GH dosage
D. Increase the hydrocortisone dosage
E. Decrease the hydrocortisone dosage

17 A 43-year-old woman is referred for management of Cushing disease manifested by typical signs and symptoms.

Laboratory test results:
Urinary free cortisol = 451 µg/24 h (4-50 µg/24 h) (SI: 1244.8 nmol/d [11.0-138.0 nmol/d])
Serum cortisol (8 AM) = 28 µg/dL (5-25 µg/dL) (SI: 772.5 nmol/L [137.9-689.7 nmol/L])
ACTH = 93 pg/mL (10-60 pg/mL) (SI: 20.5 pmol/L [2.2-13.2 pmol/L])

Following incomplete surgical removal of her 9-mm pituitary adenoma, her hormone levels remain elevated. While on medical therapy, the patient subsequently develops diabetes mellitus.

Which of the following medications is the most likely culprit?

A. Metyrapone
B. Ketoconazole
C. Pasireotide
D. Mifepristone

18 A 44-year-old woman is diagnosed with a 3.2-cm clinically nonfunctioning pituitary macroadenoma that is causing chiasmal compression. Her preoperative evaluation reveals no evidence of acromegaly, Cushing disease, or salt and water imbalance. Her laboratory testing shows normal pituitary function. She undergoes transsphenoidal surgery, which is uneventful. On postoperative day 1, she develops polyuria and polydipsia, and the following laboratory values are documented:
Serum sodium = 152 mEq/L (136-142 mEq/L) (SI: 152 mmol/L [136-142 mmol/L])
Urine osmolality = 110 mOsm/kg (150-1150 mOsm/kg) (SI: 110 mmol/kg [150-1150 mmol/kg])

She is treated with DDAVP, 0.1 mg orally as needed, and symptoms resolve by postoperative day 3, so DDAVP is discontinued. She presents to the emergency department on postoperative day 7 and describes nausea and marked fatigue. She is admitted to the intensive care unit due to the following laboratory test results:
Serum sodium = 121 mEq/L (SI: 121 mmol/L)
Urine osmolality = 373 mOsm/kg (SI: 373 mmol/kg)

Which of the following will correct her serum sodium most effectively?

A. Restrict free water intake to less than 1500 mL/24 h
B. Start demeclocycline
C. Start tolvaptan
D. Start intravenous furosemide

19 Cushing disease is diagnosed in a 33-year-old woman. MRI shows a 4-mm pituitary lesion. Following transsphenoidal surgery, her morning cortisol concentration is 1.2 µg/dL (33.1 nmol/L), and she is discharged home on glucocorticoids, which are weaned over 4 months. She loses weight, and her cushingoid appearance resolves over the next

6 months. Approximately 18 months after surgery, she returns for a clinic visit, as she is concerned that the Cushing syndrome has recurred. Her blood pressure is 133/88 mm Hg. She has a modest moon face, facial plethora, and modest supraclavicular fat.

She undergoes a 1-mg overnight dexamethasone test, and the morning cortisol concentration is 1.2 µg/dL (5-25 µg/dL) (SI: 33.1 nmol/L [137.9-689.7 nmol/L]). Other laboratory values:

Morning ACTH = 35 pg/mL (10-60 pg/mL)
(SI: 7.7 pmol/L [2.2-13.2 pmol/L])
Free T$_4$ = 1.4 ng/dL (0.8-1.8 ng/dL) (SI: 18.0 pmol/L [10.30-23.17 pmol/L])

Which of the following is the next test to perform to evaluate for Cushing syndrome?
A. 24-Hour urinary free cortisol excretion
B. Pituitary MRI
C. Morning serum cortisol measurement in 6 months
D. Late-night salivary cortisol measurement
E. Another ACTH measurement

20 A 35-year-old woman develops bothersome headaches. Despite longstanding normal menstrual cycles, she has had amenorrhea for the past 6 months. Her prolactin concentration is 188 ng/mL (4-30 ng/mL) (SI: 8.2 nmol/L [0.17-1.30 nmol/L]) and is unchanged on dilution. Head MRI shows a 2.8 x 2.8 x 2.2-cm hypoenhancing sellar and suprasellar mass, which abuts the optic chiasm. Her visual field tests show minor temporal-superior deficits. The rest of her physical examination findings are unremarkable.

Laboratory test results:
Free T$_4$ = 0.9 ng/dL (0.8-1.8 ng/dL) (SI: 11.6 pmol/L [10.30-23.17 pmol/L])
Cortisol (8 AM) = 7.1 µg/dL (5-25 µg/dL)
(SI: 195.9 nmol/L [137.9-689.7 nmol/L])
Estradiol = 22 pg/mL (10-180 pg/mL)
(SI: 81 pmol/L [36.7-660.8 pmol/L])
IGF-1 = 122 ng/mL (113-297 ng/mL)
(SI: 15.9 nmol/L [14.8-38.9 nmol/L])

On the basis of the presented information, which of the following treatments should you recommend?
A. Start bromocriptine, 5 mg orally 3 times daily
B. Start octreotide LAR, 20 mg intramuscularly monthly
C. Perform transsphenoidal surgery
D. Start cabergoline, 1.0 mg orally twice weekly
E. Perform stereotactic radiosurgery

21 A 44-year-old man is evaluated for persistent fatigue. He was previously diagnosed with a craniopharyngioma, and he underwent transsphenoidal surgery followed by fractionated radiation therapy 7 years ago. He developed hypopituitarism, and he has been taking levothyroxine, 88 mcg orally daily; hydrocortisone, 25 mg orally daily; transdermal testosterone, 5 g daily; and desmopressin, 0.3 mg orally twice daily. He notes difficulty with short-term memory and has been unable to function at work due to poor attention span. Family history and personal medical history are unremarkable (aside from his craniopharyngioma).

On physical examination, he appears fatigued and slightly depressed. His blood pressure is 115/84 mm Hg, pulse rate is 84 beats/min, and BMI is 29 kg/m^2. He has increased abdominal girth, but examination findings are otherwise normal.

Laboratory test results:
Free T$_4$ = 1.6 ng/dL (0.8-1.8 ng/dL) (SI: 20.6 pmol/L [10.30-23.17 pmol/L])
Prolactin = 7.6 ng/mL (4-23 ng/mL)
(SI: 0.33 nmol/L [0.17-1.00 nmol/L])
Testosterone = 320 ng/dL (300-900 ng/dL)
(SI: 11.1 nmol/L [10.4-31.2 nmol/L])
IGF-1 = 115 ng/dL (98-261 ng/mL) (SI: 15.1 nmol/L [12.8-34.2 nmol/L])
Comprehensive chemistry panel, normal
Complete blood cell count, normal

Which of the following is the best next step in his endocrine management?
A. Refer to a psychiatrist for management of depression
B. Perform a macimorelin-stimulation test to assess GH levels
C. Measure random GH level
D. Increase the levothyroxine dosage

22 A 52-year-old woman presents with acromegaly. Her IGF-1 concentration is 1226 ng/mL (84-233 ng/mL) (SI: 160.6 nmol/L [11.0-30.5 nmol/L]), and she has a 2.5-cm pituitary macroadenoma with invasion of the left cavernous sinus. She undergoes transsphenoidal surgery, and her 12-week postoperative IGF-1 level is 968 ng/mL (126.8 nmol/L). MRI shows 7.5-mm residual disease in the cavernous sinus. She has persistent headaches, arthralgias, and sweating. She is postmenopausal. Octreotide LAR is initiated with a dosage increase to 30 mg intramuscular monthly. On this dosage, her IGF-1 level is 770 ng/mL (100.9 nmol/L). Her symptoms persist. MRI findings remain unchanged.

Which of the following options would be most effective in controlling her acromegaly within the next 6 months?

A. Increase the octreotide LAR dosage to 40 mg every 28 days
B. Stop octreotide LAR and switch to cabergoline
C. Add pegvisomant
D. Proceed with radiation therapy
E. Refer for reoperation

23 A 37-year-old man with ACTH-dependent Cushing syndrome has an MRI finding of a 4-mm left-sided sellar lesion, adjacent to cavernous sinus. The ACTH level is 58 pg/mL (12.8 pmol/L). Inferior petrosal sinus catheterization shows central ACTH hypersecretion, and there is lateralization to the left side. The patient undergoes transsphenoidal surgery, and the left-sided lesion is determined to be an adenoma, subsequently staining positive for ACTH. The adjacent dura has tumor involvement as well. Postoperatively, the serum cortisol fails to normalize. Reoperation with left hemihypophysectomy does not result in further cortisol lowing, and no tumor is detected. The patient is hyperglycemic with a hemoglobin A_{1c} level of 7.5% (58 mmol/mol). The decision is made to start medical therapy. A medication is initiated, and over the subsequent weeks his cushingoid features improve and his plasma glucose level normalizes. His current plasma ACTH concentration is now 73 pg/mL (16.1 pmol/L). However, he has bothersome lower-extremity edema and his blood pressure is higher.

Which of the following medications is he most likely receiving?

A. Mifepristone
B. Ketoconazole
C. Pasireotide
D. Cabergoline

24 A 38-year-old woman with a history of clinically nonfunctioning pituitary macroadenoma underwent surgery and adjuvant radiotherapy 4 years ago. She has been doing well. Her medications include an oral contraceptive agent, as well as a daily multivitamin. She has been noting more fatigue, and, for the past 4 months, progressive arthralgias. She has tried to exercise, but she experiences muscle aches for at least a day following exercise.

On physical examination, she appears tired. She has normal vital signs and normal examination findings.

Laboratory test results (sample drawn at 8 AM):
Serum cortisol = 9.6 µg/dL (5-25 µg/dL) (SI: 264.8 nmol/L [137-39-689.7 nmol/L])
LH = 0.4 mIU/mL (1.0-18.0 mIU/mL [follicular]) (SI: 0.4 IU/L [1.0-18.0 IU/L])
FSH = 2.1 mIU/mL (2.0-12.0 mIU/mL [follicular]) (SI: 2.1 IU/L [2.0-12.0 IU/L])
GH = 0.1 ng/mL (0.01-3.61 ng/mL) (SI: 0.1 µg/L [0.01-3.61 µg/L])
Prolactin = 1.3 ng/mL (4-30 ng/mL) (SI: 0.06 nmol/L [0.17-1.30 nmol/L])
TSH = 0.3 mIU/L (0.5-5.0 mIU/L)
Total T_4 = 8.0 µg/dL (5.5-12.5 µg/dL) (SI: 103.0 nmol/L [94.02-213.68 nmol/L])
Serum sodium = 142 mEq/L (136-142 mEq/L) (SI: 142 mmol/L [136-142 mmol/L])

Which other pituitary hormone is most likely deficient on the basis of these lab results?

A. Gonadotropins
B. GH
C. Antidiuretic hormone
D. ACTH

25 A 37-year-old woman presents with a sellar mass and headache. She is G2, P2, and had an uneventful pregnancy until her complicated delivery 3 days ago. During the delivery, she had a massive hemorrhage and received 4 units of packed red blood cells. She had hypotension, treated with saline infusion.

Headache prompted an urgent MRI, which revealed large, heterogeneous sellar contents without chiasmal compression.

On physical examination, she appears uncomfortable. Her vital signs are stable. Examination findings, including those from neurologic examination, are normal.

Which of the following is the first manifestation of this disorder?
    A. Inability to lactate
    B. Low free T_4 concentration
    C. Vision loss
    D. Absent menses

Thyroid Board Review

Elizabeth N. Pearce, MD, MSc

1 A 52-year-old woman seeks evaluation for a thyroid nodule that was recently noted incidentally on a head CT performed after a car crash. She subsequently had thyroid ultrasonography performed in an outside hospital, which demonstrated a solitary right-sided nodule described as follows:

Size: 15 x 10 x 17 mm
Location: right mid pole
Composition: cystic or almost completely cystic (0)
Echogenicity: hypoechoic (2)
Shape: not taller-than-wide (0)
Margins: smooth (0)
Echogenic foci: punctate echogenic foci (3)
American College of Radiology TI-RADS total
   points: 5
American College of Radiology TI-RADS risk
   category: 4
Impression: recommend FNA

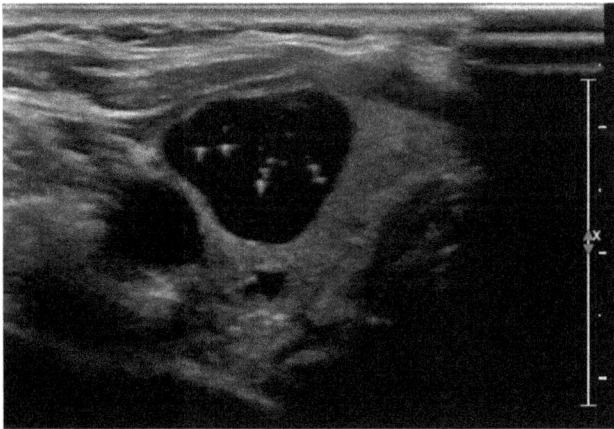

The serum TSH concentration is 2.37 mIU/L (0.5-5.0 mIU/L).

Which of the following is the best next step in this patient's management?
A. Radioactive iodine uptake and scan
B. Ultrasonography again in 12 months
C. FNA biopsy of the nodule
D. Diagnostic thyroid lobectomy

2 A 31-year-old woman presents for follow-up of thyroid cancer. She underwent left thyroid lobectomy 3 years ago for a 2.2-cm papillary thyroid cancer. Surgical margins were negative, none of the 6 resected lymph nodes were positive for tumor, and there was no extrathyroidal extension. She is taking levothyroxine, 88 mcg daily.

Recent laboratory test results:
   TSH = 0.8 mIU/L (0.5-5.0 mIU/L)
   Thyroglobulin antibodies = <0.4 IU/mL (≤4.0
      IU/mL) (SI: <4.0 kIU/L [≤4.0 kIU/L])
   Thyroglobulin = 1.6 ng/mL (SI: 1.6 µg/L) (stable
      from 6 months ago)

Neck surveillance ultrasonography 6 months ago demonstrated no evidence of recurrent or persistent tumor.

She is planning her first pregnancy and asks you about implications of her thyroid cancer during gestation.

Which of the following is the most appropriate management regarding this patient's planned pregnancy?
A. Measure serum thyroglobulin and perform thyroid ultrasonography each trimester
B. Increase the levothyroxine dosage before conception with a goal of TSH suppression
C. Perform serial fetal ultrasonography during gestation
D. Measure serum TSH as soon as pregnancy is confirmed
E. Advise the patient against conception due to a high risk of tumor progression

3 A 67-year-old man is treated with ipilimumab-nivolumab therapy for melanoma. He has no personal or family history of thyroid disease. Three weeks after therapy initiation, he is seen for a routine follow-up visit and the following thyroid laboratory values are noted:

TSH = 0.06 mIU/L (0.5-5.0 mIU/L)

Total T_3 = 240 ng/dL (70-200 ng/dL)
(SI: 3.70 nmol/L [1.08-3.08 nmol/L])

Total T_4 = 17.1 µg/dL (5.5-12.5 µg/dL)
(SI: 220.08 nmol/L [94.02-213.68 nmol/L])

Free T_4 = 3.2 ng/dL (0.8-1.8 ng/dL) (SI: 41.2 pmol/L [10.30-23.17 pmol/L])

On physical examination, his pulse rate is 92 beats/min and he has no ophthalmopathy. His thyroid gland is nontender to palpation, firm, 20 g in size, and without nodules.

After another 8 weeks, findings on thyroid examination are unchanged.

Which of the following thyroid function test patterns is now most likely in this patient?

Answer	TSH	Free T_4	Total T_3	TPO Antibody	TSH-Receptor Antibody
A.	High	Low	Low	Positive	Negative
B.	Low	Low	Low	Negative	Negative
C.	Normal	Normal	Normal	Negative	Negative
D.	Low	High	High	Positive	Positive

4 A 47-year-old woman presents for follow-up of hypothyroidism. Hashimoto thyroiditis was diagnosed 8 years ago, and she has been on levothyroxine since. Previously, her hypothyroidism was well controlled. However, over the last year, despite escalating levothyroxine dosages, her serum TSH has been elevated:

Date	TSH (reference range, 0.5-5.0 mIU/L)	Free T_4 (reference range, 0.8-1.8 ng/dL [SI: 10.30-23.17 pmol/L])	Levothyroxine Dosage
September	74 mIU/L	0.5 ng/dL (SI: 6.44 pmol/L)	112 mcg daily
November	98 mIU/L	0.4 ng/dL (SI: 5.15 pmol/L)	125 mcg daily
February	116 mIU/L	0.3 ng/dL (SI: 3.86 pmol/L)	137 mcg daily
April	84 mIU/L	0.4 ng/dL (SI: 5.15 pmol/L)	175 mcg daily
June	111 mIU/L	0.3 ng/dL (SI: 3.86 pmol/L)	200 mcg daily
August	96 mIU/L	0.3 ng/dL (SI: 3.86 pmol/L)	300 mcg daily

She reports that she is taking levothyroxine daily on an empty stomach and that she is not taking any other medications or supplements. She has gained 15 lb (6.8 kg) in the past 8 months and has developed cold intolerance and constipation.

On physical examination, her blood pressure is 144/86 mm Hg and her weight is 180 lb (81.8 kg). Her thyroid gland is firm and 20 g in size. The relaxation phase of her deep tendon reflexes is delayed.

A single oral dose of levothyroxine (1000 mcg) is administered in the office after an overnight fast, and thyroid function tests are repeated 2, 4, and 6 hours after administration:

Time	TSH	Free T_4	Total T_3
Baseline	98 mIU/L	0.40 ng/dL (SI: 5.15 pmol/L)	46 ng/dL (SI: 0.71 nmol/L)
2 hours	86 mIU/L	1.90 ng/dL (SI: 24.45 pmol/L)	51 ng/dL (SI: 0.79 nmol/L)
4 hours	74 mIU/L	1.84 ng/dL (SI: 23.68 pmol/L)	54 ng/dL (SI: 0.83 nmol/L)
6 hours	66 mIU/L	1.72 ng/dL (SI: 22.14 pmol/L)	58 ng/dL (SI: 0.89 nmol/L)

Which of the following is the best next step in this patient's management?

A. Increase the levothyroxine dosage to 400 mcg daily

B. Continue the current levothyroxine dosage and add liothyronine, 5 mcg twice daily

C. Change the levothyroxine dosage to 875 mcg weekly in an observed setting

D. Continue the current levothyroxine dosage and recommend a gluten-free diet

5 A 67-year-old woman is seen for a second opinion regarding management of papillary thyroid carcinoma. Four months ago, a thyroid nodule was incidentally noted during carotid ultrasonography. Subsequent thyroid ultrasonography revealed a solitary hypoechoic, 0.9-cm, right-sided nodule with microcalcifications located in the mid lobe, not adjacent to the thyroid capsule. Ultrasonography did not identify other thyroid abnormalities or abnormal cervical lymph nodes. FNA biopsy of the nodule was interpreted as Bethesda VI (papillary carcinoma). The serum TSH level was 1.52 mIU/L. Neither TPO nor thyroglobulin antibodies have been detected.

She lives close to the hospital and has a good history of attending medical visits. High-quality neck ultrasonography is available at your center. The patient has read about active surveillance strategies and strongly wishes to avoid thyroid surgery.

During active surveillance in this patient, which of the following circumstances would prompt surgery?
- A. Tumor size increase of at least 3 mm
- B. Tumor volume increase of 100%
- C. Increase in serum thyroglobulin of at least 0.3 ng/mL
- D. Increase in serum thyroglobulin of at least 30%

6 A 69-year-old man presents for management of a thyroid nodule. The nodule was palpated during a recent routine physical examination. Thyroid ultrasonography showed a 4.2-cm, left-sided, isoechoic nodule that is wider-than-tall, is hypervascular, has smooth borders, and has no calcifications. The remainder of the thyroid appears normal and there is no cervical lymphadenopathy.

FNA biopsy is performed. Cytopathology is interpreted as a follicular neoplasm (Bethesda IV). The cytopathologist's report notes that "although the architectural features suggest a follicular neoplasm, some nuclear features raise the possibility of an invasive follicular variant of papillary cancer or its recently described indolent counterpart, noninvasive follicular thyroid neoplasm with papillary-like nuclear features (NIFTP); definitive distinction among these entities is not possible on cytologic material."

A biopsy sample is sent for molecular marker testing and is found to be positive for a *RAS* mutation.

On the basis of the test results thus far, which of the following do you recommend as the best next step?
- A. FNA biopsy for *BRAF* V600E mutation testing
- B. Radioactive iodine scan
- C. FNA biopsy for flow cytometry
- D. Thyroid ultrasonography in 6 months
- E. Thyroid lobectomy

7 A 52-year-old woman with a history of post-ablative hypothyroidism comes to see you for the first time. She has been taking levothyroxine, 125 mcg daily, for the past several years. She describes fatigue and "brain fog" and is frustrated by her inability to lose weight. Despite adherence to dietary and exercise recommendations, her weight has increased 9 lb (4.1 kg) over the past 2 years.

On physical examination, her blood pressure is 132/76 mm Hg and weight is 170 lb (77.3 kg). Her thyroid is firm and 20 g in size. The relaxation phase of her deep tendon reflexes is normal.

Laboratory values are as follows:
TSH = 2.59 mIU/L (0.5-5.0 mIU/L)
Free T_4 = 1.6 ng/dL (0.8-1.8 ng/dL)
(SI: 20.59 pmol/L [10.30-23.17 pmol/L])

She asks you to increase her levothyroxine dosage for a goal TSH in the low-normal range (0.5-0.8 mIU/L), which she believes will help with her weight loss and improve her quality of life.

Which of the following would be most likely if this patient's levothyroxine dosage were increased as she has requested?
- A. Improved mood
- B. Decreased visceral fat mass
- C. Increased resting energy expenditure
- D. Improved cognitive function
- E. Perceived benefit of the change

8 A 66-year-old woman presented 4 months ago with a palpable right-sided thyroid nodule. Thyroid ultrasonography demonstrated a solitary hypoechoic nodule with irregular margins. FNA biopsy of the nodule was interpreted as Bethesda VI (malignant), and the patient subsequently underwent total thyroidectomy 6 weeks ago. Surgical pathology revealed a 4.1-cm papillary cancer with no vascular invasion and no extrathyroidal extension. Surgical margins were clear. Six of 17 resected right-sided cervical lymph nodes were positive for malignancy; the largest nodal metastasis was 1.2 cm. She is currently taking levothyroxine, 137 mcg daily.

Laboratory test results:
Thyroglobulin antibodies, negative
Thyroglobulin = 4.3 ng/mL (SI: 4.3 µg/L)
TSH = 0.42 mIU/L (0.5-5.0 mIU/L)

Which of the following should you advise regarding radioactive iodine treatment and levothyroxine dosing?

Answer	^{131}I Iodine Dose	Levothyroxine for Initial TSH Goal of:
A.	None	0.5-2.0 mIU/L
B.	30 mCi	0.5-2.0 mIU/L
C.	30 mCi	0.1-0.5 mIU/L
D.	150 mCi	<0.1 mIU/L
E.	200 mCi	<0.1 mIU/L

9 A 63-year-old man with stage IV medullary thyroid cancer is referred for consideration of further therapy. Medullary thyroid cancer was diagnosed 8 years earlier and he has had a persistent postoperative elevation of serum calcitonin. Distant metastases to the lungs and ribs were detected 1 year ago, with disease progression over the past 6 months. Physical examination reveals a well-healed thyroidectomy scar but findings are otherwise unremarkable.

Laboratory test results:
Serum calcitonin = 14,000 pg/mL (<10 pg/mL)
(SI: 4088 pmol/L [<2.9 pmol/L])
Carcinoembryonic antigen = 72 ng/mL
(<2.5 ng/mL) (SI: 72 µg/L [<2.5 µg/L])

Which of the following is the most appropriate next step in this patient's management?
A. Radioactive iodine treatment
B. Chemotherapy with doxorubicin and cisplatin
C. Radiotherapy to the lung and rib lesions
D. Vandetanib therapy
E. Octreotide therapy

10 A 48-year-old woman presents after a thyroid nodule is noted incidentally on CT. She has not been aware of anterior neck changes. Her serum TSH level is 2.37 mIU/L. She has no history of head or neck radiation and has no family history of thyroid cancer. Ultrasonography demonstrates the following in the right thyroid lobe (*see image*).

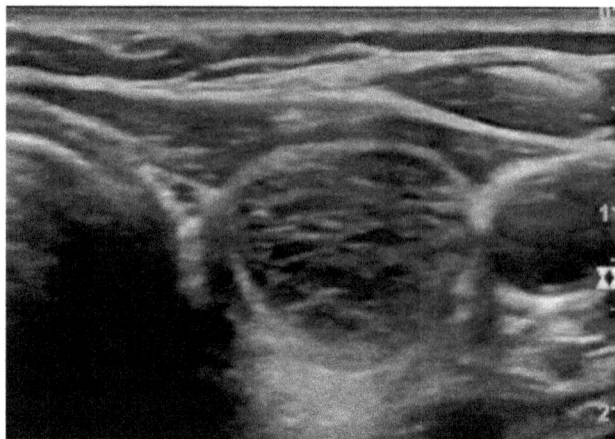

On the basis of the ultrasonographic pattern, which of the following best approximates her risk for malignancy?
A. <3%
B. 10%-20%
C. 20%-40%
D. 70%-90%

11 A 26-year-old woman presents to you for the first time for follow-up of hypothyroidism, which was diagnosed several years ago. She is currently being treated with levothyroxine, 88 mcg daily, and liothyronine, 10 mcg daily. Her regimen was changed to levothyroxine/liothyronine combination therapy 2 years ago due to persistent fatigue on levothyroxine alone; she reports that symptoms improved with this change and she is currently feeling well. Her most recent serum TSH value, measured 3 weeks ago, was 1.23 mIU/L. She reports that her period is 2 weeks late, and an in-office urine pregnancy test is positive.

Which of the following is the best option for her thyroid hormone therapy now?
A. Continue current treatment
B. Stop liothyronine and increase the levothyroxine dosage to 150 mcg daily
C. Increase both the levothyroxine and liothyronine dosages by 25%
D. Increase the levothyroxine dosage to 112 mcg daily and continue the current liothyronine dosage

12 A 34-year-old woman presents with symptoms of tachycardia, tremor, heat intolerance, and irregular menses.

On physical examination, her blood pressure is 128/77 mm Hg and pulse rate is 96 beats/min. She has a palpable, nontender, 3-cm right-sided thyroid nodule.

Laboratory test results:
TSH = <0.01 mIU/L (0.5-5.0 mIU/L)
Free T_4 = 2.9 ng/dL (0.8-1.8 ng/dL) (SI: 37.3 pmol/L [10.30-23.17 pmol/L])
Total T_3 = 320 ng/dL (70-200 ng/dL) (SI: 4.9 nmol/L [1.08-3.08 nmol/L])
TPO antibodies = 37 IU/mL (<2.0 IU/mL) (SI: 37 kIU/L [<2.0 kIU/L])
Thyroid stimulating immunoglobulin = <120% (≤120% of basal activity)

Her radioactive iodine uptake is 26% at 24 hours (*see image*). In discussing therapeutic options, she makes it clear that her primary concern is to avoid the need for lifelong medication.

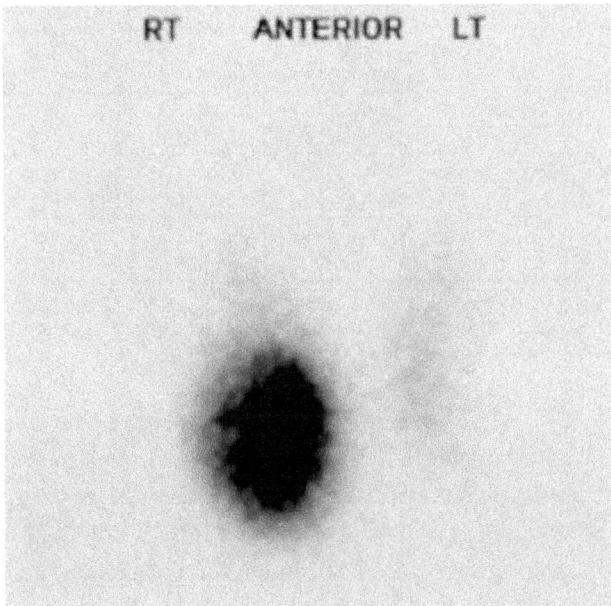

RT   ANTERIOR   LT

Which of the following therapeutic options would be most appropriate for this patient?
A. Radioactive iodine treatment
B. Methimazole
C. Thyroid lobectomy
D. Ethanol injection
E. Radiofrequency ablation

13 A 21-year-old man with attention deficit disorder is referred for palpitations and abnormal thyroid function test results. He has no compressive symptoms.

On physical examination, his pulse rate is 96 beats/min and regular. He has a diffuse goiter, without nodules or bruit. Tremor is absent, and he has normal deep tendon reflexes.

Laboratory test results:
Free T_4 = 2.7 ng/dL (0.8-1.8 ng/dL) (SI: 34.8 pmol/L [10.30-23.17 pmol/L])
TSH = 4.3 mIU/L (0.5-5.0 mIU/L)
Radioactive iodine uptake = 35% at 24 hours (15%-30% at 24 hours)
α-Subunit of pituitary glycoprotein hormones = 0.3 ng/mL (<1.2 ng/mL) (SI: 0.3 μg/L [<1.2 μg/L])
SHBG = 3.0 μg/mL (1.1-6.7 μg/mL) (SI: 26.7 nmol/L [10-60 nmol/L])

MRI shows a normal-appearing pituitary gland. Results from a test for heterophile antibodies are negative.

Which of the following is the most appropriate next step in this patient's management?
A. Start propranolol
B. Start methimazole
C. Treat with radioiodine
D. Refer for thyroidectomy
E. No intervention at this time

14 An 83-year-old man with refractory atrial fibrillation is prescribed amiodarone. Three months later, he reports increasing palpitations and diaphoresis.

On physical examination, his pulse rate is 90 beats/min and regular, his thyroid gland is of normal size and is nontender, and he has a fine tremor.

Which of the following would be the most specific indicator of thyrotoxicosis in this patient?
A. Elevated total T_4 level
B. Elevated free T_4 level (by dialysis)
C. Suppressed serum TSH level
D. Low radioactive iodine uptake
E. Clinical signs and symptoms

15 A 37-year-old woman comes to see you after recently moving to your area. She underwent transsphenoidal resection of a nonfunctional pituitary adenoma 5 years ago. There is a history of type 1 diabetes mellitus in her mother. Her medications include hydrocortisone, 10 mg in the morning and 5 mg in the afternoon, and an oral contraceptive. She describes mild fatigue and difficulty losing weight.

Laboratory test results:
TSH = 5.6 mIU/L (0.5-5.0 mIU/L)
Free T_4 = 0.6 ng/dL (0.8-1.8 ng/dL) (SI: 7.7 pmol/L [10.30-23.17 pmol/L])

Levothyroxine is initiated at a dosage of 50 mcg daily. Six week later, her fatigue is unchanged.

Laboratory test results:
TSH = 0.16 mIU/L
Free T_4 = 0.9 ng/dL (SI: 11.6 pmol/L)

Which of the following is the best next step?
  A. Discontinue levothyroxine
  B. Reduce the levothyroxine dosage to 25 mcg daily
  C. Continue the current levothyroxine dosage and add liothyronine, 5 mcg daily
  D. Continue the current levothyroxine dosage and increase the hydrocortisone dosage to 15 mg in the morning and 5 mg in the afternoon
  E. Increase the levothyroxine dosage to 88 mcg daily

16 A 52-year-old man presents for a routine physical examination. There is a family history of Hashimoto thyroiditis in his mother. The patient reports anxiety and recent hair loss, but has no other symptoms.

On physical examination, his pulse rate is 76 beats/min. He has no exophthalmos, lid lag, or stare. His thyroid gland is 20 g in size without nodules, and there is no tremor of his outstretched hands.

He is not taking any prescription medications. He reports taking a multivitamin; biotin, 4500 mcg daily; and a selenium supplement, 300 mcg daily. His serum TSH level is documented to be less than 0.01 mIU/L.

Results of repeated laboratory testing 3 days later:
TSH = <0.01 mIU/L (0.5-5.0 mIU/L)
Free T_4 = 3.2 ng/dL (0.8-1.8 ng/dL) (SI: 41.2 pmol/L [10.30-23.17 pmol/L])
Total T_3 = 374 ng/dL (70-200 ng/dL) (SI: 5.8 nmol/L [1.08-3.08 nmol/L])

Which of the following is the best next step for establishing this patient's diagnosis?
  A. Radioactive iodine uptake and scan
  B. Repeated blood tests after stopping biotin for 7 days
  C. Initiation of methimazole
  D. Measurement of serum thyroid-stimulating immunoglobulin

17 A 67-year-old man is admitted to the intensive care unit with hypotension due to sepsis. Despite aggressive therapy, the patient's condition continues to deteriorate. One month earlier, the patient had a normal thyroid laboratory panel.

Which of the following patterns is expected in this patient?

Answer	TSH	Total T_4	Total T_3	Free T_4
A.	10.0 mIU/L	7.0 µg/dL (SI: 90.1 nmol/L)	70 ng/dL (SI: 1.1 nmol/L)	0.7 ng/dL (SI: 9.0 pmol/L)
B.	7.5 mIU/L	5.5 µg/dL (SI: 70.8 nmol/L)	55 ng/dL (SI: 0.8 nmol/L)	0.8 ng/dL (SI: 10.3 pmol/L)
C.	0.2 mIU/L	2.5 µg/dL (SI: 31.2 nmol/L)	25 ng/dL (SI: 0.4 nmol/L)	0.5 ng/dL (SI: 6.4 pmol/L)
D.	5.0 mIU/L	12.0 µg/dL (SI: 154.4 nmol/L)	70 ng/dL (SI: 1.1 nmol/L)	2.2 ng/dL (SI: 28.3 pmol/L)
E.	0.01 mIU/L	12.0 µg/dL (SI: 154.4 nmol/L)	360 ng/dL (SI: 5.5 nmol/L)	2.2 ng/dL (SI: 28.3 pmol/L)

Reference ranges: TSH, 0.5-5.0 mIU/L; total T_4, 5.5-12.5 µg/dL (SI: 70.8-160.9 nmol/L); total T_3, 70-200 ng/dL (SI: 1.1-3.1 nmol/L); free T_4, 0.8-1.8 ng/dL (SI: 10.3-23.2 pmol/L).

18 A 46-year-old woman is noted to have a palpable left thyroid nodule on physical examination. No cervical adenopathy is noted. Her serum TSH concentration is 2.4 mIU/L, and thyroid ultrasonography shows a 2.7-cm solitary hypoechoic nodule without suspicious features.

Which of the following thyroid FNA biopsy findings (see accompanying images) should result in a referral for thyroidectomy?
  A. Figure A
  B. Figure B
  C. Figure C
  D. Figure D

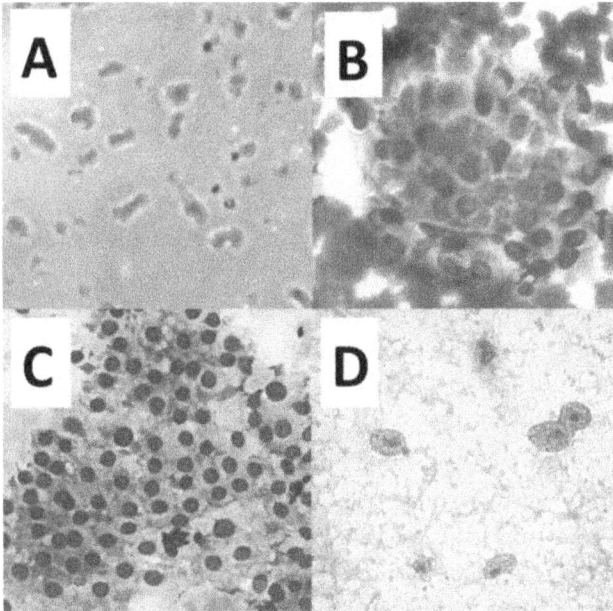

19 A 42-year-old woman is found to have a TSH concentration of 0.14 mIU/L on laboratory tests performed as part of routine physical examination. She has no hyperthyroid symptoms. She is otherwise healthy and is not currently taking any medications or supplements. There is a small goiter on examination with no bruit and no palpable nodules. She has no signs of Graves eye disease. Her resting pulse rate is 78 beats/min.

Laboratory test results 4 months later:
    TSH = 0.19 mIU/L (0.5-5.0 mIU/L)
    Free T_4 = 1.6 ng/dL (0.8-1.8 ng/dL)
       (SI: 20.59 pmol/L [10.30-23.17 pmol/L])
    Total T_3 = 166 ng/dL (70-200 ng/dL)
       (SI: 2.56 nmol/L [1.08-3.08 nmol/L])
    Thyroid-stimulating immunoglobulin = 137%
       (≤120% of basal activity)

She has 2 children and is not planning additional pregnancies.

Which of the following is the best option?
   A. Repeat thyroid function tests in 6 months
   B. Start atenolol, 25 mg daily
   C. Start methimazole, 5 mg daily
   D. Schedule radioactive iodine treatment
   E. Schedule total thyroidectomy

20 A 76-year-old Hispanic man undergoing evaluation for syncope is referred for abnormalities identified on thyroid function testing. He has hypertension and takes hydrochlorothiazide.

On physical examination, his pulse rate is 92 beats/min and he has a normal thyroid gland. He has a fine tremor, but normal deep tendon reflexes.

Thyroid function test results:
    Total T_4 = 16.8 µg/dL (5.5-12.5 µg/dL)
       (SI: 216.22 nmol/L [94.02-213.68 nmol/L])
    Free T_4 = 1.7 ng/dL (0.8-1.8 ng/dL)
       (SI: 21.88 pmol/L [10.30-23.17 pmol/L])
    Total T_3 = 170 ng/dL (70-200 ng/dL)
       (SI: 2.62 nmol/L [1.08-3.08 nmol/L])
    Free T_3 = 3.2 pg/mL (2.3-4.2 pg/mL)
       (SI: 4.92 pmol/L [3.53-6.45 pmol/L])
    TSH = 2.1 mIU/L (0.5-5.0 mIU/L)

Which of the following is the most likely diagnosis?
   A. Selenium deficiency
   B. Familial thyroxine-binding globulin excess
   C. Familial dysalbuminemic hyperthyroxinemia
   D. Thyroid hormone resistance
   E. TSH-secreting pituitary adenoma

21 A 62-year-old woman is referred for evaluation of a neck mass. The patient notes dysphagia with solid foods and positional dyspnea when lying on her right side. Medical history is noncontributory.

On physical examination, she has a large goiter extending below the clavicle on the left. Her serum TSH level is 0.5 mIU/L, and radioiodine uptake is 13% at 24 hours. Ultrasonography shows a multinodular goiter with confluent isoechoic nodules throughout. Results from FNA biopsy of the largest nodule are benign. Noncontrast CT of the neck is shown (*see image*).

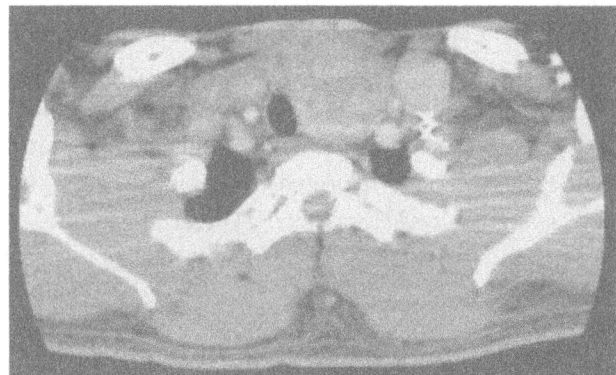

Which of the following is the best next step in this patient's management?

  A. Levothyroxine suppressive therapy
  B. Radioiodine therapy using recombinant human TSH
  C. Thermal ablation therapy
  D. Thyroidectomy from collar incision
  E. No intervention until symptoms progress

22 A 27-year-old woman with Graves hyperthyroidism has been treated with methimazole, 10 mg daily, for 14 months. On palpation, her thyroid gland is at the upper limit of normal size. There is no bruit. She does not smoke cigarettes. She is interested in stopping methimazole.

Current laboratory test results:
  TSH = 0.7 mIU/L (0.5-5.0 mIU/L)
  Total T_3 = 166 ng/dL (70-200 ng/dL)
    (SI: 2.56 nmol/L [1.08-3.08 nmol/L])
  Free T_4 = 1.6 ng/dL (0.8-1.8 ng/dL)
    (SI: 20.59 pmol/L [10.30-23.17 pmol/L])
  TPO antibodies = 594 IU/mL (<2.0 IU/mL) (SI: 594 kIU/L [<2.0 kIU/L])
  Thyroid-stimulating immunoglobulin = 396% (≤120% of basal activity)

Which of the following characteristics of this patient predicts a likelihood that her Graves hyperthyroidism will recur if methimazole is stopped?

  A. Age
  B. TPO antibody titer
  C. Thyroid-stimulating immunoglobulin level
  D. Thyroid size
  E. Smoking status

23 A 37-year-old man is found to have a left thyroid nodule. Thyroid ultrasonography shows a 4.6-cm hypoechoic nodule without calcification or hypervascularity, with no suspicious lymph nodes. The patient undergoes FNA biopsy of the dominant nodule with cytologic findings of follicular neoplasm (Bethesda class IV). Repeated FNA biopsy with molecular analysis reveals a *RET/PTC* rearrangement.

Which of the following is the most appropriate next step in this patient's management?

  A. Repeated thyroid ultrasonography in 6 months
  B. Repeated FNA biopsy in 6 months
  C. Referral for lobectomy
  D. Referral for total thyroidectomy
  E. Referral for total thyroidectomy with bilateral neck dissection

24 A 52-year-old man presents with palpitations. His weight has recently decreased from 237 to 211 lb (107.7 to 95.9 kg). He has otherwise been healthy and has had no recent illnesses. He takes no medications or supplements.

On physical examination, his thyroid is nontender and there is no goiter. He has a fine tremor of his outstretched hands, and his pulse rate is 97 beats/min. He has no stigmata of Graves disease.

Laboratory test results:
  TSH = <0.01 mIU/L (0.5-5.0 mIU/L)
  Free T_4 = 4.3 ng/dL (0.8-1.8 ng/dL)
    (SI: 55.35 pmol/L [10.30-23.17 pmol/L])
  Total T_3 = 290 ng/dL (70-200 ng/dL)
    (SI: 4.47 nmol/L [1.08-3.08 nmol/L])
  Thyroglobulin antibodies = <4.0 IU/mL (≤4.0 IU/mL) (SI: <4.0 kIU/L [≤4.0 kIU/L])
  Radioactive iodine uptake = <1% at 24 hours (15%-30%)

A spot urinary iodine concentration on the day of the radioactive iodine uptake test is 96 μg/L (while a reference range is not available, the most recent median urinary iodine concentration in adults in the United States is 144 μg/L).

Which of the following tests is most likely to reveal the diagnosis?

  A. Radioactive iodine uptake/scan after a low-iodine diet
  B. Serum thyroglobulin measurement
  C. Assessment of serum erythrocyte sedimentation rate
  D. Thyroid ultrasonography with color Doppler
  E. Thyroid-stimulating immunoglobulin measurement

25 You recently palpated a new thyroid nodule in a 42-year-old woman with a history of hypothyroidism. Ultrasound-guided FNA biopsy of her palpable nodule is interpreted as suspicious for papillary carcinoma. She undergoes total thyroidectomy without complications. Surgical pathology shows a 2.4-cm intrathyroidal, fully encapsulated papillary carcinoma with clear margins, no lymphovascular invasion, and no positive lymph nodes. Three months ago, her TSH level was 0.7 mIU/L on levothyroxine, 112 mcg daily. Her dosage was increased to 137 mcg daily at the time of her surgery.

Current laboratory test results 1 week postoperatively:
TSH = 0.3 mIU/L (0.5-5.0 mIU/L)
Thyroglobulin (measured using a radioimmunoassay) = 17 ng/mL (SI: 17 μg/L)
Thyroglobulin antibodies = <4.0 IU/mL

Which of the following is the best next step?
A. Repeated thyroglobulin measurement using an immunometric assay
B. Repeated thyroglobulin and thyroglobulin antibody measurements in 6 weeks using the same radioimmunoassay
C. Measurement of thyroglobulin in serially diluted sera
D. Measurement of thyroglobulin by mass spectroscopy
E. Radioactive iodine ablation

26 A 32-year-old woman undergoes thyroidectomy with central neck dissection for a 4.5-cm papillary thyroid cancer. The tumor shows microscopic local invasion but no aggressive histology and 2 of 11 central lymph nodes contain tumor. The patient undergoes radioiodine remnant ablation using 100 mCi of ^{131}I, and a posttreatment scan shows no uptake outside of the thyroid bed. Surveillance testing at 6 months reveals a stimulated thyroglobulin concentration of 16 ng/mL (16 μg/L) with negative thyroglobulin antibodies, no abnormal uptake on radioiodine whole-body scan, and no adenopathy on neck ultrasonography. No additional therapy is given. Six months later, a suppressed thyroglobulin level is 0.6 ng/mL (0.6 μg/L), stimulated thyroglobulin is 5 ng/mL (5 μg/L), thyroglobulin antibodies are negative, and neck ultrasonography is unchanged.

Which of the following should be the next step in this patient's management?
A. Thyroglobulin testing using a different assay
B. PET-CT scan
C. CT of the chest
D. MRI of the neck
E. Repeated surveillance testing in 1 year

27 A 79-year-old woman reports a 2-week history of left-sided neck pain and palpitations. Physical examination reveals firm enlargement (about 1.5 times normal size) and tenderness over the right thyroid lobe. Laboratory testing shows an elevated free T_4 level and suppressed TSH level. Thyroid-stimulating immunoglobulin is normal. She is prescribed prednisone.

Three weeks later the patient notes persistent pain, now accompanied by dysphagia, and a further increase in size of the right thyroid lobe (now 3 times normal size). Thyroid function test results are essentially unchanged. Ultrasonography reveals an enlarged and heterogeneous right thyroid lobe with increased vascularity.

Which of the following should be the next step in this patient's management?
A. Perform FNA biopsy
B. Start methimazole
C. Change prednisone to intravenous methylprednisolone
D. Perform contrast CT of the neck
E. Refer for thyroidectomy

28 A 28-year-old pregnant woman with Graves disease treated with propylthiouracil is referred for medication adjustment. She is in her 18th week of pregnancy.

Which of the following sets of laboratory results is within recommended targets for this patient?

Answer	TSH	Free T₄ Index	Total T₃
A.	0.05 mIU/L	5.2	400 ng/dL (SI: 6.2 nmol/L)
B.	0.1 mIU/L	4.2	350 ng/dL (SI: 5.4 nmol/L)
C.	1.5 mIU/L	3.2	330 ng/dL (SI: 5.1 nmol/L)
D.	2.5 mIU/L	2.4	280 ng/dL (SI: 4.3 nmol/L)
E.	3.5 mIU/L	1.8	210 ng/dL (SI: 3.2 nmol/L)

Reference ranges: TSH, 0.5-5.0 mIU/L; free T_4 index, 1-4; total T_3, 70-200 ng/dL (1.1-3.1 nmol/L).

29 A 62-year-old woman with hypothyroidism is admitted to the surgical intensive care unit with acute necrotizing pancreatitis. Her serum TSH level 1 month before admission was 1.8 mIU/L. Her outpatient levothyroxine dosage is 100 mcg daily. Her surgical team is concerned about poor levothyroxine absorption due to bowel edema and wishes to change to parenteral thyroid hormone therapy.

Which of the following regimens would be most appropriate?
   A. Levothyroxine, 150 mcg intravenously once daily
   B. Levothyroxine, 100 mcg intravenously once daily
   C. Levothyroxine, 1000 mcg intramuscularly once weekly
   D. Levothyroxine, 70 mcg intravenously once daily
   E. Liothyronine, 25 mcg intravenously twice daily

30 A 43-year-old woman with a history of Graves disease treated 7 months earlier with radioiodine is noted to have progressive monocular vision loss.

On physical examination, she has bilateral periorbital edema and conjunctival erythema, with Hertel measurements of 23 mm proptosis on the right side and 22 mm on the left side. Extraocular eye muscle testing shows restricted upward and lateral gaze on the left side. An afferent pupillary defect is present on the right side, and visual acuity measurement is 20/40 on the left and 20/400 on the right.

Laboratory test results:
   Serum TSH = 1.2 mIU/L (0.5-5.0 mIU/L)
   Free T_4 = 1.2 ng/dL (0.8-1.8 ng/dL)
      (SI: 15.44 pmol/L [10.3-23.2 pmol/L])
   Thyroid-stimulating immunoglobulin = 360%
      (≤120% of basal activity)

The patient is given pulse therapy with methylprednisolone with no improvement.

Which of the following is the best next step in this patient's management?
   A. Orbital radiotherapy
   B. Rituximab
   C. Strabismus surgery
   D. Teprotumumab
   E. Orbital decompression surgery

ENDOCRINE
BOARD
REVIEW

Adrenal Board Review

Richard J. Auchus, MD, PhD

1 ANSWER: B) Follicular-phase progesterone

Few women with classic 21-hydroxylase deficiency attempt to bear children (<25% of all and <10% of those with null *CYP21A2* alleles). For those who do attempt to have children, however, fecundity rates are close to that of the general population (>90%). Of the parameters that matter for achieving fertility, neither androgens nor the precursor 17-hydroxyprogesterone—which are characteristically elevated in this disease—are targets of therapy (thus, Answers A, C, D, and E are incorrect). Women with 21-hydroxylase deficiency can ovulate despite elevated adrenal-derived androgens. In contrast, high adrenal-derived progesterone in the follicular phase (Answer B) has the same effect as progestin-only contraceptives, making the cervical mucus unfavorable and thinning the endometrial lining, thus impairing sperm penetration and endometrial receptivity. The goal is a follicular-phase progesterone concentration less than 0.6 ng/mL (<2.0 nmol/L).

Educational Objective

Titrate therapy for a woman with classic 21-hydroxylase deficiency who is attempting to bear children.

Reference(s)

Auchus RJ, Arlt W. Approach to the patient: the adult with congenital adrenal hyperplasia. *J Clin Endocrinol Metab*. 2013;98(7):2645-2655. PMID: 23837188

Speiser PW, Arlt W, Auchus RJ, et al. Congenital adrenal hyperplasia due to steroid 21-hydroxylase deficiency: an Endocrine Society clinical practice guideline. *J Clin Endocrinol Metab*. 2018; 103(11):4043-4088. PMID: 30272171

Casteràs A, De Silva P, Rumsby G, Conway GS. Reassessing fecundity in women with classical congenital adrenal hyperplasia (CAH): normal pregnancy rate but reduced fertility rate. *Clin Endocrinol (Oxf)*. 2009;70(6):833-837. PMID: 19250265

2 ANSWER: E) Measure serum cortisol after 1-mg dexamethasone

Because of hypertension and hypokalemia, this patient was evaluated for primary aldosteronism, and the screening aldosterone-to-renin ratio is positive, but only modestly so. Ordinarily, one would proceed to confirmatory testing, followed by CT, and then adrenal venous sampling to localize the source(s) of aldosterone. In this case, however, the weight gain, hyperglycemia, and dermal atrophy are suggestive of hypercortisolism as well. Proximal myopathy and striae are late manifestations in the development of Cushing syndrome and are insensitive findings. Because CT was performed, we know that she has a fairly large adrenal tumor—significantly larger than those that usually cause primary aldosteronism. Also, the contralateral (right) adrenal gland is somewhat atrophic, suggesting hypercortisolism from the left adrenal tumor. When the diameter of adrenal cortical tumors is greater than 2.4 cm, the risk of hypercortisolism rises, and if the tumor is removed without testing cortisol dynamics, adrenal crisis might occur postoperatively. In addition, the CT scan in this vignette was done only with contrast, so one cannot use density to determine whether the tumor is lipid-rich, which would exclude pheochromocytoma. However, plasma metanephrines would be elevated if a mass this large were a pheochromocytoma.

Spironolactone (Answer A) would treat the mineralocorticoid excess but not glucocorticoid manifestations, and this patient needs further evaluation before starting therapy. Left adrenalectomy or biopsy (Answers B and C) is incorrect because the possibilities of hypercortisolism (and pheochromocytoma) must be excluded before performing surgery or biopsy for a tumor of this size. Adrenal venous sampling (Answer D) is the gold standard for lateralizing aldosterone production in primary aldosteronism, but if the tumor is cosecreting cortisol—which is used to correct adrenal vein aldosterone concentrations for dilution with mixed venous blood—the suppression of cortisol from the contralateral adrenal will artifactually raise the aldosterone-to-cortisol ratio on the contralateral side. With the concern of hypercortisolism and the presence of a large adrenal tumor, performing a 1-mg overnight dexamethasone suppression test (Answer E) before deciding whether to refer for surgery or venous sampling is the correct next step.

In this case, the overnight dexamethasone suppression test resulted in a cortisol concentration of 4.4 μg/dL (121 nmol/L). Subsequent testing documented an ACTH concentration of 6.0 pg/mL (1.3 pmol/L), DHEA-S concentration of 22 μg/dL (0.6 μmol/L) (reference range, 44-352 μg/dL [1.2-9.5 μmol/L]), and normal urinary free cortisol excretion. Thus, the diagnosis of ACTH-independent hypercortisolism was established, which overrides the evaluation of primary aldosteronism and indicates that the large left adrenal tumor should be removed with perioperative glucocorticoid coverage. Coproduction of aldosterone and cortisol from adrenal cortical adenomas, particularly larger tumors, is well described. It is possible, although unlikely, that the primary aldosteronism is bilateral and unrelated to the adrenal tumor, so the patient should be rescreened for primary aldosteronism after adrenalectomy. If it persists, spironolactone would be an appropriate treatment. After adrenalectomy, this patient had resolution of hypercortisolemia, hyperaldosteronism, and hypertension.

Educational Objective
Suspect cortisol coproduction in large aldosterone-producing adenomas.

Reference(s)
Spath M, Korovkin S, Antke C, Anlauf M, Willenberg HS. Aldosterone- and cortisol-co-secreting adrenal tumors: the lost subtype of primary aldosteronism. *Eur J Endocrinol*. 2011; 164(4):447-455. PMID: 21270113

Morelli V, Reimondo G, Giordano R, et al. Long-term follow-up in adrenal incidentalomas: an Italian multicenter study. *J Clin Endocrinol Metab*. 2014;99(3):827-834. PMID: 24423350

Fallo F, Bertello C, Tizzani D, et al. Concurrent primary aldosteronism and subclinical cortisol hypersecretion: a prospective study. *J Hypertens*. 2011;29(9):1773-1777. PMID: 2170261

ANSWER: A) Metoclopramide
Patients with known or suspected pheochromocytomas are vulnerable to catecholamine crises, and certain medications precipitate an abrupt burst of catecholamine secretion. For example, pregnant women with pheochromocytoma are particularly vulnerable to such crises, and this population often requires treatment for nausea. Perhaps the most consistently dangerous agents are dopamine (D2-receptor) antagonists such as metoclopramide (Answer A). Intravenous glucocorticoid administration has been documented to precipitate crises, and a few cases of crises have occurred during oral dexamethasone suppression testing for evaluation of an adrenal mass. Other drugs that can precipitate crises and should be avoided include glucagon, inhalational anesthetics, monoamine oxidase inhibitors, phenothiazines, and cosyntropin, as all of these agents have been associated with crises. Low-osmolar contrast media is safe to use even before α-adrenergic blockade. H1-blockers (Answer B), benzodiazepines (Answer C), H2-blockers (Answer D), and serotonin 5-HT3 receptor antagonists such as ondansetron (Answer E) are all safe to administer.

Educational Objective
List the drugs and diagnostic agents that should be avoided in patients with suspected pheochromocytoma.

Reference(s)
Eisenhofer G, Rivers G, Rosas AL, Quezado Z, Manger WM, Pacak K. Adverse drug reactions in patients with phaeochromocytoma: incidence, prevention and management. *Drug Saf*. 2007; 30(11):1031-1062. PMID: 17973541

Baid SK, Lai EW, Wesley RA, et al. Brief communication: radiographic contrast infusion and catecholamine release in patients with pheochromocytoma [published correction appears in *Ann Intern Med*. 2009;150(4):292]. *Ann Intern Med*. 2009;150(1):27-32. PMID: 19124817

Barrett C, van Uum SH, Lenders JW. Risk of catecholaminergic crisis following glucocorticoid administration in patients with an adrenal mass: a literature review. *Clin Endocrinol (Oxf)*. 2015; 83(5):622-628. PMID: 25940577

4 ANSWER: D) Serum DHEA-S concentration = 360 µg/dL (38-523 µg/dL) (SI: 9.8 µmol/L [1.0-14.2 µmol/L])

The hypothalamic-pituitary-adrenal axis displays a prominent circadian rhythm, and these diurnal fluctuations in ACTH and cortisol production both guide and impede testing. A random serum cortisol measurement can be used to exclude adrenal insufficiency when it is above roughly 14 µg/dL (>386 nmol/L). ACTH is high in primary adrenal insufficiency and low in secondary adrenal insufficiency, and hence ACTH alone cannot diagnose adrenal insufficiency. Chances are best for obtaining a convincingly high value for cortisol in the early morning. Lower random values in the afternoon are typical, and while the laboratory might report a "normal range" for cortisol and ACTH in the afternoon, this normal range cannot be used to conclusively exclude adrenal insufficiency. Because cortisol has a short half-life of 30 to 60 min, dynamic testing is most commonly used to exclude adrenal insufficiency in the afternoon. Alternatively, DHEA-S is also a measure of adrenal cortex function because it is produced in parallel with cortisol under ACTH stimulation. In contrast to cortisol, the half-life of DHEA-S is long (approximately 1 day), so little diurnal fluctuation is observed. Consequently, it is more likely that a conclusively normal DHEA-S value will be obtained in the afternoon (as opposed to cortisol), and a normal DHEA-S value in the absence of DHEA consumption excludes both primary and secondary adrenal insufficiency (thus, Answer D is correct). A single dose of dexamethasone will not suppress adrenal function for more than a few days, so random testing 10 days later is an appropriate screen. The caveat with DHEA-S testing is that an age-related decline occurs, such that normal values are low when patients are older than about 64 years.

An afternoon serum cortisol value of 5.0 µg/dL (138 nmol/L) (Answer A) might be in the "normal range" for that time of day, but the value would have to exceed roughly 14.0 µg/dL (>386 nmol/L) to exclude adrenal insufficiency. Random afternoon salivary cortisol testing (Answer B) has not been validated as a test of adrenal function, and ACTH values alone (Answer C) cannot be used to exclude adrenal insufficiency.

Educational Objective
Use DHEA-S measurement in the evaluation of adrenal function.

Reference(s)
Fischli S, Jenni S, Allemann S, et al. Dehydroepiandrosterone sulfate in the assessment of the hypothalamic-pituitary-adrenal axis. *J Clin Endocrinol Metab*. 2008; 93(2):539-542. PMID: 17986637

Al-Aridi R, Abdelmannan D, Arafah BM. Biochemical diagnosis of adrenal insufficiency: the added value of dehydroepiandrosterone sulfate measurements. *Endocr Pract*. 2011;17(2):261-270. PMID: 21134877

Stewart PM, Corrie J, Seckl JR, Edwards CR, Padfield PL. A rational approach for assessing the hypothalamo-pituitary-adrenal axis. *Lancet*. 1988;1(8596):1208-1210. PMID: 2897016

5 ANSWER: A) Administer α-adrenergic blockade and refer for left adrenalectomy

The classic presentation of pheochromocytoma involves paroxysmal hypertension with sweating and palpitations. In order to produce such symptoms, however, the tumor must be fairly large, and catecholamine production (as assessed with plasma or urine metanephrines) must be at least 5- or 10-fold elevated. Today, up to 60% of pheochromocytomas are discovered incidentally as adrenal nodules found on cross-sectional imaging performed for other reasons. The imaging features of pheochromocytomas include higher-than-lipid density (>10 Hounsfield units) on precontrast CT scans and low (<60% absolute) contrast washout at 15 minutes, as is the case for this patient's tumor. Measurement of plasma metanephrines is a very sensitive test for pheochromocytoma, although fraught with false-positive results. A typical false-positive result is a plasma normetanephrine concentration less than 1.5 times the upper normal limit, whereas any elevation of plasma metanephrine must be taken seriously. This patient's screening metanephrines are convincingly positive and of the magnitude that does not typically result in symptoms. He received α-adrenergic blockade and underwent adrenalectomy (Answer A), and the tumor was documented to be a pheochromocytoma.

For a patient with an incidental adrenal nodule, renin and aldosterone measurement (Answer B) are indicated only if hypertension and/or hypokalemia are present, which is not the case here. Neither adrenal MRI (Answer C) nor additional biochemical testing is needed as the diagnosis is already established. Pheochromocytomas grow and can be malignant, so waiting to perform a repeated CT scan in 12 months (Answer D), as is often done when biochemical testing is negative, is unwise. Biopsy of an adrenal mass (Answer E) is rarely indicated, except in a patient with suspected adrenal metastasis from an occult or recurrent malignancy, and biopsy should never be performed without adrenergic blockade when plasma or urine metanephrines are elevated because of the potential for precipitating a catecholamine crisis.

Educational Objective
Diagnose an incidentally discovered pheochromocytoma.

Reference(s)
Young WF Jr. Endocrine hypertension: then and now. *Endocr Pract.* 2010;16(5):888-902. PMID: 20713331

Sawka AM, Jaeschke R, Singh RJ, Young WF Jr. A comparison of biochemical tests for pheochromocytoma: measurement of fractionated plasma metanephrines compared with the combination of 24-hour urinary metanephrines and catecholamines. *J Clin Endocrinol Metab.* 2003;88(2):553-558. PMID: 12574179

Eisenhofer G, Goldstein DS, Walther MM, et al. Biochemical diagnosis of pheochromocytoma: how to distinguish true- from false-positive test results. *J Clin Endocrinol Metab.* 2003;88(6):2656-2666. PMID: 12788870

Gruber LM, Hartman RP, Thompson GB, et al. Pheochromocytoma characteristics and behavior differ depending on method of discovery. *J Clin Endocrinol Metab.* 2019;104(5):1386-1393. PMID: 30462226

6 ANSWER: C) Change the hydrocortisone dosage to 20 mg 3 times daily

Mitotane therapy is typically prescribed for residual adrenal cancer following debulking surgery or as adjuvant therapy for high-risk disease. Mitotane has a number of adverse effects and alters endocrine laboratory tests through a variety of mechanisms, including direct adrenal cytotoxicity. This patient had Cushing syndrome before surgery, and debulking has left him with adrenal insufficiency due to a temporarily suppressed hypothalamic-pituitary-adrenal axis, as evidenced by the undetectable plasma ACTH. At the same time, mitotane markedly increases corticosteroid-binding globulin and potently induces expression of P450 3A4, a major enzyme in cortisol catabolism. As a consequence, the dosage requirement and frequency for oral hydrocortisone increases markedly with concomitant mitotane therapy, and this patient's symptoms of adrenal insufficiency are due to inadequate cortisol exposure (thus, Answer C is correct).

Mitotane rarely causes aldosterone deficiency, and he is not volume depleted, so fludrocortisone at the dosage of 0.1 mg daily (Answer A) will not provide benefit. This patient is at high risk of cancer recurrence, and reducing the mitotane dosage (Answer B) will result in subtherapeutic drug levels, which is unwise. Hypogonadism and gynecomastia can occur with mitotane therapy, due to a rise in SHBG and some inhibition of testosterone synthesis, but his testosterone and inferred bioavailable testosterone are normal and do not account for his symptoms. Thus, both testosterone enanthate (Answer D) and anastrozole (Answer E) are incorrect.

Educational Objective
Adjust the dosage of hydrocortisone during mitotane therapy for adrenal carcinoma.

Reference(s)
Chortis V, Taylor AE, Schneider P, et al. Mitotane therapy in adrenocortical cancer induces CYP3A4 and inhibits 5α-reductase, explaining the need for personalized glucocorticoid and androgen replacement. *J Clin Endocrinol Metab.* 2013;98(1):161-171. PMID: 23162091

Kroiss M, Quinkler M, Lutz WK, Allolio B, Fassnacht M. Drug interactions with mitotane by induction of CYP3A4 metabolism in the clinical management of adrenocortical carcinoma. *Clin Endocrinol (Oxf).* 2011;75(5):585-591. PMID: 21883349

Else T, Kim AC, Sabolch A, et al. Adrenocortical carcinoma. *Endocr Rev.* 2014;35(2):282-326. PMID: 24423978

7 ANSWER: C) Normal serum potassium

Mifepristone is a competitive antagonist for both the glucocorticoid receptor and the progesterone receptor, but it does not block cortisol action on the mineralocorticoid receptor. Mifepristone is used for the treatment of Cushing syndrome in patients with glucose intolerance or diabetes mellitus. Because mifepristone also antagonizes the feedback inhibition of cortisol on the adenoma, ACTH and cortisol production often rise in patients with Cushing disease on treatment, but not enough to offset the beneficial effects of glucocorticoid receptor blockade in peripheral tissues. Consequently, serum cortisol and plasma ACTH tend to rise and exert even greater effects on the mineralocorticoid receptor, which can cause hypokalemia and hypertension. For this reason, serum potassium must be corrected before starting mifepristone (Answer C).

Blood pressure occasionally rises, but it more commonly decreases after several weeks of treatment. This patient's degree of blood pressure control is acceptable for starting therapy (thus, Answer A is incorrect). When elevated, serum glucose decreases rapidly with mifepristone treatment, and the improved glycemic control is a reliable indicator of therapeutic effect. In fact, patients treated with insulin and hypoglycemic agents other than metformin should reduce their dosages before commencing mifepristone, and normalizing blood glucose with these agents before starting therapy can lead to dangerous hypoglycemia (thus, Answer B is incorrect). Plasma triglycerides also tend to improve slightly with mifepristone and do not worsen (thus, Answer E is incorrect). Additional parameters to monitor as indications of therapeutic response include weight loss, improvement in cognition and depression (when present), and regression of cushingoid features, but these changes take much longer than the immediate reduction in glucose.

Because of potent progesterone receptor antagonism, menses cease and pregnancy is not possible during mifepristone therapy. Mifepristone will cause abortion in a pregnant woman. Therefore, a negative pregnancy test was documented in this patient before starting therapy, but additional contraception is unnecessary. In addition, endometrial hypertrophy and vaginal bleeding can occur weeks to months after starting therapy and should be monitored.

Educational Objective
Identify contraindications and precautions when using mifepristone therapy for Cushing disease.

Reference(s)
Castinetti F, Fassnacht M, Johanssen S, et al. Merits and pitfalls of mifepristone in Cushing's syndrome. *Eur J Endocrinol.* 2009;160(6):1003-1010. PMID: 19289534

Fleseriu M, Biller BM, Findling JW, Molitch ME, Schteingart DE, Gross C; SEISMIC Study Investigators. Mifepristone, a glucocorticoid receptor antagonist, produces clinical and metabolic benefits in patients with Cushing's syndrome. *J Clin Endocrinol Metab.* 2012;97(6):2039-2049. PMID: 22466348

8 ANSWER: E) No changes

Primary aldosteronism causes more end-organ damage than equivalent degrees of essential hypertension, particularly on the kidney, heart, and vasculature. Proteinuria and renal insufficiency are common complications that improve with targeted treatment, either surgery or mineralocorticoid receptor antagonist therapy. Similar to the early stages of diabetic nephropathy, primary aldosteronism is a state of renal hyperfiltration, and targeted therapy often uncovers occult renal damage, manifest as a rise in serum creatinine. In an older individual with longstanding hypertension and evidence of renal damage, a rise in creatinine is expected with surgical cure or medical treatment of primary aldosteronism with a mineralocorticoid receptor antagonist. The goals of medical therapy are to normalize blood pressure and serum potassium and to stabilize renal deterioration. Most authorities also target to increase plasma renin at least to measurable levels, but the increase in renin can take months to years. Consequently, given normal blood pressure and serum potassium on this regimen, the rise in creatinine to a new stable value is expected, and no changes should be made (Answer E).

Reducing the eplerenone dosage to 50 mg daily (Answer A), which did not previously adequately control his blood pressure, is a mistake. Dosage adjustments of a mineralocorticoid receptor antagonist should be made slowly, with gradual up-titration (as was done in this case), as several weeks are required to observe steady-state changes in blood pressure. Spironolactone is, if anything, more potent than eplerenone on a milligram-for-milligram basis, and the dosage of 100 mg daily (Answer B) might be excessive and cause hyperkalemia. In addition, there is no reason to change. Given his age and duration of hypertension, he is most likely to have a degree of fixed hypertension even with proper treatment of the primary aldosteronism, and his blood pressure would probably rise if amlodipine were discontinued (Answer C). Eplerenone should not be discontinued (Answer D). A β-adrenergic blocker such as atenolol, which lowers plasma renin, is often used in high-renin hypertension.

Educational Objective
Titrate medical therapy for primary aldosteronism.

Reference(s)

Reincke M, Rump LC, Quinkler M, et al; Participants of German Conn's Registry. Risk factors associated with a low glomerular filtration rate in primary aldosteronism. *J Clin Endocrinol Metab.* 2009;94(3):869-875. PMID: 19116235

Fourkiotis V, Vonend O, Diederich S, et al; Mephisto Study Group. Effectiveness of eplerenone or spironolactone in preserving renal function in primary aldosteronism. *Eur J Endocrinol.* 2012;168(1):75-81. PMID: 23033260

Sechi LA, Colussi G, Di Fabio A, Catena C. Cardiovascular and renal damage in primary aldosteronism: outcomes after treatment. *Am J Hypertens.* 2010;23(12):1253-1260. PMID: 20706195

Byrd JB, Turcu AF, Auchus RJ. Primary aldosteronism. *Circulation.* 2018;138(8):823-835. PMID: 30359120

9 ANSWER: C) Laparoscopic right adrenalectomy

This patient has fairly significant ACTH-independent hypercortisolism with low ACTH, abnormal cortisol suppression with dexamethasone, and even mildly elevated urinary free cortisol. Macronodular adrenocortical hyperplasia is observed on CT imaging. Unlike what is observed with unilateral adenomas, progression to overt hypercortisolism is common in macronodular hyperplasia. Cortisol production in this condition roughly correlates with adrenal size, and when there is significant asymmetry, unilateral adrenalectomy of the larger side (Answer C) often induces remission and clinical improvement. However, recurrence of hypercortisolism from further hyperplasia of the remaining gland might occur in the future.

Observation (Answer A) would not be appropriate for a patient with this degree of hypercortisolism who has a clear etiology and marked symptoms. Pasireotide (Answer B) is a pan-somatostatin receptor agonist that is approved for the treatment of Cushing disease but not ACTH-independent hypercortisolism. Spironolactone and metformin (Answer E) would treat the blood pressure and hyperglycemia but not the cushingoid features and the catabolic actions of cortisol. MRI of the adrenal glands (Answer D) would only confirm the fact that these are lipid-rich cortical adenomas and would not provide additional diagnostic or therapeutic value. A few studies have attempted to define useful parameters for adrenal venous sampling that quantify the amount of cortisol coming from each adrenal. Unlike in the setting of primary aldosteronism, both sides are always producing cortisol, although not always symmetrically, and nearly always proportionate to size.

Educational Objective
Manage macronodular adrenocortical hyperplasia.

Reference(s)

Debillon E, Velayoudom-Cephise FL, Salenave S, et al. Unilateral adrenalectomy as a first-line treatment of Cushing's syndrome in patients with primary bilateral macronodular adrenal hyperplasia. *J Clin Endocrinol Metab.* 2015; 100(12):4417-4424. PMID: 26451908

Xu Y, Rui W, Qi Y, et al. The role of unilateral adrenalectomy in corticotropin-independent bilateral adrenocortical hyperplasias. *World J Surg.* 2013;37(7):1626-1632. PMID: 23592061

Acharya R, Dhir M, Bandi R, Yip L, Challinor S. Outcomes of adrenal venous sampling in patients with bilateral adrenal masses and ACTH-independent Cushing's syndrome. *World J Surg.* 2019;43(2):527-533. PMID: 30232569

Ueland GÅ, Methlie P, Jøssang DE, et al. Adrenal venous sampling for assessment of autonomous cortisol secretion. *J Clin Endocrinol Metab.* 2018; 103(12):4553-4560. PMID: 30137397

Young WF Jr, du Plessis H, Thompson GB, et al. The clinical conundrum of corticotropin-independent autonomous cortisol secretion in patients with bilateral adrenal masses. *World J Surg.* 2008;32(5):856-862. PMID: 18074172

10 ANSWER: A) Insufficient hydrocortisone dosage

This woman had severe Cushing disease for a prolonged period. Pituitary surgery was successful with histologic confirmation that the resected adenoma was the source of ACTH, and Crooke hyaline change in the pituitary cells is a specific histologic feature seen only in Cushing syndrome. Furthermore, laboratory testing documented undetectable cortisol and ACTH, as well as DHEA-S. Her hypothalamic-pituitary-adrenal axis will remain suppressed for many months, and she requires cortisol replacement therapy. Not surprisingly, she is suffering from cortisol withdrawal syndrome. Laboratory testing confirms central adrenal insufficiency, and residual disease (Answer C) is excluded. Instead, her hydrocortisone dosage should be increased, as the current dosage is insufficient (Answer A). While the current dosage might seem supraphysiologic, it is still very low relative to her cortisol exposure when she had Cushing disease. Patients even experience cortisol withdrawal syndrome when Cushing disease is not cured but ACTH and cortisol production is significantly lowered.

Because her cortisol deficiency is central, her renin-angiotensin-aldosterone axis is functional, and both standing blood pressure and serum potassium are normal. Her problem is not insufficient mineralocorticoid replacement, which would cause hyperkalemia and orthostasis but not her current symptoms (Answer B). DHEA-S decreases following cure of Cushing disease and can remain low for years despite recovery of cortisol production. Some literature suggests that adrenal androgen deficiency in women can contribute to sexuality difficulties, but adrenal androgen deficiency (Answer D) does not cause these classic cortisol withdrawal symptoms. Adrenal medulla dysfunction (Answer E) has been documented in patients with classic 21-hydroxylase deficiency, but epinephrine deficiency causes subtle disturbances with exercise and not fatigue and myalgias.

Ancillary medications to aid symptoms include selective serotonin reuptake inhibitors for mood problems and nonsteroidal antiinflammatory drugs for myalgias. The hydrocortisone dosage is gradually tapered as symptoms abate to allow axis recovery. For those with severe glucocorticoid-induced myopathy, physical therapy is very important from the middle of the recovery phase.

Educational Objective
Manage the cortisol withdrawal syndrome following cure of Cushing disease.

Reference(s)
Bhattacharyya A, Kaushal K, Tymms DJ, Davis JR. Steroid withdrawal syndrome after successful treatment of Cushing's syndrome: a reminder. *Eur J Endocrinol.* 2005;153(2):207-210. PMID: 16061825

Kleiber H, Rey F, Temler E, Gomez F. Dissociated recovery of cortisol and dehydroepiandrosterone sulphate after treatment for Cushing's syndrome. *J Endocrinol Invest.* 1991;14(6):489-492. PMID: 1663528

El Asmar N, Rajpal A, Selman WR, Arafah BM. The value of perioperative levels of ACTH, DHEA, and DHEA-S and tumor size in predicting recurrence of Cushing disease. *J Clin Endocrinol Metab.* 2018;103(2):477-445. PMID: 29244084

Nieman LK, Biller BM, Findling JW, et al; Endocrine Society. Treatment of Cushing's syndrome: an Endocrine Society Clinical Practice Guideline. *J Clin Endocrinol Metab.* 2015;100(8):2807-2831. PMID: 26222757

11 ANSWER: A) Cosyntropin-stimulation test measuring 17-hydroxyprogesterone and cortisol

The evaluation of chronic, nonprogressive androgen excess without virilization in a young woman is primarily to distinguish polycystic ovary syndrome (PCOS) from secondary causes of PCOS: Cushing syndrome, hyperprolactinemia, and nonclassic congenital adrenal hyperplasia. This patient has no clinical features of Cushing syndrome (and no directed tests are necessary or given as options) and a normal serum prolactin level. Her history and physical examination findings are atypical for PCOS in that she had onset of androgen excess in childhood before menses, she is not obese, and she has a normal glucose concentration without evidence of insulin resistance. Thus, nonclassic 21-hydroxylase deficiency should be considered. A morning follicular-phase 17-hydroxyprogesterone concentration less than

200 ng/dL (<6.1 nmol/L) excludes nonclassic 21-hydroxylase deficiency, and a value greater than 1000 ng/dL (>30.3 nmol/L) establishes the diagnosis. Serum 17-hydroxyprogesterone varies with the time of day and across the menstrual cycle. Given this patient's suspicious history and an equivocal random value of 300 ng/dL (9.1 nmol/L), a formal cosyntropin-stimulation test for 17-hydroxyprogesterone (Answer A) is warranted.

Adrenal-directed CT (Answer C) is recommended if the testosterone concentration is markedly elevated (>150 ng/dL [>5.2 nmol/L]). Nonclassic 3β-hydroxysteroid dehydrogenase/isomerase type 2 (3β-HSD2) deficiency is exceedingly rare and is only considered in unusual cases after nonclassic 21-hydroxylase deficiency has been excluded. Furthermore, 17-hydroxyprogesterone is also elevated in 3β-HSD2 deficiency because of the type 1 enzyme, and the most discriminatory parameter for this condition is the 17-hydroxypregnenolone-to-cortisol ratio (thus, Answer B is incorrect). Plasma ACTH measurement (Answer D) will not aid in this patient's diagnosis. In a patient with childhood-onset androgen excess sufficient to advance bone age, a diagnosis should be pursued. Thus, no further testing (Answer E) is incorrect.

Educational Objective
Guide the biochemical evaluation of adrenal androgen excess.

Reference(s)
Auchus RJ. The classic and nonclassic congenital adrenal hyperplasias. *Endocr Pract.* 2015;21(4):383-389. PMID: 25536973

Witchel SF. Nonclassic congenital adrenal hyperplasia. *Curr Opin Endocrinol Diabetes Obes.* 2012;19(3):151-158. PMID: 22499220

Carbunaru G, Prasad P, Scoccia B, et al. The hormonal phenotype of nonclassic 3β-hydroxysteroid dehydrogenase (HSD3B) deficiency in hyperandrogenic females is associated with insulin-resistant polycystic ovary syndrome and is not a variant of inherited HSD3B2 deficiency. *J Clin Endocrinol Metab.* 2004;89(2):783-794. PMID: 14764797

Speiser PW, Arlt W, Auchus RJ, et al. Congenital adrenal hyperplasia due to steroid 21-hydroxylase deficiency: an Endocrine Society clinical practice guideline. *J Clin Endocrinol Metab.* 2018;103(11):4043-4088. PMID: 30272171

12 ANSWER: D) Low plasma renin activity and low serum aldosterone

For many years, licorice consumption has been appreciated as a cause of hypertension and hypokalemic metabolic alkalosis. The state of mineralocorticoid excess is clinically similar to that in patients with primary aldosteronism; however, patients with primary aldosteronism could be expected to have an elevated aldosterone level and low plasma renin activity (Answer B). In licorice-induced hypertension and hypokalemia, normal amounts of cortisol act as a mineralocorticoid. Licorice contains glycyrrhizic acid, which is hydrolyzed to glycyrrhetinic acid after ingestion. Glycyrrhetinic acid inhibits 11β-hydroxysteroid dehydrogenase type 2, an enzyme that reversibly catalyzes the conversion of cortisol to cortisone in the distal renal tubule. This conversion of cortisol to its inactive metabolite cortisone protects the mineralocorticoid receptor from cortisol. The inhibition of this enzyme by glycyrrhetinic acid raises intrarenal cortisol levels, providing free access to the mineralocorticoid receptor and causing potassium wasting, sodium retention, hypertension, and suppression of the renin-angiotensin-aldosterone system (thus, Answer D is correct).

Not unexpectedly, urinary cortisol measurements may also be increased in patients consuming licorice. It is a common misconception that licorice-flavored products (confections, dietary supplements, chewing tobacco) sold in the United States do not contain glycyrrhizic acid; on the contrary, many products contain variable amounts of the active ingredients of licorice.

Renovascular hypertension with secondary hyperaldosteronism may present in this fashion but would be associated with elevations of aldosterone and plasma renin activity (thus, Answer A is incorrect). The use of an ACE inhibitor or an angiotensin-receptor blocker would induce an elevation of plasma renin activity and a decrease in serum aldosterone (Answer C). Of course, normal levels of plasma renin activity and aldosterone (Answer E) would not provide any insight into the cause of the hypertension and hypokalemia in this patient.

Educational Objective
Explain the biochemical mechanism of licorice-induced hypertension and hypokalemia.

Reference(s)

Walker BR, Edwards CR. Licorice-induced hypertension and syndromes of apparent mineralocorticoid excess. *Endocrinol Metab Clin North Am.* 1994;23(2):359-377. PMID: 8070427

Epstein MT, Espiner EA, Donald RA, Hughes H, Cowles RJ, Lun S. Licorice raises urinary cortisol in man. *J Clin Endocrinol Metab.* 1978;47(2):397-400. PMID: 233669

Lalande BM, Findling JW. Amelioration of licorice-induced hypokalemic rhabdomyolysis with dexamethasone: a case report and review of the literature. *Endocrinologist.* 1998;8:359-363.

13 ANSWER: E) Serum cortisol and 11-deoxycortisol measurements by tandem mass spectrometry

Metyrapone inhibits several enzymes in cortisol biosynthesis, most importantly 11β-hydroxylase (P450 11B1). As a result, 11-deoxycortisol rises. In addition, steroids more proximal to the block in the pathway increase, including mineralocorticoids such as 11-deoxycorticosterone and androgen precursors. The cortisol immunoassays used in most hospital laboratories show significant cross-reactivity with 11-deoxycortisol. Consequently, when serum 11-deoxycortisol concentrations are markedly elevated as in patients with Cushing syndrome who are treated with metyrapone, the serum cortisol value can be artifactually elevated, and the tendency to increase the dosage to lower the cortisol further can lead to symptoms of adrenal insufficiency. Measuring cortisol and 11-deoxycortisol by mass spectrometry (Answer E) obviates the cross-reactivity and affords true values.

Serum DHEA-S (Answer B) can be increased with metyrapone, but it is not used in dosage adjustment. Likewise, the accumulation of 11-deoxycorticosterone can cause volume expansion and suppress plasma renin activity (Answer C), but this parameter is also not used to monitor therapy. A cosyntropin-stimulation test (Answer D) is of no value in diagnosing or monitoring Cushing syndrome, and measurement of late-night salivary cortisol (Answer A) is not useful to assess for cortisol deficiency.

Educational Objective
Interpret results of serum cortisol testing in patients taking metyrapone.

Reference(s)

Valassi E, Crespo I, Gich I, Rodriguez J, Webb SM. A reappraisal of the medical therapy with steroidogenesis inhibitors in Cushing's syndrome. *Clin Endocrinol (Oxf).* 2012;77(5):735-742. PMID: 22533782

Monaghan PJ, Owen LJ, Trainer PJ, Brabant G, Keevil BG, Darby D. Comparison of serum cortisol measurement by immunoassay and liquid chromatography-tandem mass spectrometry in patients receiving the 11β-hydroxylase inhibitor metyrapone. *Ann Clin Biochem.* 2011;48(Pt 5):441-446. PMID: 21813575

14 ANSWER: B) Perform bilateral adrenalectomy

This woman has a metastatic, low-grade foregut neuroendocrine tumor with a pancreatic primary tumor. Originally, this tumor showed only features of gastrinoma, and predictably, she showed slow progression and good hormonal control with depot octreotide. With time, clones from this tumor can acquire the capacity to produce other hormones, and this patient has rapidly progressive hypercortisolism typical of ectopic ACTH syndrome. Pancreatic neuroendocrine tumors that produce ACTH often cosecrete gastrin, so the index of suspicion for ectopic ACTH syndrome is quite high, and the history, physical examination findings, and laboratory findings corroborate the diagnosis. The most important point in this patient's management is that the tumor burden is not her most pressing immediate problem; rather, it is her hypercortisolism. She is at high risk for psychosis, opportunistic infections, and venous thrombosis. Prompt control of her Cushing syndrome is indicated with medical and/or surgical management. Bilateral adrenalectomy (Answer B) is the best step now.

Biopsy of the liver mass (Answer A) will only reveal a low-grade neuroendocrine tumor. Given the delayed onset of Cushing syndrome with the preexisting tumor, it is likely that not all of the cells will stain for ACTH, and the biopsy findings would not add to the management plan.

Although octreotide dose-response spans a wide range, ACTH production this high is very likely not to respond to a 33% increase in dosage (Answer C). Anthracycline-based chemotherapy (Answer D) for neuroendocrine tumors is reserved for high-grade neuroendocrine tumors, including small cell lung cancer, and is not indicated for this low-grade malignancy. Liver MRI (Answer E) is better than CT for demonstrating subtle metastases, but metastatic disease is already documented in this case. In addition, the primary objective is to control the hypercortisolism. In the case of ectopic ACTH syndrome with an occult tumor source, ^{111}In-pentetreotide scintigraphy can be useful, but it rarely identifies tumors smaller than 1 cm in diameter and is rarely positive if the CT is non-diagnostic. A newer somatostatin analogue imaging agent, ^{68}Ga-DOTATATE, provides high-resolution PET-CT images and is generally considered more sensitive than ^{111}In-pentetreotide scintigraphy.

Educational Objective

Manage ectopic ACTH syndrome resulting from a metastatic neuroendocrine tumor.

Reference(s)

Kamp K, Alwani RA, Korpershoek E, Franssen GJ, de Herder WW, Feelders RA. Prevalence and clinical features of the ectopic ACTH syndrome in patients with gastroenteropancreatic and thoracic neuroendocrine tumors. *Eur J Endocrinol*. 2016;174(3):271-280. PMID: 26643855

Ejaz S, Vassilopoulou-Sellin R, Busaidy NL, et al. Cushing syndrome secondary to ectopic adrenocorticotropic hormone secretion: the University of Texas MD Anderson Cancer Center Experience. *Cancer*. 2011;117(19):4381-4389. PMID: 21412758

Isidori AM, Kaltsas GA, Pozza C, et al. The ectopic adrenocorticotropin syndrome: clinical features, diagnosis, management, and long-term follow-up. *J Clin Endocrinol Metab*. 2006;91(2):371-377. PMID: 16303835

Ilias I, Torpy DJ, Pacak K, Mullen N, Wesley RA, Nieman LK. Cushing's syndrome due to ectopic corticotropin secretion: twenty years' experience at the National Institutes of Health. *J Clin Endocrinol Metab*. 2005;90(8):4955-4962. PMID: 15914534

15 ANSWER: E) Adrenal CT

This patient's clinical presentation with hyponatremia, hypokalemia, nausea, and vomiting suggests primary adrenal insufficiency of acute onset. The differential diagnosis for this condition is narrow and includes adrenal infarction or hemorrhage, pituitary apoplexy, and withdrawal of long-term pharmacologic glucocorticoids. Although she was on long-term prednisone treatment, the dosage was small and given on alternate days, which should not suppress ACTH. Indeed, her ACTH is high, not low. Thus, a urine synthetic glucocorticoid screen (Answer C) and pituitary MRI (Answer B) are incorrect. Risk factors for adrenal hemorrhage include the antiphospholipid syndrome, anticoagulation, and sepsis, especially meningococcemia. She has 2 of these risk factors, and adrenal CT (Answer E) will reveal enlarged and poorly enhancing adrenal glands (*see image*). Serum DHEA-S measurement (Answer A) might be confirmatory, but it is unnecessary given the high ACTH and low cortisol. Autoimmune adrenalitis is of gradual onset and is not more common in patients with lupus, so assessment for 21-hydroxylase antibodies (Answer D) is incorrect.

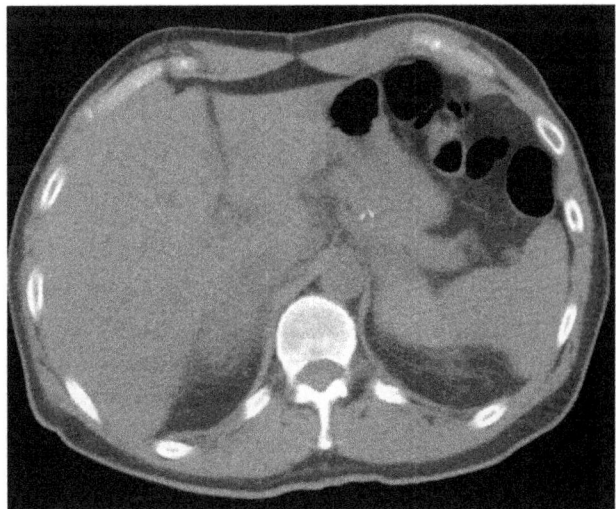

Educational Objective

Identify risk factors for bilateral adrenal hemorrhage and guide the evaluation.

Reference(s)

Bornstein SR, Allolio B, Arlt W, et al. Diagnosis and treatment of primary adrenal insufficiency: an Endocrine Society Clinical Practice Guideline. *J Clin Endocrinol Metab*. 2016;101(2):364-389. PMID: 26760044

Charmandari E, Nicolaides NC, Chrousos GP. Adrenal insufficiency. *Lancet.* 2014;383(9935): 2152-2167. PMID: 24503135

Ramon I, Mathian A, Bachelot A, et al. Primary adrenal insufficiency due to bilateral adrenal hemorrhage-adrenal infarction in the antiphospholipid syndrome: long-term outcome of 16 patients. *J Clin Endocrinol Metab.* 2013; 98(8):3179-3189. PMID: 23783099

16 ANSWER: C) Successful study: both adrenal glands are sources (bilateral hyperaldosteronism)

For adrenal venous sampling, the cortisol concentrations in the adrenal vein samples are used to determine whether the adrenal veins were accessed and to correct for the fractional dilution of the adrenal vein blood with mixed venous blood. This ratio of cortisol in the adrenal vein blood to the cortisol in the mixed venous blood is often called the selectivity index. The selectivity index on both sides should be greater than 2 if adrenal venous sampling is performed without cosyntropin infusion and greater than 4 if performed with cosyntropin. Otherwise, the sample does not contain sufficient adrenal vein blood to interpret the results. The study should not be interpreted unless both selectivity indices are greater than these minimum values, with the one exception discussed below. The right side, which is more difficult to access, more often fails the selectivity test than the left side. When access to the right side is successful, the steroids in the right-side sample are usually more concentrated than in the left-side sample due to the dilution of the left adrenal vein specimen from the inferior phrenic vein. In this case, the selectivity index on the right side is 37.5, and although the selectivity index on the left side is only 6, this value is sufficient for a valid study (thus, Answers A, D, and E are incorrect).

Although the absolute value of aldosterone in the right adrenal vein sample is much higher than in the left adrenal vein sample, the cortisol-corrected aldosterone (aldosterone-to-cortisol ratio) is well within a factor of 2 (4.0/3.8 = 1.05) (thus, Answer C is correct and Answer B is incorrect). If the aldosterone-to-cortisol ratio in one adrenal vein is much lower than in the mixed venous blood, which is called "contralateral suppression," aldosterone production can usually be confidently localized to the other adrenal, even if that implicated adrenal vein was not accessed adequately.

Educational Objective
Interpret results of adrenal venous sampling.

Reference(s)

Rossi GP, Auchus RJ, Brown M, et al. An expert consensus statement on the use of adrenal vein sampling for the subtyping of primary aldosteronism. *Hypertension.* 2014;63(1):151-160. PMID: 24218436

Funder JW, Carey RM, Mantero F, et al. The management of primary aldosteronism: case detection, diagnosis, and treatment: an Endocrine Society Clinical Practice Guideline. *J Clin Endocrinol Metab.* 2016;101(5):1889-1916. PMID: 26934393

Vaidya A, Malchoff CD, Auchus RJ; AACE Adrenal Scientific Committee. An individualized approach to the evaluation and management of primary aldosteronism. *Endocr Pract.* 2017; 23(6):680-689. PMID: 28332881

17 ANSWER: A) Perform ^{18}F-fluorodeoxyglucose PET

The evaluation of an incidental adrenal nodule most often involves small tumors (<2 cm) and a focus on detecting subtle autonomous hormone excess. Thus, the recommended initial screening is for hypercortisolism (1-mg overnight dexamethasone suppression test), pheochromocytoma (measurement of urinary or plasma metanephrines), and, if the patient is hypertensive or hypokalemic, measurement of serum aldosterone and plasma renin activity. In this vignette, the situation is a little different because the patient has a history of colon cancer and an adrenal mass that appeared over the last year. Her blood pressure is normal, and the imaging characteristics (25 Hounsfield units, 30% washout) are not typical of a lipid-rich cortical neoplasm. Thus, one should be suspicious of metastasis to the adrenal.

Right adrenalectomy (Answer C) is premature until a diagnosis is made. For example, if metastatic cancer is found in the adrenal, then she could have disease elsewhere, and additional chemotherapy would be the treatment of choice, rather than adrenalectomy. MRI (Answer B) might provide additional evidence for or against a lipid-rich adenoma, but the CT results cannot be ignored and MRI would not rule out metastatic disease. Waiting a year to repeat the CT (Answer D) is inappropriate given the imaging characteristics and recent appearance of the mass in a patient with a history of cancer. Because she does not have hypertension or hypokalemia, there is no need to screen for primary aldosteronism (Answer E). An ^{18}F-fluorodeoxyglucose PET scan (Answer A) would determine whether the mass has high metabolic activity typical of malignancy. Because it is a whole-body imaging study, it would screen for disease elsewhere. Biopsy of the right adrenal mass would also be an appropriate option in this setting, but the ^{18}F-fluorodeoxyglucose PET scan has the added benefit of screening for disease elsewhere.

Educational Objective
Recommend appropriate use of PET scanning in the evaluation of an adrenal mass.

Reference(s)
Kandathil A, Wong KK, Wale DJ, et al. Metabolic and anatomic characteristics of benign and malignant adrenal masses on positron emission tomography/computed tomography: a review of literature. *Endocrine.* 2015;49(1):6-26. PMID: 25273320

Boland GW, Blake MA, Holalkere NS, Hahn PF. PET/CT for the characterization of adrenal masses in patients with cancer: qualitative versus quantitative accuracy in 150 consecutive patients. *AJR Am J Roentgenol.* 2009;192(4):956-962. PMID: 19304700

18 ANSWER: C) Low progesterone, low 17-hydroxyprogesterone, and low androstenedione

This patient has a history of adrenal insufficiency at birth with enlarged adrenal glands, consistent with some form of congenital adrenal hyperplasia (CAH). While many forms of CAH feature menstrual irregularity, this patient's poor estrogen production suggests a defect that also involves the ovaries. The absence of androgen excess excludes classic 21-hydroxylase deficiency and 11-hydroxylase deficiency (consistent with Answer A). Genital virilization is seen in girls with P450-oxidoreductase deficiency as well, although postnatal androgens are low, and isolated 17,20-lyase deficiency would not cause adrenal insufficiency (consistent with Answer B). There is no disease that would cause low progesterone and 17-hydroxyprogesterone yet have elevated androstenedione (consistent with Answer D). For the patient to have both adrenal insufficiency and hypogonadism, all steroids would have to be low.

The diagnosis is lipoid congenital adrenal hyperplasia (LCAH), in which all steroid production is low or absent (Answer C). All children with LCAH have adrenal insufficiency, large adrenals laden with cholesterol esters, and female phenotype due to absent gonadal steroidogenesis. In 46,XX adolescents with LCAH, some estrogen production and ovulation can occur, but the ovaries later fail due to cholesterol ester accumulation. Pregnancy with live births has been achieved twice in a 46,XX woman with LCAH. LCAH is an autosomal recessive condition due to pathogenic variants in the *STAR* gene, which encodes the steroidogenic acute regulatory protein that is required for movement of cholesterol from the outer mitochondrial membrane to the inner mitochondrial membrane and the cholesterol side-chain cleavage enzyme (P450 11A1). A nonclassic form of LCAH exists in which cortisol deficiency dominates and sex steroid production is variably reduced, and often these patients are labeled as having familial glucocorticoid deficiency. Rare classic or nonclassic pathogenic variants exist in the gene encoding the side-chain cleavage enzyme. In the classic form, the disorder is indistinguishable from LCAH except that the adrenals are not engorged with cholesterol esters. In 17-hydroxylase deficiency, cortisol and androgens are also low, but progesterone is high. Corticosterone and 11-deoxycorticosterone accumulate, which prevent adrenal insufficiency and cause hypertension with hypokalemia, respectively, unlike this case.

Educational Objective
Identify the pattern of steroids in lipoid congenital adrenal hyperplasia.

Reference(s)
Bose HS, Sugawara T, Strauss JF 3rd, Miller WL; International Congenital Lipoid Adrenal Hyperplasia Consortium. The pathophysiology and genetics of congenital lipoid adrenal hyperplasia. *N Engl J Med.* 1996;335(25):1870-1878. PMID: 8948562

Miller WL. Disorders in the initial steps of steroid hormone synthesis. *J Steroid Biochem Mol Biol.* 2017;165(Pt A):18-37. PMID: 26960203

Baker BY, Lin L, Kim CJ, Raza J, Smith CP, Miller WL, Achermann JC. Nonclassic congenital lipoid adrenal hyperplasia: a new disorder of the steroidogenic acute regulatory protein with very late presentation and normal male genitalia. *J Clin Endocrinol Metab.* 2006;91(12):4781-4785. PMID: 16968793

Khoury K, Barbar E, Ainmelk Y, Ouellet A, Lehoux JG. Gonadal function, first cases of pregnancy, and child delivery in a woman with lipoid congenital adrenal hyperplasia. *J Clin Endocrinol Metab.* 2009;94(4):1333-1337. PMID: 19158201

19 ANSWER: D) Testicular ultrasonography

An alarming number of young adults with classic 21-hydroxylase deficiency, especially men, become partially or completely nonadherent to their adrenal replacement therapy after leaving pediatric endocrinology care. His story is not unusual, and the consequences of prolonged poor disease control should be assessed. His mineralocorticoid replacement is adequate, and serum aldosterone measurement (Answer A) is uninformative and will not change his treatment. Although his serum testosterone value is in the normal male range, most is derived from his adrenals, because his androstenedione is much higher than his testosterone. On the basis of these 2 tests alone, his disease control is poor despite resuming treatment after a lapse of 3.5 years, and his treatment should be intensified. His 17-hydroxyprogesterone level (Answer C) would be predictably high, and his semen analysis (Answer E) would be expected to show azoospermia.

About half of young men with classic 21-hydroxylase deficiency develop testicular adrenal rest tumors (TARTs). These are ACTH-responsive masses that are either ectopic adrenal tissue or reprogrammed steroidogenic stem cells in the testes that grow and produce a pattern of steroids similar to that of the adrenal cortex of these patients. TARTs are firm, irregular masses arising from the rete testis posteriorly and are typically bilateral. In 21-hydroxylase deficiency, the adrenals produce abundant androstenedione and inefficiently convert this precursor to testosterone, so the major laboratory feature is elevated androstenedione, disproportionate to the testosterone, which is typically "normal," but not derived from the normal testicular Leydig cells. The high adrenal androgen production suppresses LH. Initially, FSH is also low, but with time the masses compromise blood flow to the normal testis and cause irreversible damage to the Sertoli and germ cells, and FSH rises. The presence of TARTs and high FSH are poor prognostic factors for fertility in men with classic 21-hydroxylase deficiency. Intensification of glucocorticoid therapy can allow regression of the rests and restoration of fertility, but this can take many months. Surgical removal of TARTs often provides long-term control of the tumors, but it does not restore testicular function. Thus, testicular ultrasonography (Answer D) is indicated. A physical examination should be performed first, but this was not given as an option. Although adrenal enlargement, nodular hyperplasia, and myelolipomas are common in adults with classic 21-hydroxylase deficiency, routine adrenal imaging (Answer B) is not recommended and will not assess his more pressing issue of testicular dysfunction.

Educational Objective

Evaluate testicular adrenal rest tumors in men with congenital adrenal hyperplasia.

Reference(s)

Speiser PW, Arlt W, Auchus RJ, et al; Congenital Adrenal Hyperplasia Due to Steroid 21-Hydroxylase Deficiency: An Endocrine Society Clinical Practice Guideline. *J Clin Endocrinol Metab.* 2018;103(11):4043-4088. PMID: 30272171.

Auchus RJ, Arlt W. Approach to the patient: the adult with congenital adrenal hyperplasia. *J Clin Endocrinol Metab.* 2013;98(7):2645-2655. PMID: 23837188

Reisch N, Rottenkolber M, Greifenstein A, et al. Testicular adrenal rest tumors develop independently of long-term disease control: a longitudinal analysis of 50 adult men with congenital adrenal hyperplasia due to classic 21-hydroxylase deficiency. *J Clin Endocrinol Metab.* 2013;98(11):E1820-E1826. PMID: 23969190

Claahsen-van der Grinten HL, Otten BJ, Takahashi S, et al. Testicular adrenal rest tumors in adult males with congenital adrenal hyperplasia: evaluation of pituitary-gonadal function before and after successful testis-sparing surgery in eight patients. *J Clin Endocrinol Metab.* 2007; 92(2):612-615. PMID: 17090637

King TF, Lee MC, Williamson EE, Conway GS. Experience in optimizing fertility outcomes in men with congenital adrenal hyperplasia due to 21 hydroxylase deficiency. *Clin Endocrinol (Oxf)*. 2016;84(6):830-836. PMID: 26666213

20 ANSWER: C) Add fludrocortisone acetate, 0.1 mg daily

Adrenal replacement therapy is guided primarily on clinical grounds with limited laboratory testing. In particular, the plasma ACTH does not normalize with physiologic replacement doses and should not be used to titrate glucocorticoid as the TSH is used for thyroxine replacement. Weight regain is a good sign that glucocorticoid dosing is adequate, and lack of cushingoid stigmata suggests that he is not overtreated. Fatigue persists in some patients, and if it is due to glucocorticoid deficiency, this will transiently improve following each dose, which is not the case in this man. Consequently, a more distributed dose of methylprednisolone (Answer A) is not going to help, and a bedtime dose of glucocorticoid is generally unnecessary for patients with adrenal insufficiency—other than in congenital adrenal hyperplasia to lower cortisol precursor production. A single morning dose of hydrocortisone (Answer B) is sometimes sufficient for partial secondary adrenal insufficiency, but it is most likely not going to provide adequate exposure through the day in a patient with primary adrenal insufficiency.

Chronic volume depletion is another cause of fatigue in patients with adrenal insufficiency. This patient has constant fatigue, a mild increase in heart rate, and borderline-low blood pressure. More importantly, the plasma renin activity is quite elevated and the serum potassium value is high-normal. The patient was asked to stand for 2 minutes, and his blood pressure fell to 88/66 mm Hg and pulse rate rose to 115 beats/min. Hydrocortisone (cortisol) is a mineralocorticoid, but the enzyme 11β-hydroxysteroid dehydrogenase type 2 inactivates most of the cortisol before it binds to the mineralocorticoid receptor. Hydrocortisone doses of roughly 25 mg per day or more provide a variable amount of mineralocorticoid activity, and in this patient, 30 mg daily was sufficient to maintain his volume status. In contrast, neither methylprednisolone nor dexamethasone (Answer D) provides much mineralocorticoid activity. With the switch from hydrocortisone to methylprednisolone, he has become volume depleted (thus, recommending no changes [Answer E]

is incorrect), and he now needs fludrocortisone acetate therapy (Answer C). This scenario is often encountered in the setting of congenital adrenal hyperplasia, where the use of glucocorticoids other than hydrocortisone is common. For many patients with primary adrenal insufficiency, the "standard" fludrocortisone dosage of 0.1 mg daily is inadequate, and he might require a higher dosage to restore volume status and normalize plasma renin activity and serum potassium.

Educational Objective
Characterize the differences in mineralocorticoid activity of cortisol replacement therapies.

Reference(s)
Bornstein SR, Allolio B, Arlt W, et al. Diagnosis and treatment of primary adrenal insufficiency: an Endocrine Society Clinical Practice Guideline. *J Clin Endocrinol Metab*. 2016;101(2):364-389. PMID: 26760044

Bancos I, Hahner S, Tomlinson J, Arlt W. Diagnosis and management of adrenal insufficiency. *Lancet Diabetes Endocrinol*. 2015;3(3):216-226. PMID: 25098712

Esposito D, Pasquali D, Johannsson G. Primary adrenal insufficiency: managing mineralocorticoid replacement therapy. *J Clin Endocrinol Metab*. 2018;103(2):376-387. PMID: 29156052

21 ANSWER: B) Serum 17-hydroxyprogesterone measurement

Androgen-deprivation therapy is a cornerstone of prostate cancer therapy. Long-acting GnRH agonists and antagonists suppress gonadotropins and thus eliminate testicular testosterone production. If the treatment was ineffective and the testes were the source of testosterone, LH and FSH would not be suppressed, as is the case in this man. The adrenal glands are a second source of testosterone, which is ordinarily a minor contribution in men. The bizarre finding in this patient is that he has sustained testosterone production despite suppressed gonadotropins. The most common cause of adrenal-derived androgen excess in men is nonclassic 21-hydroxylase deficiency (an incidence of 1 in 1000 or greater). Boys and men are rarely diagnosed with this condition (<1% of genetically affected males), and over time, the adrenals develop bilateral nodularity as in this octogenarian. His serum 17-hydroxyprogesterone concentration (Answer B) was 5000 ng/dL (152 nmol/L), and the diagnosis of nonclassic 21-hydroxylase deficiency was confirmed. Additional clues to the diagnosis are his short stature and "normal" DHEA-S concentration, which is ordinarily very low in men of this age.

If the masses were bilateral pheochromocytomas, plasma metanephrines would be markedly elevated—not a modestly elevated normetanephrine value of 202 pg/mL (1 nmol/L), which is a typical false-positive result. Hence, the MIBG scan (Answer A) is unnecessary and would not address the source of androgens. Bilateral adrenocortical cancer is extraordinarily rare, and the minimal growth over 3 years rules out adrenal cancer. Adrenal biopsy (Answer C) would only show adrenal cortex cells, and MRI (Answer E) would demonstrate lipid-rich adrenal cortex hyperplasia, but it would not yield a specific diagnosis. While elevated SHBG (Answer D) might be used to calculate the serum free testosterone from the total testosterone, the result would not determine the mechanism of testosterone production or the diagnosis.

The patient was treated with abiraterone acetate (a P450 17A1 inhibitor that blocks testosterone production) and prednisone, and his PSA concentration fell to less than 1.0 ng/mL (<1.0 μg/L) with improvement in his bone pain.

Educational Objective
Diagnose occult nonclassic 21-hydroxylase deficiency.

Reference(s)

Falhammar H, Torpy DJ. Congenital adrenal hyperplasia due to 21-hydroxylase deficiency presenting as adrenal incidentaloma: a systematic review and meta-analysis. *Endocr Pract.* 2016;22(6):736-752. PMID: 26919651

Arlt W, Willis DS, Wild SH, et al; United Kingdom Congenital Adrenal Hyperplasia Adult Study Executive (CaHASE). Health status of adults with congenital adrenal hyperplasia: a cohort study of 203 patients. *J Clin Endocrinol Metab.* 2010;95(10):5110-5121. PMID: 20719839

Auchus RJ, Arlt W. Approach to the patient: the adult with congenital adrenal hyperplasia. *J Clin Endocrinol Metab.* 2013;98(7):2645-2655. PMID: 23837188

22 ANSWER: E) Inferior petrosal sinus sampling

There is no question that this woman has severe ACTH-dependent hypercortisolism, both clinically and biochemically, so additional screening tests such as late-night salivary cortisol measurement (Answer D) are unnecessary. Statistically, the most common cause of Cushing disease is a pituitary adenoma, but ectopic ACTH syndrome due to foregut neuroendocrine tumors is also in the differential diagnosis. In this case, factors that favor Cushing disease are the modest magnitude of the ACTH and urinary cortisol elevations and statistical considerations. Factors that favor ectopic ACTH syndrome are the hypokalemia, myopathy, and fairly rapid onset. Nevertheless, none of these features is conclusive or reliable in distinguishing Cushing disease from ectopic ACTH syndrome, and the 8-mg dexamethasone suppression test (Answer B) does not reliably distinguish the 2 types of Cushing syndrome. In fact, the test was done in this patient, and her serum cortisol concentration fell to 6.0 μg/dL (166 nmol/L). Incidental pituitary adenomas are found in up to 10% of imaging studies, and up to half of patients with Cushing disease do not have a tumor visible on MRI. Her sella is somewhat inhomogeneous on this MRI image, and a tumor cannot be excluded.

Somatostatin receptor imaging (Answer A) might be used as further evidence that the pancreatic mass is a neuroendocrine tumor, but incidental pancreatic neuroendocrine tumors are not rare, and the study will not determine whether that tumor is producing ACTH. A fluorodeoxyglucose PET-CT (Answer C) images tumors of high metabolic activity, but neuroendocrine tumors often do not have high metabolic activity, and again the study would not localize the source of ACTH. Only inferior petrosal sinus sampling (Answer E) can consistently distinguish Cushing disease from ectopic ACTH syndrome. This patient was found to have the ectopic ACTH syndrome, but it was not the pancreatic tumor. A small lung mass was the source, and she was cured with removal of the lung tumor.

Educational Objective
Evaluate ACTH-dependent hypercortisolism.

Reference(s)

Nieman LK, Biller BM, Findling JW, et al. The diagnosis of Cushing's syndrome: an Endocrine Society clinical practice guideline. *J Clin Endocrinol Metab.* 2008;93(5):1526-1540. PMID: 18334580

Ilias I, Torpy DJ, Pacak K, Mullen N, Wesley RA, Nieman LK. Cushing's syndrome due to ectopic corticotropin secretion: twenty years' experience at the National Institutes of Health. *J Clin Endocrinol Metab.* 2005;90(8):4955-4962. PMID: 15914534

23 ANSWER: B) Left adrenal gland is the source (left adenoma)

For adrenal venous sampling, the cortisol concentrations in the adrenal vein samples are used to determine whether the adrenal veins were accessed and to correct for the fractional dilution of the adrenal vein blood with mixed venous blood. This ratio of cortisol in the adrenal vein blood to cortisol in the mixed venous blood is often called the selectivity index. The selectivity index on both sides should be greater than 2 if adrenal venous sampling is performed without cosyntropin infusion and greater than 4 if performed with cosyntropin. Otherwise, the sample does not contain sufficient adrenal vein blood to interpret the results, and the study should not be interpreted unless both selectivity indices are greater than these minimum values. Usually, the right side, which is more difficult to access, is more likely to fail the selectivity index test. In this case, although the cortisol in the right adrenal vein is much lower than the left, the selectivity index is 300/22 = 13.6 (more than adequate). Thus, the study is successful, and all the information is available for interpretation (thus, Answer E is incorrect).

Next, the lateralization indices are calculated, dividing aldosterone by cortisol to obtain aldosterone-to-cortisol (A/C) ratios or cortisol-corrected aldosterone values (*see table*). If the adrenal vein A/C ratios differ by a factor of 4 or more for a cosyntropin-stimulated study (>2 without cosyntropin), the study is interpreted as lateralization to the higher (dominant) adrenal vein. When the A/C ratio in the lower (nondominant) adrenal vein is lower than in the inferior vena cava, also called "contralateral suppression," there is even greater confidence that aldosterone production is lateralized to the dominant adrenal. Note that contralateral suppression is not always observed in studies with convincing lateralization, so lack of contralateral suppression does not equate to bilateral aldosterone production. Contralateral suppression can also be used to lateralize aldosterone production to the other adrenal when only one adrenal vein is accessed successfully. In this case, the quotient of A/C ratios is 10/1 = 10, favoring the left adrenal, and contralateral suppression (1 < 2) is observed for the right adrenal. Thus, aldosterone production lateralizes to the left (thus, Answer B is correct and Answers C and D are incorrect).

Guidelines for performing adrenal venous sampling recommend discontinuing mineralocorticoid receptor antagonists for several weeks before performing the study. The concern is that if the dose is sufficient to antagonize the aldosterone, volume depletion will occur, and renin will rise. Renin will stimulate aldosterone production from both adrenal glands and could obscure a lateralizing gradient. Thus, if the results showed bilateral aldosterone production, the study might be invalid because of spironolactone exposure. However, lateralization in the presence of spironolactone or eplerenone can still be interpreted with confidence (thus, Answer A is incorrect).

Educational Objective

Interpret results of adrenal venous sampling.

Reference(s)

Haase M, Riester A, Kröpil P, et al. Outcome of adrenal vein sampling performed during concurrent mineralocorticoid receptor antagonist therapy. *J Clin Endocrinol Metab.* 2014;99(12):4397-4402. PMID: 25222758

Nanba AT, Wannachalee T, Shields JJ, et al. Adrenal vein sampling lateralization despite mineralocorticoid receptor antagonists exposure in primary aldosteronism. *J Clin Endocrinol Metab.* 2019;104(2):487-492. PMID: 30239792

Funder JW, Carey RM, Mantero F, et al. The management of primary aldosteronism: case detection, diagnosis, and treatment: an Endocrine Society clinical practice guideline. *J Clin Endocrinol Metab.* 2016;101(5):1889-1916. PMID: 26934393

Rossi GP, Auchus RJ, Brown M, et al. An expert consensus statement on the use of adrenal vein sampling for the subtyping of primary aldosteronism. *Hypertension.* 2014;63(1):151-160. PMID: 24218436

24 ANSWER: D) MRI imaging characteristics

Incidentally discovered adrenal nodules are common on CT and MRI, and imaging characteristics are helpful is assessing the origin and probable behavior of the tumor. Most commonly, the tumors are adenomas of the adrenal cortex, which can be nonfunctional, weakly functional, or highly functional in producing aldosterone or cortisol. These cells are lipid-rich, and on CT they have low density and rapid contrast washout. On MRI, lipid-rich tumors have loss of signal on out-of-phase images and low signal on T2-weighted images (Answer D). Medullary tumors (pheochromocytomas), adrenal cancers, metastatic cancers, and infectious processes lack these features.

Up to 60% of pheochromocytomas are incidentally discovered in patients with normal blood pressure, and these tumors tend to be small (<3 cm). Thus, the size of the mass (Answer A), the patient's normal blood pressure (Answer B), and the fact that the tumor was found incidentally (Answer C) do not necessarily support that the mass is a benign cortical adenoma. Many patients with mild cortisol excess from cortical adenomas do not have cushingoid stigmata, so absence of these findings (Answer E) is not discriminatory.

Educational Objective
Use imaging characteristics to identify cortical adenomas.

Reference(s)
Mendiratta-Lala M, Avram A, Turcu AF, Dunnick NR. Adrenal imaging. *Endocrinol Metab Clin North Am.* 2017;46(3):741-759. PMID: 28760236

Wale DJ, Wong KK, Viglianti BL, Rubello D, Gross MD. Contemporary imaging of incidentally discovered adrenal masses. *Biomed Pharmacother.* 2017;87:256-262. PMID: 28063406

Ioachimescu AG, Remer EM, Hamrahian AH. Adrenal incidentalomas: a disease of modern technology offering opportunities for improved patient care. *Endocrinol Metab Clin North Am.* 2015;44(2):335-354. PMID: 26038204

Fassnacht M, Arlt W, Bancos I, et al. Management of adrenal incidentalomas: European Society of Endocrinology clinical practice guideline in collaboration with the European Network for the Study of Adrenal Tumors. *Eur J Endocrinol.* 2016;175(2):G1-G34. PMID: 27390021

25 ANSWER: D) Hypoparathyroidism

The combination of mucocutaneous candidiasis, ectodermal dysplasia, and autoimmune adrenal insufficiency establishes a diagnosis of polyglandular autoimmune syndrome (APS) type 1. APS type 1 is an autosomal recessive disorder due to pathogenic variants in the autoimmune regulatory (*AIRE*) gene, which is necessary for the thymus to eliminate autoreactive T cells. About 60% of patients with APS type 1 develop adrenal insufficiency, usually in adolescence or adulthood after first acquiring mucocutaneous candidiasis, ectodermal dysplasia, and hypoparathyroidism as children. Hypoparathyroidism (Answer D) develops in more than 80% of patients with pathologic variants in the *AIRE* gene, often as a first or second manifestation, although rarely patients develop adrenal insufficiency before hypoparathyroidism. In patients with apparently isolated adrenal insufficiency, genetic testing for *AIRE* pathogenic variants or testing for autoantibodies against cytokines, including interleukin-22, interferon α2, and interferon-ω, can identify patients with APS type 1. Positive 21-hydroxylase antibodies in a patient with APS type 1 predict current or future adrenal insufficiency in nearly 100% of cases.

The horizontal bands on teeth develop because of enamel hypoplasia, part of the ectodermal dysplasia in this syndrome, which also involves the nails. The syndrome is also called APECED (autoimmune polyendocrinopathy–candidiasis–ectodermal dysplasia).

In contrast to APS type 2, autoimmune thyroid diseases (Answers A and E) and type 1 diabetes (Answer B) occur in only 10% of patients with APS type 1. Gonadal failure (Answer C) occurs in approximately 50% and almost exclusively in females. Other frequent autoimmune manifestations in APS type 1 include hepatitis, alopecia, vitiligo, pernicious anemia, and chronic diarrhea.

Note: Image in stem is reproduced with permissions from Orlova EM, Sozaeva LS, Kareva MA, et al. Expanding the phenotypic and genotypic landscape of autoimmune polyendocrine syndrome type 1. *J Clin Endocrinol Metab.* 2017;102(9):3546-3556. PMID: 28911151

Educational Objective
List the endocrinopathies associated with polyglandular autoimmune syndrome type 1.

Reference(s)

Eriksson D, Dalin F, Eriksson GN, et al. Cytokine autoantibody screening in the Swedish Addison Registry identifies patients with undiagnosed APS1. *J Clin Endocrinol Metab.* 2018;103(1):179-186. PMID: 29069385

Orlova EM, Sozaeva LS, Kareva MA, et al. Expanding the phenotypic and genotypic landscape of autoimmune polyendocrine syndrome type 1. *J Clin Endocrinol Metab.* 2017;102(9): 3546-3556. PMID: 28911151

Bruserud Ø, Oftedal BE, Landegren N, et al. A longitudinal follow-up of autoimmune polyendocrine syndrome type 1. *J Clin Endocrinol Metab.* 2016;101(8):2975-2783. PMID: 27253668

Calcium & Bone Board Review

Carolyn B. Becker, MD

1 ANSWER: A) Urinary calcium-to-creatinine clearance ratio

Does this patient have familial hypocalciuric hypercalcemia (FHH) or primary hyperparathyroidism? Answering this question might be easier if she had documentation of previous serum calcium measurements (normal serum calcium values in the past would make FHH unlikely) or relatives in whom serum calcium measurements could be obtained. She is young (<50 years), so surgery would be recommended if she has primary hyperparathyroidism. However, surgery (Answer C) should not be performed until her diagnosis is confirmed, particularly given her very mild presentation. Similarly, bone mineral densitometry (DXA) of the one-third distal radius (Answer B) is not required for recommending surgery in those younger than 50 years. A sestamibi parathyroid scan (Answer D) or some other form of parathyroid imaging is the best next step once FHH has been ruled out. Continued annual monitoring (Answer E) is not appropriate in a young patient with primary hyperparathyroidism or in a patient with FHH. The correct response is to obtain and calculate the urinary calcium-to-creatinine clearance ratio (Answer A).

The 24-hour urine calcium-to-creatinine clearance ratio in FHH is generally less than 0.01 and is calculated using the following formula:

[urine calcium (mg/24 h) x serum creatinine (mg/dL)] / [urine creatinine (mg/24 h) x serum calcium (mg/dL)]

The most common form of FHH, known as FHH type 1, is caused by inactivating pathogenic variants in the gene encoding the calcium-sensing receptor (*CASR*). If the 24-hour urine calcium-to-creatinine clearance ratio is suggestive of FHH, confirmatory genetic testing for pathogenic variants in *CASR* would be the next step. Recently, mutations in the *GNA11* gene and pathogenic variants affecting codon 15 in the *AP2S1* gene have been documented to cause FHH type 2 and FHH type 3, respectively. FHH types 2 and 3 are

much more rare than FHH type 1. Persons with FHH continue to secrete PTH because the inactivated calcium-sensing receptor is reading a low serum calcium level. This also occurs in the renal tubular calcium-sensing receptor where it leads to renal calcium conservation (decreased renal calcium excretion). The end result is hypercalcemia and hypocalciuria.

If the patient has FHH, one of her parents most likely had the same mutation, as transmission is autosomal dominant (although this cannot be confirmed because her family history is unknown). Because primary hyperparathyroidism is much more common than FHH, should the diagnosis still be unclear after *CASR* genetic testing, parathyroid surgery could be considered.

Educational Objective

Distinguish familial hypocalciuric hypercalcemia from primary hyperparathyroidism in a young patient.

Reference(s)

Hovden S, Rejnmark L, Ladefoged SA, Nissen PH. AP2S1 and NA11 mutations – not a common cause of familial hypocalciuric hypercalcemia. *Eur J Endocrinol.* 2017;176(2):177-185. PMID: 27913609

Christensen SE, Nissen PH, Vestergaard P, Mosekilde L. Familial hypocalciuric hypercalcaemia: a review. *Curr Opin Endocrinol Diabetes Obes.* 2011;18(5):359-370. PMID: 21986511

Shinall MC Jr, Dahir KM, Broome JT. Differentiating familial hypocalciuric hypercalcemia from primary hyperparathyroidism. *Endocr Pract.* 2013;19(4):697-702. PMID: 23425644

2 ANSWER: C) Serum alkaline phosphatase

This man has hypophosphatasia, a rare metabolic bone disorder in which tissue nonspecific alkaline phosphatase (TNSALP) deficiency in osteoblasts and chondrocytes impairs mineralization, leading to a rickets-like syndrome in children and osteomalacia in adults. The pathognomonic finding is subnormal serum activity of the TNSALP enzyme, which may result from any one of hundreds of pathogenic variants in the gene encoding TNSALP (ALPL). Genetic inheritance is autosomal recessive for the infantile forms but either autosomal recessive or autosomal dominant for the milder, adult forms with variable penetrance. The prevalence of severe hypophosphatasia is approximately 1 in 100,000 among Anglo-Saxon populations and is particularly prevalent among the Mennonites in Manitoba, Canada, where 1 in every 25 persons is a carrier.

The clinical presentation depends on the age at presentation. Adult hypophosphatasia can be associated with premature loss of deciduous teeth or early loss of adult teeth. Osteomalacia results in painful feet with poor healing of metatarsal stress fractures, as well as thigh or hip pain from femoral pseudofractures located in the lateral cortices of the femora. Some patients experience attacks of arthritis (pseudogout from calcium pyrophosphate crystal deposition), cartilage degeneration, and pyrophosphate arthropathy.

TNSALP is tethered to osteoblasts and chondrocytes and hydrolyzes inorganic pyrophosphate and 5′-phosphate, a major form of vitamin B_6. When TNSALP is low, inorganic pyrophosphate inhibits formation of hydroxyapatite, causing rickets or osteomalacia.

Characteristic laboratory findings include low serum activity of alkaline phosphatase (Answer C). In general, the lower the alkaline phosphatase level, the more severe the symptoms. The decrease in alkaline phosphatase activity leads to an increase in pyridoxal 5′-phosphate; thus, once the condition is suspected, serum 5′phophate or vitamin B_6 should be measured. Genetic testing for pathogenic variants in the ALPL gene is confirmatory. Since 2015, enzyme replacement with asfotase alfa for hypophosphatasia has been available. Indications for enzyme treatment and duration of treatment are not well established.

Measuring 24-hour urinary calcium excretion (Answer A) would not be useful. This patient does not have a history of kidney stones to suggest hypercalciuria or calcium/vitamin D deficiency to suggest hypocalciuria from malabsorption. Serum C-telopeptide (Answer B), a marker of bone resorption, would not be diagnostic, as it may be high after a fracture or low in men with idiopathic osteoporosis. It would not be useful for the diagnosis of hypophosphatasia. Serum 1,25-dihydroxyvitamin D measurement (Answer D) is generally not useful in the differential diagnosis of fractures. In osteomalacia, 1,25-dihydroxyvitamin D can be low, normal, or high depending on renal function, 25-hydroxyvitamin D, PTH, phosphate, and renal function. In this patient, it should be normal. Finally, FGF-23 (Answer E) is useful in the differential diagnosis of hypophosphatemia, particularly in X-linked hypophosphatemic rickets or tumor-induced osteomalacia, but in this patient, the serum phosphate level is normal.

Educational Objective
Identify the clinical features of hypophosphatasia and select the best test to diagnose this condition.

Reference(s)
Whyte MP. Hypophosphatasia: an overview for 2017. Bone. 2017;102:15-25. PMID: 28238808

Whyte MP, Mumm S, Deal C. Adult hypophosphatasia treated with teriparatide. J Clin Endocrinol Metab. 2007;92(4):1203-1208. PMID: 17213282

3 ANSWER: D) Stop cinacalcet

This patient's PTH level is lower than the goal in patients undergoing dialysis and that, coupled with the low alkaline phosphatase level and multiple fragility fractures, is most consistent with adynamic bone disease. Adynamic bone disease, a type of renal osteodystrophy (now called chronic kidney disease–mineral bone disorder [CKD-MBD]), is present in at least one-third of patients receiving dialysis. Adynamic bone disease is characterized by markedly low bone turnover, reduction of both osteoclast and osteoblast activity, no accumulation of osteoid, and high fracture risk. Serum PTH levels in adynamic bone disease are relatively low (usually <150 pg/mL [<150 ng/L]) compared with levels in patients undergoing dialysis who have other forms of CKD-MBD. This patient's low alkaline phosphatase level is also consistent with a low bone turnover state.

In patients with end-stage kidney disease, there is PTH resistance due at least in part to increased N-terminal truncated PTH (7-84), which counteracts the effect of the 1-84 whole molecule on bone. This can be exacerbated by the use of cinacalcet, as well as overly aggressive treatment with calcitriol, both of which reduce PTH secretion. Excessive use of calcium-containing phosphate binders can also contribute. Stopping the cinacalcet (Answer D) would allow PTH to rise again and restore some bone turnover. This will help improve bone quality and reduce the risk of future fractures. Surgical removal of the remaining parathyroid tissue (Answer A) will result in permanent hypoparathyroidism and worsening adynamic bone disease. Antiresorptive therapy with either denosumab (Answer B) or pamidronate (Answer C) is contraindicated in patients with adynamic bone disease and may lead to more bone fragility. Finally, stopping or reducing the calcitriol (Answer E) is not the best option given that his serum calcium level is already low and this will decrease further if calcitriol reduction precedes cinacalcet reduction. Thus, the best sequence would be to reduce or stop cinacalcet, then, if PTH and calcium rise, consider reducing calcitriol. In some cases, anabolic therapy with teriparatide is used to stimulate bone turnover and bone formation in severe cases of adynamic bone disease, but this is an off-label indication.

In general, patients with both type 1 diabetes and type 2 diabetes tend to have low bone turnover. In a systematic review and meta-analysis of 66 studies evaluating bone metabolism in patients with diabetes, markers of both bone formation (osteocalcin) and resorption (C-telopeptide) were decreased in patients with type 1 and type 2 diabetes compared with controls.

Similar changes have been noted in patients with diabetes who progress to end-stage renal disease. Compared with participants without diabetes, patients with diabetes are more likely to have adynamic bone disease, whereas hyperparathyroid bone disease is infrequent, occurring in less than 10% of cases.

The mechanism causing reduced bone turnover in diabetes is multifactorial. Because the anabolic effects of insulin may be mediated through the IGF-1 pathway, low levels of insulin and IGF-1 can impair osteoblast function in type 1 diabetes. In contrast, obesity-induced insulin resistance in type 2 diabetes leads to increased levels of insulin and IGF-1, with a possible anabolic effect on bone, resulting in higher-than-average bone mineral density.

The accumulation of advanced glycation end products in collagen as a result of hyperglycemia also may contribute to reduced bone formation. Low bone turnover, with a reduction in unmineralized bone matrix, and increased collagen glycosylation may contribute to increased bone fragility in patients with diabetes, independent from bone mineral density.

Educational Objective

Diagnose adynamic bone disease in a patient with diabetes mellitus who has end-stage renal disease.

Reference(s)

Cannata-Andía JB, Rodriguez García M, Gómez Alonso C. Osteoporosis and adynamic bone in chronic kidney disease. *J Nephrol.* 2013;26(1): 73-80. PMID: 23023723

Hygum K, Starup-Linde J, Harsløf T, Vestergaard P, Langdahl BL. Mechanisms in endocrinology: diabetes mellitus, a state of low bone turnover - a systematic review and meta-analysis. *Eur J Endocrinol.* 2017;176(3):R137-R157. PMID: 28049653

Ketteler M, Block GA, Evenepoel P, et al. Diagnosis, evaluation, prevention, and treatment of chronic kidney disease-mineral and bone disorder: synopsis of the kidney disease: improving global outcomes 2017 clinical practice guideline update. *Ann Intern Med.* 2018;168(6):422-430. PMID: 29459980

4 ANSWER: B) 24,25-Dihydroxyvitamin D deficiency

In the 1950s, a small group of infants who received supplemental vitamin D (4000 IU daily) to prevent rickets developed infantile hypercalcemia, hypercalciuria, and nephrolithiasis. The cause remained elusive until 2010. At that time, a group of infants and adults with elevated 25-hydroxyvitamin D and 1,25-dihydroxyvitamin D levels were noted to have undetectable or very low 24,25-dihydroxyvitamin D levels (Answer B). Eventually the findings were linked to inactivating pathogenic variants in the gene encoding the 24-hydroxylase enzyme (*CYP24A1*). This enzyme inactivates vitamin D and prevents vitamin D toxicity. Thus, this young man has an inherited form of vitamin D toxicity due to an inactivating pathogenic variant in the *CYP24A1* gene (*see image*).

The hallmarks of the syndrome are kidney stones, nephrocalcinosis, low bone mineral density, and renal failure. Laboratory studies show elevated serum and urine calcium levels with suppressed PTH along with usually normal or occasionally elevated 25-hydroxy-vitamin D and frankly elevated 1,25-dihydroxyvitamin D levels. Low bone mineral density results from the resorptive effects of chronically activated vitamin D on bone along with hypercalciuria. Confirmatory tests include measuring the 24,25-hydroxyvitamin D metabolites (which will be very low or undetectable) and sequencing the *CYP24A1* gene. Inheritance is autosomal recessive with variable penetrance. Rare autosomal dominant cases have been described. Treatment includes a low-calcium diet, avoidance of sunlight, and ketoconazole, which inhibits the conversion of 25-hydroxyvitamin D to 1,25-dihydroxyvitamin D.

Renal leak hypercalciuria (Answer A) would not present with hypercalcemia or suppressed PTH. Familial sarcoidosis (Answer C) is a rare condition that would typically include pulmonary symptoms and/or hilar lymphadenopathy (his chest x-ray was normal), along with other extrapulmonary symptoms involving joints, skin, eyes, etc. Although 1,25-dihydroxyvitamin D levels may be elevated in sarcoidosis, 25-hydroxyvitamin D levels tend to be normal or low. Elevated vitamin D–binding protein (Answer D) could account for the high vitamin D levels, but it would not explain the other clinical findings since "free" unbound vitamin D levels would be normal. Finally, an inactivating pathogenic variant in the vitamin D receptor gene causing vitamin D resistance (Answer E) could be associated with elevated vitamin D levels, but would result in rickets, not hypercalcemia, kidney stones, and hypercalciuria.

Loss of CYP24A1 Enzyme Function

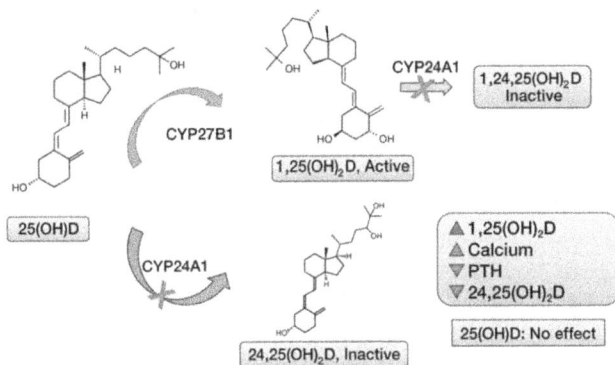

Figure is reprinted from Mayo Clinic.org. Ratio of 25(OH)D-to-24,25(OH)2D: a new test to confirm 24-hydroxylase (CUP24A1) deficiency as the cause of hypercalcemia (Used with permission of Mayo Foundation for Medical Education and Research. All rights reserved. https://www.mayoclinic.org/medical-professionals/endocrinology/news/ratio-of-25OHD-to-24-25OH2D-a-new-test-to-confirm-24-hydroxylase-CYP24A1-deficiency-as-the-cause-of-hypercalcemia/MAC-20430939)

Educational Objective

Diagnose 24,25-dihydroxyvitamin D deficiency as a cause of hypercalcemia and kidney stones.

Reference(s)

Jones G, Kottler ML, Schlingmann KP. Genetic diseases of vitamin D metabolizing enzymes. *Endocrinol Metab Clin North Am.* 2017;46(4): 1095-1117. PMID: 29080636

Molin A, Baudoin R, Kaufmann M, et al. CYP24A1 mutations in a cohort of hypercalcemic patients: evidence for a recessive trait. *J Clin Endocrinol Metab.* 2015;100(10):E1343-E1352. PMID: 26214117

5 ANSWER: A) Stop calcitonin and continue current intravenous hydration

This is a case of humoral hypercalcemia of malignancy from a squamous cell carcinoma of the lung. Squamous cell carcinoma, renal cell carcinoma, and other solid tumors can secrete PTHrP and cause symptomatic hypercalcemia. Dehydration reduces renal blood flow and calcium excretion, so intravenous hydration with normal saline is critical. There is no role for furosemide (Answer B) except in cases of congestive heart failure or volume overload. Methylprednisolone (Answer E) is appropriate in cases of vitamin D–associated malignant hypercalcemia (eg, lymphoma or granulomatous disease), usually with elevated or "nonsuppressed" 1,25-dihydroxyvitamin D levels, but there is no evidence of vitamin D–mediated hypercalcemia in this case.

Zoledronic acid (Answer D) is a potent bisphosphonate that can stop or slow bone resorption in hypercalcemia of malignancy. Maximal hypocalcemic effect begins at 48 hours and peaks at 5 to 6 days. Since the patient is improving clinically, there is no need to administer another dose of any antiresorptive therapy. Therefore, zoledronic acid (Answer D) and denosumab (Answer C) are both incorrect. Calcitonin has antiresorptive effects at the bone and induces calciuresis at the kidneys but loses effectiveness after 24 to 48 hours (calciphylaxis). Therefore, it should be stopped and intravenous hydration should be continued (Answer A).

Educational Objective

Manage hypercalcemic crisis in a patient with humoral hypercalcemia of malignancy (PTHrP-mediated).

Reference(s)

Goldner W. Cancer-related hypercalcemia. *J Oncol Pract.* 2016;12(5):426-432. PMID: 27170690

Minisola S, Pepe J, Piemonte S, Cipriani C. The diagnosis and management of hypercalcaemia. *BMJ.* 2015;350:h2723. PMID: 26037642

Zagzag J, Hu MI, Fisher SB, Perrier ND. Hypercalcemia and cancer: differential diagnosis and treatment. *CA Cancer J Clin.* 2018;68(5):377-386. PMID: 30240520

6 ANSWER: D) Calcium gluconate, 2 ampules (186 mg elemental calcium) in 50 cc D5W over 20 minutes intravenously, followed by elemental calcium, 1 mg/mL at 50 mL/h

Severe, acute, and symptomatic hypocalcemia with a corrected serum calcium value less than 7.5 mg/dL (<1.9 mmol/L) is a medical emergency that requires intravenous calcium administration in order to prevent tetany. Oral elemental calcium and calcitriol given alone (Answer A), with a loading dose of ergocalciferol (Answer B), or with recombinant human PTH (Answer C) are not appropriate in this emergency setting. Between the 2 intravenous options provided, Answer D is the recommended treatment, as the doses in Answer E are too high.

The recommended approach to patients with acute hypocalcemia is as follows:

1) If symptomatic with carpopedal spasm, seizures, tetany, or prolonged QT interval → begin intravenous calcium immediately
2) If symptomatic with milder signs/symptoms (eg, paresthesias), but the corrected total serum calcium is ≤7.5 mg/dL (≤1.9 mmol/L) (or the ionized calcium is ≤3 mg/dL [≤0.8 mmol/L]) → begin intravenous calcium immediately
3) If the corrected total serum calcium is >7.5 mg/dL (>1.9 mmol/L), but the patient is unable to take or absorb oral medications → begin intravenous calcium immediately; if the patient can take and absorb oral medications, oral calcium and activated vitamin D may be used

The standard intravenous regimen for treating acute, symptomatic hypocalcemia is as follows:

1) Initially, 1 to 2 g of calcium gluconate, equivalent to 93 mg (1 ampule) – 186 mg (2 ampules) of elemental calcium in 50 mL of D5W or normal saline is infused intravenously over 10 to 20 minutes. This may be repeated in 10 to 60 minutes if symptoms persist (equivalent dose, SI units: 2.25 to 4.5 mmol calcium in 50 mL D5W or normal saline infused over 10 to 20 minutes)
2) This should be followed by a slow infusion of calcium consisting of 1 mg/mL of elemental calcium. To prepare this, add 11 g of calcium gluconate (~1000 mg elemental calcium) to D5W or normal saline to provide a final volume of 1 L (equivalent dose, SI units: add 24.75 mmol calcium to normal saline or D5W to provide a final volume of 1000 mL [final concentration of 0.025 mmol/mL])
3) Begin the infusion at 50 mL/h (50 mg elemental calcium per hour)

The most likely etiology of this patient's hypocalcemia is hungry bone syndrome following removal of the large parathyroid adenoma. Exogenous recombinant PTH (Answer C) is not approved for treatment in acute postsurgical hypoparathyroidism, nor will it address the underlying pathophysiology of hungry bone syndrome.

Hungry bone syndrome was first described by Albright and Reifenstein in 1950 in patients with hyperparathyroidism who presented with severe and prolonged hypocalcemia after parathyroidectomy. Typically, hungry bone syndrome is characterized by postoperative hypocalcemia (<8.5 mg/dL [<2.1 mmol/L]), a simultaneous inorganic phosphate value less than 3.0 mg/dL (<10.0 mmol/L), and hypocalcemia lasting longer than 4 days requiring high doses of calcium supplementation despite optimization of vitamin D. In the case of patients with end-stage renal disease, treatment with activated vitamin D (calcitriol) is always necessary.

PTH and calcitriol (1α,25[OH]2D3) regulate calcium and phosphate homeostasis. PTH is secreted in response to hypocalcemia after being sensed by the parathyroid calcium-sensing receptor. PTH receptors are mainly present in kidney and bone tissue, and when activated, they increase calcium efflux from bone and decrease renal excretion of calcium to restore normal serum calcium concentrations. Hungry bone syndrome pathophysiology begins with elevated PTH production (primary, secondary, or tertiary hyperparathyroidism), which augments bone and calcium turnover. Surgical treatment of primary or tertiary hyperparathyroidism with resection of 1 or more overactive parathyroid glands causes a sudden cessation of bone resorption. Consequently, a marked depletion of serum circulating calcium, phosphate, and magnesium is seen as the "hungry bones" remineralize.

Patients at highest risk for hungry bone syndrome are those with the most severe hyperparathyroidism preoperatively, and they often have elevated alkaline phosphatase levels and areas of osteitis fibrosa cystica (brown tumors) visible on skeletal radiographs. Some have advocated use of intravenous bisphosphonates preoperatively to prevent hungry bone syndrome even though this could also delay skeletal remineralization. In severe cases of hungry bone syndrome, intravenous or high-dosage oral calcium and vitamin D may be needed for many weeks or months. Patients with primary hyperparathyroidism are also at risk for hungry bone syndrome after parathyroidectomy, but these cases are usually much less severe.

Educational Objective
Manage acute symptomatic hypocalcemia following surgery for primary hyperparathyroidism (need for intravenous calcium).

Reference(s)
Yang G, Zha X, Mao H, Yu X, Wang N, Xing C. Hypocalcemia-based prediction of hungry bone syndrome after parathyroidectomy in hemodialysis patients with refractory secondary hyperparathyroidism. *J Int Med Res.* 2018;46(12): 4985-4994. PMID: 30064280

Witteveen JE, van Thiel S, Romijn JA, Hamdy NA. Hungry bone syndrome: still a challenge in the post-operative management of primary hyperparathyroidism: a systematic review of the literature. *Eur J Endocrinol.* 2013;168(3): R45-R53. PMID: 23152439

Cooper MS, Gittoes NJ. Diagnosis and management of hypocalcaemia [published correction appears in *BMJ.* 2008;336(7659)]. *BMJ.* 2008;336(7656): 1298-1302. PMID: 18535072

7 ANSWER: D) Exogenous glucocorticoid exposure

This patient presents with a spontaneous vertebral fracture due to exogenous glucocorticoids from multiple orthopedic steroid injections (Answer D). She shows signs of Cushing syndrome with osteoporosis, ruddy face, and striae, yet she has undetectable 24-hour urinary free cortisol excretion. The key is to recognize the presentation of exogenous Cushing syndrome and to realize that she may also be at risk for adrenal insufficiency if the injections are stopped. Many exogenous glucocorticoids are not measured as part of the urinary free cortisol assay. The key to the diagnosis is to ask about all possible sources, including nasal sprays, inhalers, topical creams, herbal supplements, and injections.

Severe postmenopausal bone loss (Answer A) is possible, but this would not explain her physical findings and 24-hour urinary free cortisol excretion. Moreover, loss of 30% of bone mineral density at the spine over 3 years would be atypically high for menopausal bone loss alone. Cyclical Cushing syndrome (Answer B) is characterized by repeated episodes of cortisol excess interspersed by periods of normal cortisol secretion. This should not result in undetectable urinary free cortisol levels as observed in this patient. Pseudo-Cushing syndrome (Answer C) is a condition in which many of the signs, symptoms, and abnormal hormone levels seen in true Cushing syndrome are found, but without hypothalamic-pituitary-adrenal pathology. Again, urinary free cortisol levels would tend to be elevated, not suppressed. Finally, surreptitious hydrocortisone administration (Answer E) would result in elevated urinary free cortisol excretion.

Educational Objective
Diagnose exogenous glucocorticoid injections as a cause of osteoporosis and vertebral fractures.

Reference(s)
Kerezoudis P, Rinaldo L, Alvi MA, et al. The effect of epidural steroid injections on bone mineral density and vertebral fracture risk: a systematic review and critical appraisal of current literature. *Pain Med.* 2018;19(3):569-579. PMID: 29304236

8 ANSWER: D) Cholecalciferol, 1000 IU orally daily

This patient has osteoporosis, renal insufficiency, and both primary and secondary hyperparathyroidism. She meets surgical criteria for parathyroidectomy by virtue of her osteoporosis and low glomerular filtration rate, but she has declined this as an option. Raloxifene (Answer A) is not a good choice for her because it offers no protection against nonvertebral fractures for which she is at great risk. Alendronate (Answer B) is contraindicated given her low glomerular filtration rate (alendronate and zoledronate are contraindicated for glomerular filtration rate <35 mL/min per 1.73 m^2, and risedronate is contraindicated for glomerular filtration rate <30 mL/min per 1.73 m^2). Cinacalcet (Answer C) would control her primary hyperparathyroidism, but it would not improve her bone mineral density or reduce her fracture risk. Denosumab (Answer E) is safe to give to patients with renal insufficiency and may be useful in women with osteoporosis and primary hyperparathyroidism, but it could precipitate hypocalcemia in the setting of renal insufficiency and vitamin D deficiency.

Therefore, the best choice is vitamin D repletion first with cholecalciferol (Answer D) by recommending approximately 800 to 1000 IU daily. This will treat any underlying osteomalacia and will ameliorate her secondary hyperparathyroidism. A number of studies have shown that repletion with cholecalciferol up to 2800 IU daily is both safe and effective, although more modest dosages are often recommended. Following vitamin D repletion, up to a 25-hydroxyvitamin D level of 30 ng/mL (74.9 nmol/L), denosumab therapy could be considered. A recent study suggests that women with primary hyperparathyroidism respond well to denosumab in terms of bone mineral density.

Educational Objective

Recommend vitamin D repletion in patients with primary hyperparathyroidism, vitamin D deficiency, and osteoporosis.

Reference(s)

Eller-Vainicher C, Palmieri S, Cairoli E, et al. Protective effect of denosumab on bone in older women with primary hyperparathyroidism. *J Am Geriatr Soc.* 2018;66(3):518-524. PMID: 29364518

Vélayoudom-Céphise FL, Wémeau JL. Primary hyperparathyroidism and vitamin D deficiency [published correction appears in *Ann Endocrinol (Paris).* 2015;76(3):289]. *Ann Endocrinol (Paris).* 2015;76(2):153-162. PMID: 25916759

Das G, Eligar V, Govindan J, Bondugulapati LN, Okosieme O, Davies S. Impact of vitamin D replacement in normocalcoemic and hypercalcoemic primary hyperparathyroidism and coexisting vitamin D deficiency. *Ann Clin Biochem.* 2015;52(Pt 4):462-469. PMID: 25468998

Marcocci C, Bollerslev J, Khan AA, Shoback DM. Medical management of primary hyperparathyroidism: proceedings of the fourth International Workshop on the Management of Asymptomatic Primary Hyperparathyroidism. *J Clin Endocrinol Metab.* 2014;99(10):3607-3618. PMID: 25162668

Rolighed L, Rejnmark L, Sikjaer T, et al. Vitamin D treatment in primary hyperparathyroidism: a randomized placebo controlled trial. *J Clin Endocrinol Metab.* 2014;99(3):1072-1080. PMID: 24423366

9 ANSWER: C) 21-Hydroxylase antibodies

This patient has autoimmune polyendocrine syndrome type 1 (APS type 1) due to a pathogenic variant in the autoimmune regulator gene (*AIRE*). APS type 1 is also known by the acronym APECED (autoimmune polyendocrinopathy-candidiasis-ectodermal dystrophy). The classic presentation includes at least 2 of the following 3 major clinical components: chronic mucocutaneous candidiasis, primary hypoparathyroidism, and autoimmune adrenal insufficiency. Premature ovarian insufficiency occurs in about 60% of patients. Malabsorption and other gastrointestinal issues occur in 25% of patients with APS type 1. Studies have shown that primary adrenal insufficiency may be diagnosed before clinical symptoms by checking for antibodies against the 21-hydroxylase enzyme (Answer C). Note that screening with an 8-AM serum cortisol level is not sensitive enough to detect preclinical disease, although inclusion of an ACTH measurement with the morning cortisol might show early adrenal insufficiency.

Antiphospholipid antibodies (Answer A) are found in the antiphospholipid antibody syndrome, an autoimmune disorder occurring mainly in young women. Clinical presentations include deep vein thrombosis, stroke, pregnancy complications, and recurrent miscarriage. Glutamic acid decarboxylase (GAD-65) antibodies (Answer B) are often present in patients with APS type 1, but they have not been shown to predict the development of type 1 diabetes mellitus, which occurs in about 18% of those with the syndrome. Islet-cell antibodies are a better predictor. Tissue transglutaminase antibodies (Answer D) are used to diagnose celiac disease, which is not a feature of APS type 1. TPO antibodies (Answer E) as a predictor of autoimmune thyroid disease is not the best answer. About 12% of patients with APS type 1 develop hypothyroidism in contrast to 60% who develop Addison disease. Screening for adrenal insufficiency is much more critical.

Educational Objective

Diagnose autoimmune polyendocrine syndrome type 1 as a cause of hypoparathyroidism and recommend appropriate adrenal screening.

Reference(s)

Weiler FG, Dias-da-Silva MR, Lazaretti-Castro M. Autoimmune polyendocrine syndrome type 1: case report and review of literature. *Arq Bras Endocrinol Metabol.* 2012;56(1):54-66. PMID: 22460196

Akirav EM, Ruddle NH, Herold KC. The role of AIRE in human autoimmune disease. *Nat Rev Endocrinol.* 2011;7(1):25-33. PMID: 21102544

Eisenbarth GS, Gottlieb PA. Autoimmune polyendocrine syndromes. *N Engl J Med.* 2004; 350(20):2068-2079. PMID: 15141045

10 ANSWER: E) Raloxifene

This patient is an ideal candidate for raloxifene therapy (Answer E). She is a relatively young, healthy, and active postmenopausal woman with spinal osteoporosis, no prevalent fractures, no severe menopausal symptoms, and a positive family history of estrogen receptor–positive breast cancer. Her fasting serum C-telopeptide level suggests that the rate of bone resorption is not excessive. Raloxifene, although a much weaker antiresorptive agent than the other ones listed, can provide both skeletal and nonskeletal benefits. It decreases spinal fracture risk by 30% and estrogen receptor–positive breast cancer risk by 70%. Raloxifene is not approved for treatment of women with breast cancer, but it is approved for prevention of estrogen receptor–positive breast cancer in postmenopausal women at high risk.

Bisphosphonates (both oral and intravenous) (Answer A) have been associated with lower rates of breast cancer in some studies, but they are not approved for that purpose. Denosumab (Answer C) and zoledronate (Answer B) are approved as adjuvant therapies for women with early and advanced breast cancer and have beneficial effects on the skeleton by preventing bone loss (zoledronate and denosumab) and significantly reducing fractures (denosumab) in women on aromatase inhibitor therapy. Some studies show improvements in breast cancer mortality and/or recurrences with bisphosphonates. Anabolic therapy (Answer D) with either teriparatide or abaloparatide would not be indicated in a patient with mild spinal osteoporosis and no prevalent fractures.

Educational Objective

Explain the role of raloxifene in postmenopausal osteoporosis management (breast cancer prevention).

Reference(s)

Bouvard B, Chatelais J, Soulié P, et al. Osteoporosis treatment and 10 years' oestrogen receptor+ breast cancer outcome in postmenopausal women treated with aromatase inhibitors. *Eur J Cancer.* 2018;101:87-94. PMID: 30036740

Early Breast Cancer Trialists' Collaborative Group (EBCTCG). Adjuvant bisphosphonate treatment in early breast cancer: meta-analyses of individual patient data from randomised trials [published correction appears in *Lancet.* 2016; 387(10013):30]. *Lancet.* 2015;386(10001):1353-1361. PMID: 26211824

Gnant M, Pfeiler G, Dubsky PC, et al; Austrian Breast and Colorectal Cancer Study Group. Adjuvant denosumab in breast cancer (ABCSG-18): a multicentre, randomized, double-blind, placebo-controlled trial. *Lancet.* 2015;386(9992): 433-443. PMID: 26040499

Nelson HD, Smith ME, Griffin JC, Fu R. Use of medications to reduce risk for primary breast cancer: a systematic review by the U.S. Preventive Services Task Force. *Ann Intern Med.* 2013;158(8):604-614. PMID: 23588749

11 ANSWER: C) Begin an oral bisphosphonate

A major fragility fracture warrants treatment, irrespective of bone mineral density or FRAX score, after ruling out secondary causes. Repeating the DXA and recalculating FRAX scores (Answer A) is not necessary in the presence of an acute fracture. Anabolic therapy (Answer B) is contraindicated in this patient due to history of pelvic irradiation. Kyphoplasty (Answer D) should be reserved for pain that persists for 6 or more weeks despite conservative measures. Testosterone therapy (Answer E) poses risks without clear symptomatic or antifracture benefits for this older man with a history of prostate cancer and probable high risk for cardiovascular disease. The best step is to begin bisphosphonate therapy (Answer C).

Because there are no large randomized controlled trials showing antifracture efficacy for testosterone in men with osteoporosis, testosterone therapy should be considered only for hypogonadal men who are symptomatic, have an organic cause for the hypogonadism, have testosterone levels less than 200 ng/dL (<6.9 nmol/L), and/or are not candidates for other therapies. Due to reports of cardiovascular complications, testosterone is not an ideal therapy for a 71-year-old man. Men with marked hypogonadism have good skeletal responses to bisphosphonate therapy without correction of the hypogonadism.

Educational Objective

Manage osteoporosis in a man with acute vertebral fracture.

Reference(s)

Watts NB, Adler RA, Bilezikian JP, et al; Endocrine Society. Osteoporosis in men: an Endocrine Society clinical practice guideline. *J Clin Endocrinol Metab.* 2012;97(6):1802-1822. PMID: 22675062

Cosman F, de Beur SJ, LeBoff MS, et al; National Osteoporosis Foundation. Clinician's guide to prevention and treatment of osteoporosis. *Osteoporos Int.* 2014;25(10):2359-2381. PMID: 25182228

12 ANSWER: E) Physical therapy

This patient has X-linked hypophosphatemic rickets (XLH) which is complicated by enthesopathy. XLH is an X-linked dominant form of rickets that is relatively unresponsive to vitamin D. The hypophosphatemia arises as a consequence of a defective *PHEX* gene product (phosphate-regulating gene with homology to endopeptidases on the X chromosome), which ultimately results in elevated FGF-23 levels and impaired renal proximal tubule phosphate reabsorption. In addition, despite severe hypophosphatemia, 1,25-dihydroxyvitamin D_3 production is not appropriately enhanced due to FGF-23–mediated suppression of 1α-hydroxylase activity. Thus, the "normal" level of 1,25-dihydroxyvitamin D_3 is inappropriate in the setting of elevated PTH and low serum phosphate.

Although children with XLH receive treatment with calcitriol and oral phosphate, it is controversial whether adults with fused epiphyses should continue to be treated. The goal of therapy in adults is to minimize bone pain and to enhance mobility. Calcitriol and oral phosphate (Answer A) reduce bone pain and dental abscesses in XLH, but they do not improve radiographically proven enthesopathy (calcification of tendons, ligaments, and joint capsules, which is what this patient has). Thus, the best recommendation for this patient is physical therapy (Answer E) for passive stretching and other nonpharmacologic treatments.

Oral calcitriol alone (Answer B) would enhance calcium and phosphate absorption from the gut and inhibit PTH secretion, but it would not be effective for the enthesopathy. Phosphate alone (Answer C) would worsen hyperparathyroidism and therefore is not recommended. Cinacalcet (Answer D) can be useful in patients with elevated PTH levels to reduce the phosphaturic effects of PTH at the renal tubule and prevent the secondary hyperparathyroidism resulting from phosphate administration. However, cinacalcet alone has not been shown to reduce bone pain, improve osteomalacia, or reduce enthesopathy in XLH. Two important complications from standard treatment of XLH include nephrocalcinosis and hyperparathyroidism. Up to 80% of patients with XLH have radiographic evidence of nephrocalcinosis, secondary to renal tubular acidosis and deposition of calcium phosphate in the renal tubules. Intermittent hypercalcemia and hypercalciuria are believed to contribute to the development of nephrocalcinosis. Thiazide diuretics and amiloride may be useful in the prevention of nephrocalcinosis in these patients. Hyperparathyroidism usually occurs after years of treatment, but may be present early in the disease course. When calcium forms a complex with oral phosphate supplements, this can result in intermittent hypocalcemia and stimulation of PTH release despite the suppressive effects of calcitriol. When this secondary hyperparathyroidism is not adequately controlled, autonomous (tertiary) hyperparathyroidism can occur, necessitating surgical intervention.

On April 17, 2018, the human monoclonal antibody burosumab received US FDA approval for treatment of patients age 1 year and older with XLH. This drug targets FGF-23. The role of burosumab in the management of adults with symptomatic XLH awaits further studies and recommendations. The recent pivotal trial leading to approval of burosumab for adults with XLH showed marked biochemical improvements and fracture healing in those receiving the active drug. However, neither osteoarthritis nor enthesopathy-related pain would be expected to improve with burosumab based on its mechanism of action.

Note: Images in the stem are reproduced from Karaplis AC, Bai X, Falet JP, Macica CM. Mineralizing enthesopathy is a common feature of renal phosphate-wasting disorders attributed to FGF23 and is exacerbated by standard therapy in hyp mice. *Endocrinology.* 2012;153(12):5906-5917.

Educational Objective
Manage enthesopathy in an adult with X-linked hypophosphatemic rickets.

Reference(s)
Alizadeh Naderi AS, Reilly RF. Hereditary disorders of renal phosphate wasting. *Nat Rev Nephrol.* 2010;2(11):657-665. PMID: 20924400

Connor J, Olear EA, Insogna KL, et al. Conventional therapy in adults with X-linked hypophosphatemia: effects on enthesopathy and dental disease. *J Clin Endocrinol Metab.* 2015; 100(10):3625-3632. PMID: 26176801

Yavropoulou MP, Kotsa K, Gotzamani Psarrakou A, et al. Cinacalcet in hyperparathyroidism secondary to X-linked hypophosphatemic rickets: case report and brief literature review. *Hormones (Athens).* 2010;9(3):274-278. PMID: 20688626

Insogna KL, Briot K, Imel EA, et al; AXLES 1 Investigators. A randomized, double-blind, placebo-controlled phase 3 trial evaluating the efficacy of burosumab, an anti-FGF23 antibody, in adults with X-linked hypophoshatemia: week 24 primary analysis. *J Bone Miner Res.* 2018; 33(8):1383-1393. PMID: 29947083

Liang G, Katz LD, Insogna KL, Carpenter TO, Macica CM. Survey of the enthesopathy of X-linked hypophosphatemia and its characterization in Hyp mice. *Calcif Tissue Int.* 2009;85(3):235-246. PMID: 19609735

Karaplis AC, Bai X, Falet JP, Macica CM. Mineralizing enthesopathy is a common feature of renal phosphate-wasting disorders attributed to FGF23 and is exacerbated by standard therapy in hyp mice. *Endocrinology.* 2012;153(12):5906-5917. PMID: 23038738

13 ANSWER: C) Adjust the FRAX scores upward for both major osteoporotic and hip fracture risks

Patients taking any dosage of glucocorticoid with an anticipated duration of 3 months or longer require a metabolic bone evaluation. The goal is to identify patients at high risk for fracture who would benefit from possible pharmacologic intervention. Within 6 months of initiating glucocorticoids, clinical risk factors for fracture should be assessed and, in selected patients, DXA of the hip and spine should be performed. For this patient who does not have osteoporosis on DXA or a personal history of fracture, use of the FRAX calculator can help determine whether he is likely to benefit from pharmacologic treatment.

It is important to realize, however, that FRAX assumes that the glucocorticoid dosage is between 2.5 and 7.5 mg prednisone daily. For patients on dosages higher than 7.5 mg daily, the recommendation is to adjust the FRAX scores upward for both major osteoporotic and hip fracture risks (Answer C). Currently, it is recommended that the major osteoporotic fracture risk be increased by 15% and the hip fracture risk be increased by 20% for those taking higher steroid dosages. In this patient, a 20% increase in his FRAX hip fracture risk would place him above the treatment threshold of 3% (ie, 2.70% + 0.54 = 3.24%). Some experts also recommend imaging the spine (lateral spine radiographs or vertebral fracture assessments on DXA) to further identify patients at higher risk in whom intervention is warranted if, for example, silent spinal fractures were identified.

Measuring fasting serum C-telopeptide (Answer A) has not been shown to help predict fractures in glucocorticoid-induced osteoporosis. Initially, bone resorption increases in glucocorticoid-induced osteoporosis, but with time, the major defect is suppression of osteoblast function and reduced bone formation. The bone formation marker procollagen type 1 N-terminal propeptide (Answer B) will predictably decline once glucocorticoids have been started and it is not useful for monitoring. The decrease in bone formation is due to direct inhibition of osteoblast proliferation and differentiation and to increased apoptosis of mature osteoblasts and osteocytes.

Two oral bisphosphonates, alendronate and risedronate (Answer D), and the intravenous bisphosphonate, zoledronate, are approved by the US FDA for treatment of glucocorticoid-induced osteoporosis. Among anabolic therapies (Answer E), teriparatide is approved for management of glucocorticoid-induced osteoporosis. Bisphosphonates are considered first-line agents for glucocorticoid-induced osteoporosis unless there are contraindications or previous intolerance. Recently, alendronate was documented to be associated with decreased hip fractures in elderly patients on long-term glucocorticoid therapy. Denosumab was approved for treatment of glucocorticoid-induced osteoporosis in 2018. However, the first step is to recalculate FRAX scores and determine whether the patient meets criteria for pharmacologic intervention.

Educational Objective
Adjust FRAX scores in patients on glucocorticoid dosages greater than 7.5 mg daily.

Reference(s)
Kanis JA, Johansson H, Oden A, McCloskey EV. Guidance for the adjustment of FRAX according to the dose of glucocorticoids. *Osteoporos Int.* 2011;22(3):809-816. PMID: 21229233

Buckley L, Guyatt G, Fink HA, et al. 2017 American College of Rheumatology guideline for the prevention and treatment of glucocorticoid-induced osteoporosis. *Arthritis Rheumatol.* 2017;69(8): 1521-1537. PMID: 28585373

Axelsson KF, Nilsson AG, Wedel H, Lundh D, Lorentzon M. Association between alendronate use and hip fracture risk in older patients using oral prednisolone. *JAMA.* 2017;318(2):146-155. PMID: 28697254

14 ANSWER: E) Denosumab combined with teriparatide

This patient has multiple issues that place her at a high risk for future fractures: she is an elderly woman with low bone mineral density and she has 3 prevalent vertebral fractures, gait instability, and a history of frequent falls resulting from her neurologic disorder. The relatively high fasting serum C-telopeptide level suggests that she would benefit from an antiresorptive agent. However, the spinal fractures and very low bone mineral density at the spine suggest that she would benefit from an anabolic agent. Clearly, she needs agents that will improve bone mineral density optimally at the spine and hip. Of the listed answer choices, the best recommendation would be denosumab combined with teriparatide (Answer E).

Results from the DATA study (Denosumab and Teriparatide Administration), a 24-month randomized controlled trial, demonstrated that the combination of denosumab and teriparatide increased bone mineral density at the femoral neck, total hip, and posteroanterior spine significantly more than either drug alone. Moreover, the increases observed in the combination group (spine = 12.9%, femoral neck = 6.8%, total hip = 6.3%) were greater than increases seen with any currently available treatment. The DATA study has many limitations, including its small size and lack of fracture data, but there is a growing consensus that for patients at high risk for both vertebral and nonvertebral/hip fractures, combination therapy may be optimal. Whether denosumab plus abaloparatide would lead to even greater improvements in bone mineral density is unknown. Neither an oral bisphosphonate alone (Answer A), teriparatide alone (Answer B), an oral bisphosphonate combined with teriparatide (Answer C), nor denosumab alone (Answer D) would increase bone mineral density to the same degree.

Alendronate was the first bisphosphonate studied in combination with PTH analogues in humans. In the PATH study (Parathyroid Hormone and Alendronate for Osteoporosis), postmenopausal osteoporotic women were randomly assigned to receive PTH (1-84), alendronate, or the combination for 12 months. Lumbar spine bone mineral density increased similarly in the groups taking combination therapy, PTH monotherapy, and alendronate monotherapy, whereas hip bone mineral density increased more in women receiving both medications than in those receiving PTH alone, but less than in those receiving alendronate alone.

In a 12-month randomized controlled trial, postmenopausal women with osteoporosis were randomly assigned to a single infusion of zoledronic acid, 5 mg, teriparatide, or the combination of both medications. Lumbar spine bone mineral density increased similarly in the group taking combination therapy and the group taking teriparatide monotherapy (and more than the zoledronic acid monotherapy group), while total hip and femoral neck bone mineral density increased similarly in the combination group and the zoledronic acid monotherapy group (and more than the teriparatide monotherapy group). When these bisphosphonate/PTH analogue studies are considered together with additional combination therapy studies, including those performed in men, the data suggest that the coadministration of bisphosphonates and PTH analogues does not provide substantial clinical benefits compared with monotherapy.

Educational Objective

Explain the role of combination therapy vs monotherapy for patients with osteoporosis who are at very high risk for fracture.

Reference(s)

Black DM, Greenspan SL, Ensrud KE, et al; PaTH Study Investigators. The effects of parathyroid hormone and alendronate alone or in combination in postmenopausal osteoporosis. *N Engl J Med.* 2003;349(13):1207-1215. PMID: 14500804

Leder BZ, Tsai JN, Uihlein AV, et al. Two years of denosumab and teriparatide administration in postmenopausal women with osteoporosis (the DATA Extension Study): a randomized controlled trial. *J Clin Endocrinol Metab.* 2014;99(5):1694-1700. PMID: 24517156

Tsai JN, Uihlein AV, Lee H, et al. Teriparatide and denosumab, alone or combined, in women with postmenopausal osteoporosis: the DATA study randomised trial. *Lancet.* 2013;382(9886):50-56. PMID: 23683600

Cosman F, Eriksen EF, Recknor C, et al. Effects of intravenous zoledronic acid plus subcutaneous teriparatide [rhPTH(1-34)] in postmenopausal osteoporosis. *J Bone Miner Res.* 2011;26(3):503-511. PMID: 20814967

15 ANSWER: A) Bone mineral density at the lumbar spine, decrease; bone mineral density at the femoral neck and total hip, decrease; markers of bone turnover, increase

Recent studies have shown that cessation of denosumab results in a marked increase in bone turnover markers, rapid decline in bone mineral density at all sites, and, in a subgroup of patients, an increased risk of multiple spontaneous vertebral fractures within 12 to 18 months after the last injection (Answer A). Even after 10 consecutive years of treatment with denosumab, bone mineral density at the hip sites may rapidly decline below baseline after the drug is stopped. Due to this "rebound" in bone resorption, bone loss and vertebral fragility, denosumab "holidays" are not recommended. It is possible that treating with a bisphosphonate or other potent antiresorptive agent may stop this decline, but optimal postdenosumab treatment regimens are still being investigated.

In contrast, a frequent clinical question is when or if to recommend a "bisphosphonate holiday" to patients with osteoporosis who have been on either oral or intravenous bisphosphonates for several years. Because bisphosphonates have a long retention in the skeleton, they may continue to exhibit antifracture effectiveness even after therapy is stopped. The decision to stop bisphosphonate therapy must be individualized. Studies have shown that after 3 years of annual intravenous zoledronic acid or 5 years of oral bisphosphonate therapy, it is reasonable to reassess each patient and determine whether a bisphosphonate holiday should be considered. Patients and physicians worry about the risk of rare but devastating adverse effects (such as osteonecrosis of the jaw and atypical femur fractures) that seem to be correlated with duration of bisphosphonate therapy.

Data from the FLEX and HORIZON extension trials (Fracture Intervention Trial Long-Term Extension and Zolendronic Acid in the Treatment of

Postmenopausal Osteoporosis) show that many patients can stop bisphosphonate therapy temporarily after 3 to 5 years without loss of bone mineral density or increased fracture risk. However, some patient subgroups appear to be at higher risk for bone loss or fractures after stopping therapy. Patients at highest risk include those with a history of hip or vertebral fractures, multiple fractures, T-score of –2.5 or lower at the hip, or other factors placing them "at high risk" for fractures.

For these high-risk patients, experts recommend continuing oral bisphosphonates for up to 10 years, continuing intravenous bisphosphonate for up to 6 years, or switching to nonbisphosphonate therapy.

Educational Objective

Explain the bone mineral density and vertebral fracture risks involved in cessation of denosumab.

Reference(s)

Black DM, Schwartz AV, Ensrud KE, et al; FLEX Research Group. Effects of continuing or stopping alendronate after 5 years of treatment: the Fracture Intervention Trial Long-term Extension (FLEX): a randomized trial. *JAMA*. 2006;296(24): 2927-2938. PMID: 17190893

Black DM, Reid IR, Boonen S, et al. The effect of 3 versus 6 years of zoledronic acid treatment of osteoporosis: a randomized extension to the HORIZON-Pivotal Fracture Trial (PFT) [published correction appears in *J Bone Miner Res*. 2012;27(12):2612]. *J Bone Miner Res*. 2012;27(2): 243-254. PMID: 22161728

Adler RA, El-Hajj Fuleihan G, Bauer DC, et al. Managing osteoporosis in patients on long-term bisphosphonate treatment: report of a Task force of the American Society for Bone and Mineral Research. *J Bone Miner Res*. 2016;31(1):16-35. PMID: 26350171

Tripto-Shkolnik L, Rouach V, Marcus Y, Rotman-Pikielny P, Benbassat C, Vered I. Vertebral fractures following denosumab discontinuation in patients with prolonged exposure to bisphosphonates. *Calcif Tissue Int*. 2018;103(1): 44-49. PMID: 29396698

Popp AW, Varathan N, Buffat H, Senn C, Perrelet R, Lippuner K. Bone mineral density changes after 1 year of denosumab discontinuation in postmenopausal women with long-term denosumab treatment for osteoporosis. *Calcif Tissue Int*. 2018;103(1):50-54. PMIDL 29380013

Anastaskilakis AD, Polyzos SA, Makras P, Aubry-Rozier B, Kaouri S, Lamy O. Clinical features of 24 patients with rebound-associated vertebral fractures after denosumab discontinuation: systematic review and additional cases. *J Bone Miner Res*. 2017;32(6):1291-1296. PMID: 28240371

Cummings SR, Ferrari S, Eastell R, et al. Vertebral fractures after discontinuation of denosumab: a post hoc analysis of the randomized placebo-controlled FREEDOM trial and its extension. *J Bone Miner Res*. 2018;33(2):190-198. PMID: 29105841

16 **ANSWER: A) Milk-alkali syndrome**

This is a classic case of milk-alkali syndrome (Answer A) leading to a hypercalcemic crisis. The triad of hypercalcemia, renal failure, and metabolic alkalosis results from ingestion of excessive amounts of calcium and absorbable alkali over a short period. In this case, the patient was taking very large doses (bottles) of calcium carbonate and aspirin, sodium bicarbonate, and anhydrous citric acid for gastrointestinal distress following an alcohol binge. Taking a careful history and recognizing the triad are keys to making the diagnosis.

Dehydration (Answer C) can certainly be part of all types of severe hypercalcemia, but it is not the primary etiology in this patient. Pancreatitis (Answer B) has been associated with primary hyperparathyroidism, but this patient's PTH level is low. Vitamin D intoxication (Answer D) is much slower to resolve and would possibly require glucocorticoids and bisphosphonates. Acute renal failure (Answer E) is clearly a factor in the development of the hypercalcemia, but this does not best explain the precipitating factor.

In the setting of excess calcium/alkali ingestion, hypercalcemia causes renal vasoconstriction, decreases the glomerular filtration rate, and increases bicarbonate reabsorption. Metabolic alkalosis further increases renal tubular reabsorption of calcium, and hypovolemia from nausea/vomiting further reduces the glomerular filtration rate. A vicious cycle can occur with rapid clinical deterioration and death. Hyperphosphatemia may also be seen with excessive ingestion of milk as the calcium source.

Acute management of a hypercalcemic crisis generally involves saline hydration, subcutaneous calcitonin for 24 to 48 hours, intravenous bisphosphonate (or subcutaneous denosumab in selected cases), and treatment of the underlying disease. Furosemide should be added only when there is clinical evidence of volume overload or congestive heart failure. In cases of vitamin D–mediated hypercalcemia, prednisone, 40 to 60 mg daily, or another glucocorticoid equivalent may be useful, but it should not be given without biochemical evidence of inappropriate vitamin D levels. Finally, in patients with hypercalcemic crisis due to primary hyperparathyroidism, cinacalcet can be a "bridge" to parathyroidectomy.

In milk-alkali syndrome, simply stopping the exogenous calcium and alkali and providing vigorous saline hydration to increase the glomerular filtration rate and help clear the calcium and bicarbonate can rapidly reverse the metabolic disarray. In those with acute milk-alkali syndrome, treatment can lead to an acute drop in serum calcium to hypocalcemic levels (with rebound increase in PTH). More chronic cases with nephrocalcinosis take much longer to resolve.

Educational Objective
Diagnose milk-alkali syndrome.

Reference(s)
Beall DP, Scofield RH. Milk-alkali syndrome associated with calcium carbonate consumption. Report of 7 patients with parathyroid hormone levels and an estimate of prevalence among patients hospitalized with hypercalcemia. *Medicine (Baltimore)*. 1995;74(2):89-96. PMID: 7891547

Fiorino AS. Hypercalcemia and alkalosis due to the milk-alkali syndrome: a case report and review. *Yale J Biol Med*. 1996;69(6):517-523. PMID: 9436295

Picolos MK, Lavis VR, Orlander PR. Milk-alkali syndrome is a major cause of hypercalcaemia among non-end-stage renal disease (non-ESRD) inpatients. *Clin Endocrinol (Oxf)*. 2005;63(5):566-576. PMID: 16268810

Bazari H, Palmer WE, Baron JM, Armstrong K. Case records of the Massachusetts General Hospital. Case 24-2016. A 66-year-old man with malaise, weakness, and hypercalcemia. *N Engl J Med*. 2016;375(6):567-574. PMID: 27509105

17 ANSWER: E) Ionized calcium
Fifty percent of circulating calcium is bound to serum proteins, primarily to albumin. In this patient with nephrotic syndrome, serum albumin is almost certainly low. The correction factor is to adjust the serum calcium up or down by 0.8 mg/dL (0.2 mmol/L) for each 1.0 g/dL (10 g/L) deviation of serum albumin below 4 mg/dL (<40 g/L). If her albumin level were 2.0 g/dL (20 g/L) (lower range of normal 3.5 g/dL [35 g/L]), then her adjusted serum calcium level would be 8.6 mg/dL (2.2 mmol/L). Ionized calcium measurement (Answer E) would be another excellent choice. She could also have low magnesium (Answer D) in addition to low albumin, but the first step in her evaluation is to determine whether there is any calcium problem at all, and this requires correcting the measured serum calcium for the hypoalbuminemia or measuring ionized calcium. If she is truly hypocalcemic with low corrected total or ionized serum calcium, then measuring 25-hydroxyvitamin D (Answer B) and PTH (Answer A) would be appropriate. Measuring 1,25-dihydroxyvitamin D (Answer C) would not be helpful in this situation.

Educational Objective
Investigate the etiology of hypocalcemia and correct for hypoalbuminemia by measuring ionized serum calcium.

Reference(s)
Ariyan CE, Sosa JA. Assessment and management of patients with abnormal calcium. *Crit Care Med*. 2004;32(Suppl 4):S146-S154. PMID: 15064673

Shoback D. Hypocalcemia: definition, etiology, pathogenesis, diagnosis, and management. In: Rosen CJ, Compston JE, Lian JB, eds. *Primer on the Metabolic Bone Diseases and Disorders of Mineral Metabolism*. Washington, DC: The American Society for Bone and Mineral Research; 2008:313-317.

18 ANSWER: C) Hyperphosphatemia

This is a classic presentation of tumor lysis syndrome in a patient with lymphoma. Typically, tumor lysis syndrome occurs in patients with lymphoma or leukemia, but it also occurs with some solid tumors. Tumor lysis syndrome may be spontaneous, particularly in individuals with large tumor burdens, but most often it occurs as an adverse effect of cancer treatment. Tumor cells are rich in purines, potassium, and phosphorus, so as large numbers of tumor cells are destroyed or "lysed," contents of the malignant cells are released into the bloodstream. Major features include hyperkalemia, hyperuricemia, acute renal failure, hyperphosphatemia, and secondary hypocalcemia due to phosphate complexing to calcium (Answer C). Phosphate levels can be remarkably elevated and when bound to calcium, calcium-phosphate crystals can form that precipitate in the renal tubules, contributing to the acute renal failure.

Acute rhabdomyolysis (Answer A), from the rapid breakdown of skeletal muscle, can lead to many of the symptoms exhibited in this patient, as well as muscle pain and dark urine from myoglobinuria. However, the creatine kinase level would be well over 1000 U/L (>16.7 μkat/L) to cause this degree of metabolic disarray. Splenic sequestration of calcium (Answer B), acute renal failure (Answer D), and severe metabolic acidosis (Answer E) cannot explain the hypocalcemia even though they may be part of the syndrome.

Educational Objective

Identify hyperphosphatemia as the cause of acute hypocalcemia (tumor lysis syndrome).

Reference(s)

Belay Y, Yirdaw K, Enawgaw B. Tumor lysis syndrome in patients with hematological malignancies. *J Oncol.* 2017;2017:9684909. PMID: 29230244

Agarwala R, Batta A, Suryadevera V, Kumar V, Sharma V, Rana SS. Spontaneous tumour lysis syndrome in hepatocellular carcinoma presenting as hypocalcemic tetany: an unusual case and systematic literature review. *Clin Res Hepatol Gastroenterol.* 2017;41(3):e29-e31. PMID: 27743982

19 ANSWER: A) Large areas of unmineralized osteoid

This 40-year-old woman has classic signs and symptoms of osteomalacia from profound vitamin D deficiency. In some countries in the Middle East (particularly Saudi Arabia), a very high proportion of women are vitamin D deficient due to nutritional deficiencies and clothing that blocks the sunlight. The histomorphometric findings on bone biopsy of such patients include large areas of unmineralized or undermineralized osteoid (Answer A) due to inadequate vitamin D (*see image and table*). In contrast, patients with osteoporosis have normal mineralization but thin, widely separated trabecular plates and microarchitectural damage (Answer B). Biopsies of bone affected by Paget disease show excessive bone resorption and dysregulated, disorganized bone formation (Answer C). Excessive bone resorption, fibrosis, and osteoclast-lined cysts containing pigmented blood products (Answer D) is a description of a "brown tumor" found in osteitis fibrosa cystica, typically in patients with severe hyperparathyroidism.

Vitamin D Deficiency Osteomalacia
Before (A) and After (B) Treatment with Vitamin D

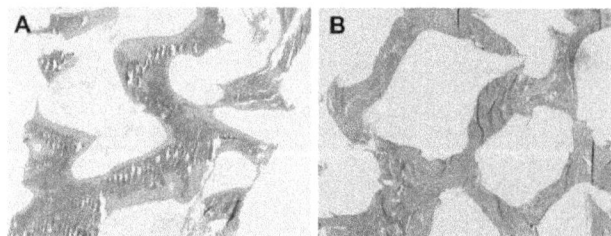

Figure reproduced from Parfitt A.M. Osteomalacia and related disorders. In: Avioli L.V., Krane S.M., editors. *Metabolic Bone Disease and Clinically Related Disorders. 3rd ed.* Academic Press; New York: 1998. pp. 327–386.

Table 3

Contrasting biochemical and bone histomorphometric features of vitamin D and phosphate deficiency osteomalacia

Measurement	Vitamin D deficiency	Phosphate deficiency
Serum calcium	Normal or low	Almost always normal[b]
Serum phosphate	Normal or low[a]	By definition < 2.5 mg/dl
Serum PTH	↑ or ↑↑	Normal[b]
Serum alkaline phosphatase	Almost always elevated	Almost always elevated
Osteoclast surface	↑↑	Normal[b]
Marrow fibrosis	Frequent	Almost never[b]
Cortical thickness	↓↓	Normal or ↑ or ↓[c]
Cancellous bone volume	Normal or ↓	Normal or ↑ or ↓[c]

Table reproduced under a Creative Commons License from Bhan, Arti & Qiu, Shijing & Rao, Sudhaker. (2018). Bone histomorphometry in the evaluation of osteomalacia. *Bone Reports.* 8. 10.1016/j.bonr.2018.03.005 under Creative Commons License.

Educational Objective

Identify the characteristic bone biopsy findings in osteomalacia due to vitamin D deficiency.

Reference(s)

Bhan A, Qui S, Rao SD. Bone histomorphometry in the evaluation of osteomalacia. *Bone Rep.* 2018;8: 125-134. PMID: 29955631

Gifre L, Peris P, Monegal A, Martinez de Osaba MJ, Alvarez L, Guañabens N. Osteomalacia revisited: a report on 28 cases. *Clin Rheumatol.* 2011;30(5): 639-645. PMID: 20949298

Bhan A, Rao AD, Rao DS. Osteomalacia as a result of vitamin D deficiency. *Endocrinol Metab Clin North Am.* 2010;39(2):321-331. PMID: 20511054

20 ANSWER: D) Cessation of breastfeeding

This case illustrates pregnancy- and lactation-associated osteoporosis, defined as one or more fragility fractures occurring within 6 months after delivery. Most cases of pregnancy- and lactation-associated osteoporosis occur in primiparous women in their 30s. About two-thirds of affected patients have predisposing risk factors for osteoporosis, including positive family history, preexisting illnesses, or pregnancy-related risk factors, such as heparin use or prolonged bedrest. Most fractures occur around the time of delivery or within 2 months postpartum during lactation. The mean number of fractures is 3 to 4, with vertebral fractures being most common.

During the first 6 months of lactation, bone mineral density at the spine and hip can decline by 10%; therefore, stopping breastfeeding (Answer D) can have very positive and immediate effects on bone mineral density. Even without pharmacologic treatment, bone mineral density gradually improves within 12 to 18 months after delivery. Longitudinal studies have shown that most women with pregnancy- and lactation-associated osteoporosis continue to have back pain and disability for 3 or more years following the fractures, so starting a potent opioid such as the fentanyl patch (Answer E) may result in addiction. These studies have also demonstrated an increased risk for fractures both during and independent of subsequent pregnancies, a risk that is not eliminated by treatment with antiosteoporosis agents after the first fracture. About 25% of women with pregnancy- and lactation-associated osteoporosis sustain subsequent fractures within 6 years of follow-up.

In addition to conservative methods such as cessation of breastfeeding and optimizing calcium plus vitamin D intake, bisphosphonates (Answer B) have been given to women with pregnancy- and lactation-associated osteoporosis. In one study, bisphosphonates resulted in a 23% increase in spinal bone mineral density after 2 years compared with an 11% improvement in untreated patients. Teriparatide (Answer A) has also been used for pregnancy- and lactation-associated osteoporosis. In a group of 27 women from Korea, bone mineral density responses to 12 months of teriparatide ranged greatly from 4.5% to 34%. On average, bone mineral density gains were doubled in the treatment group compared with results in the control group (15.5% vs 7.5%). Similarly, in a group of 52 women with pregnancy- and lactation-associated osteoporosis, treatment with teriparatide increased spinal bone mineral density by approximately 15% and increased hip bone mineral density by approximately 6% in 11 women; untreated women had bone mineral density increases that were about 50% lower over 2.5 years.

All of the therapeutic choices (teriparatide [Answer A], oral bisphosphonates [Answer B], and denosumab [Answer C]) can improve bone mineral density, but they do not seem to result in long-term benefits with respect to future fracture reduction. Moreover, calcium and vitamin D should be optimized before any pharmacologic therapies are introduced.

Educational Objective

Manage pregnancy- and lactation-associated osteoporosis by recommending cessation of breastfeeding.

Reference(s)

Kyvernitakis I, Reuter TC, Hellmeyer L, Hars O, Hadji P. Subsequent fracture risk of women with pregnancy and lactation-associated osteoporosis after a median of 6 years of follow-up. *Osteoporos Int.* 2018;29(1):135-142. PMID: 28965212

O'Sullivan SM, Grey AB, Singh R, Reid IR. Bisphosphonates in pregnancy and lactation-associated osteoporosis. *Osteoporos Int.* 2006; 17(7):1008-1012. PMID: 16758139

Hong N, Kim JE, Lee SJ, Kim SH, Rhee Y. Changes in bone mineral density and bone turnover markers during treatment with teriparatide in pregnancy- and lactation-associated osteoporosis. *Clin Endocrinol (Oxf).* 2018;88(5): 652-658. PMID: 29389010

Laroche M, Talibart M, Cormier C, Roux C, Guggenbuhl P, Degboe Y. Pregnancy-related fractures: a retrospective study of a French cohort of 52 patients and review of the literature. *Osteoporos Int.* 2017;28(11):3135-3142. PMID: 28879474

21 ANSWER: B) A formal hearing test

This patient has the mildest form of osteogenesis imperfecta, known as type 1. Inheritance is autosomal dominant, but many mutations occur de novo, so family history may be negative. Patients with osteogenesis imperfecta type 1 have normal stature and little or no skeletal deformity. Fractures occur in childhood or adolescence and decrease markedly after puberty. Affected patients may then present in middle age with "osteoporosis." In 50% of patients, there is early-onset hearing loss before age 40 years, so it is important to screen for this with a formal hearing test (Answer B).

On physical examination, affected patients may have blue sclerae and evidence of easy bruising. Joint laxity can be present, but dentinogenesis imperfecta is usually absent, so a complete dental examination (Answer A) is not necessary now. Because there is no increased risk for cardiac disease, echocardiography (Answer C) is not indicated. Young women with osteogenesis imperfecta type 1 who become pregnant should be considered to have high-risk pregnancies and require a team approach, but pregnancy is not contraindicated. Therefore, referral for tubal ligation (Answer D) is incorrect. Finally, bisphosphonates may need to be restarted in the future, particularly at the time of menopause or perimenopause given the risk for bone loss and fractures. However, there is no need to restart bisphosphonates now (Answer E).

The main therapy for osteogenesis imperfecta remains bisphosphonates (intravenous pamidronate, zoledronic acid, and oral bisphosphonates). Current limited evidence demonstrates that oral or intravenous bisphosphonates increase bone mineral density in adults with osteogenesis imperfecta. It is unclear whether oral or intravenous bisphosphonate treatment consistently decreases fractures, although multiple studies report this independently and no studies report an increased fracture rate with treatment. A systematic Cochrane database review did not show that bisphosphonates conclusively improve clinical status (reduce pain or improve growth and functional mobility) in persons with osteogenesis imperfecta. Denosumab has been used

in rare case reports. Teriparatide does not dramatically change clinical outcomes.

Educational Objective
Screen for nonskeletal risks associated with osteogenesis imperfecta type 1 such as hearing loss.

Reference(s)
Van Dijk FS, Sillence DO. Osteogenesis imperfecta: clinical diagnosis, nomenclature and severity assessment [published correction appears in *Am J Med Genet A.* 2015;167A(5):1178]. *Am J Med Genet A.* 2014;164A(6):1470-1481. PMID: 24715559

Thomas IH, DiMeglio LA. Advances in the classification and treatment of osteogenesis imperfecta. *Curr Osteoporos Rep.* 2016;14(1):1-9. PMID: 26861807

Shapiro JR, Thompson CB, Wu Y, Nunes M, Gillen C. Bone mineral density and fracture rate in response to intravenous and oral bisphosphonates in adult osteogenesis imperfecta. *Calcif Tissue Int.* 2010;87(2):120-129. PMID: 20544187

Cozzolino M, Perelli F, Maggio L, et al. Management of osteogenesis imperfecta type 1 in pregnancy: a review of literature applied to clinical practice. *Arch Gynecol Obstet.* 2016; 293(6):1153-1159. PMID: 26781260

Dwan K, Phillipi CA, Steiner RD, Basel D. Bisphosphonate therapy for osteogenesis imperfecta. *Cochrane Database Syst Rev.* 2016;10: CD005088. PMID: 27760454

22 ANSWER: C) Cholecalciferol, 5000 IU daily, plus calcitriol, 0.5 mcg twice daily

This patient has profound calcium and vitamin D deficiencies following gastric bypass surgery, which is not unusual. However, instead of developing secondary hyperparathyroidism, his PTH level is inappropriately normal, resulting in symptomatic hypocalcemia. The key to answering this question is to recognize that patients with subclinical surgical hypoparathyroidism from previous neck surgery or other parathyroid insult may become frankly hypocalcemic when an additional stress is added. This stress can be a potent antiresorptive agent for osteoporosis or cancer, calcium/vitamin D deficiency from poor intake or malabsorption, or both. Supplementing vitamin D alone (Answers A and B) will not reverse his hypocalcemia, nor will oral magnesium (Answer E), which will give him diarrhea and not address the underlying cause. Calcitriol alone (Answer D) would be helpful, but ultimately, this patient needs both vitamin D substrate and activated vitamin D (Answer C). Given that his symptoms are relatively mild and he retains some PTH activity, he can be managed as an outpatient with very close monitoring.

Educational Objective

Diagnose and treat postsurgical hypocalcemia in the setting of gastric bypass surgery.

Reference(s)

Parrott J, Frank L, Rabena R, Craggs-Dino L, Isom KA, Greiman L. American Society for Metabolic and Bariatric Surgery integrated health nutritional guidelines for the surgical weight loss patient 2016 Update: micronutrients. *Surg Obes Relat Dis.* 2017;13(5):727-741. PMID: 28392254

Mechanick JI, Youdim A, Jones DB, et al. Clinical practice guidelines for the perioperative nutritional, metabolic, and nonsurgical support of the bariatric surgery patient--2013 update: cosponsored by American Association of Clinical Endocrinologists, the Obesity Society, and American Society for Metabolic & Bariatric Surgery. *Surg Obes Relat Dis.* 2013;9(2):159-191. PMID: 23537696

Allo Miguel G, García Fernández E, Martínez Díaz-Guerra G, et al. Recalcitrant hypocalcaemia in a patient with post-thyroidectomy hypoparathyroidism and Roux-en-Y gastric bypass. *Obes Res Clin Pract.* 2016;10(3):344-347. PMID: 26387060

Panazzolo DG, Braga TG, Bergamim A, Pires B, Almeida H, Kraemer-Aguiar LG. Hypoparathyroidism after Roux-en-Y gastric bypass--a challenge for clinical management: a case report. *J Med Case Rep.* 2014;28;8:357. PMID: 25348653

23 ANSWER: D) Plain radiographs showing a transverse linear lucency extending medially through a thickened lateral cortex on one or both femurs

Atypical femur fractures after long-term bisphosphonate treatment for osteoporosis are rare but have a number of common features. They are bilateral in approximately 50% of cases. Bone turnover markers such as low C-telopeptide (Answer A) have not been shown to predict or correlate well with atypical femur fractures, and a fasting C-telopeptide level less than 200 pg/mL would not be uncommon in a patient on zoledronate therapy. In atypical femur fractures, plain radiographs of the femurs show thick, not thin (Answer B), cortices. Nuclear bone scan is the most sensitive way to evaluate both femurs and show early stress reactions or stress fractures, but these discrete hot spots occur on the lateral, not medial (Answer C), surfaces. These can progress to complete transverse fractures and may require urgent placement of rods within the femur(s) to stabilize. Iliac crest bone biopsy results tend to show low bone formation and changes in bone composition (ie, higher degree of mineralization, increased collagen maturity, and decreased heterogeneity of the degree of mineralization). Biopsies do not tend to show increased numbers of giant multinucleated osteoclasts (Answer E).

One of the most specific signs of impending transverse femur fracture is the so-called dreaded black line that appears on plain radiographs, usually associated with a thickened lateral cortex (site of a stress reaction or stress fracture) (Answer D). This should prompt cessation of the bisphosphonate and urgent orthopedic referral.

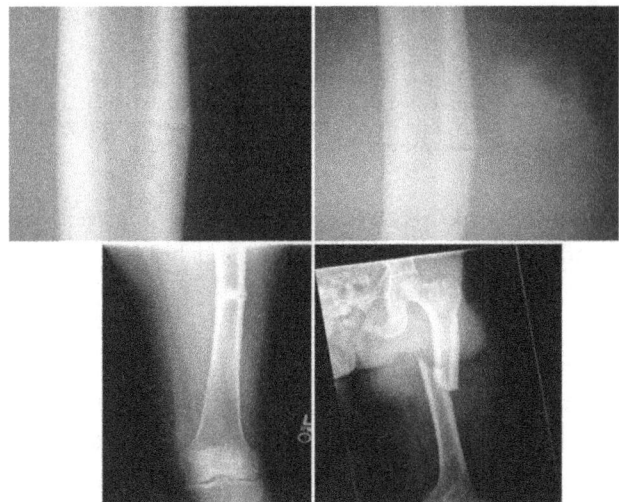

Stages of evolution of an atypical femur fracture from initial "dreaded black line" to stress fracture to full atypical femur fracture (reproduced from Black DM, Abrahamsen B, Bouxsein ML, Einhorn T, Napoli N. Atypical femur fractures: review of epidemiology, relationship to bisphosphonates, prevention, and clinical management. *Endocr Rev.* 2019;40[2]:333-368.)

A task force of the American Society for Bone and Mineral Research released case definitions for atypical femur fractures that include 4 of 5 major features:

- Fracture is associated with minimal or no trauma (eg, fall from standing height)
- Fracture line originates at the lateral cortex and is substantially transverse in orientation, although it may become oblique as it traverses medially across the femur
- Complete fractures extend through both cortices and may be associated with a medial spike; incomplete fractures include only the lateral cortex
- Fractures are noncomminuted or only minimally comminuted
- Localized periosteal or endosteal thickening of the lateral cortex is present at the fracture site ("beaking" or "flaring")

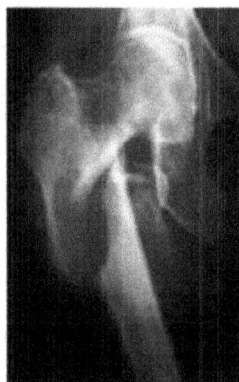

TYPICAL Subtrochanteric Fracture
- Spiral pattern
- Substantial comminution
- Thin cortices

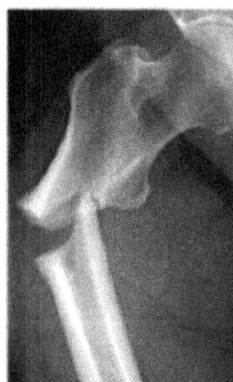

ATYPICAL Subtrochanteric Fracture
- Transverse or short oblique orientation
- No comminution
- Thick cortices – focal or generalized

The 2 images above illustrate the differences between "typical" and "atypical" femur fractures (reproduced with permission from Khosla S, Bilezikian JP, Dempster DW, et al. Benefits and risks of bisphosphonate therapy for osteoporosis. *J Clin Endocrinol Metab.* 2012;97:2272-2282.).

Educational Objective
Identify the early radiographic features of bisphosphonate-related atypical femur fractures.

Reference(s)
Khosla S, Bilezikian JP, Dempster DW, et al. Benefits and risks of bisphosphonate therapy for osteoporosis. *J Clin Endocrinol Metab.* 2012; 97(7):2272-2282. PMID: 22523337

Png MA, Koh JS, Goh SK, Fook-Chong S, Howe TS. Bisphosphonate-related femoral periosteal stress reactions: scoring system based on radiographic and MRI findings. *AJR Am J Roentgenol.* 2012; 198(4):869-877. PMID: 22451554

Shane E, Burr D, Ebeling PR, et al; American Society for Bone and Mineral Research. Atypical subtrochanteric and diaphyseal femoral fractures: report of a task force of the American Society for Bone and Mineral Research [published correction appears in *J Bone Miner Res.* 2011;26(8):1987]. *J Bone Miner Res.* 2010;25(11): 2267-2294. PMID: 20842676

Shaikh W 3rd, Morris D, Morris S 4th. Signs of insufficiency fractures overlooked in a patient receiving chronic bisphosphonate therapy. *J Am Board Fam Med.* 2016;29(3):404-407. PMID: 27170798

Starr J, Tay YKD, Shane E. Current understanding of epidemiology, pathophysiology, and management of atypical femur fractures. *Curr Osteoporos Rep.* 2018;16(4):519-529. PMID: 29951870

Koh JS, Goh SK, Png MA, Kwek EB, Howe TS. Femoral cortical stress lesions in long-term bisphosphonate therapy: a herald of impending fracture? *J Orthop Trauma.* 2010;24(2):75-81. PMID: 20101130

Black DM, Abrahamsen B, Bouxsein ML, Einhorn T, Napoli N. Atypical femur fractures: review of epidemiology, relationship to bisphosphonates, prevention, and clinical management. *Endocr Rev.* 2019;40(2):333-368. PMID: 30169557

24 ANSWER: D) Measure calcium and PTH after stopping hydrochlorothiazide for 3 months

In this vignette, the dilemma is to decide whether the patient's laboratory values reflect true primary hyperparathyroidism or a drug effect from the thiazide diuretic. The best way to distinguish these possibilities is to stop hydrochlorothiazide for several weeks or months and repeat the calcium and PTH measurement (Answer D).

Calculation of the calcium-to-creatinine clearance ratio (Answer A) to rule out familial hypocalciuric hypercalcemia could be considered given the mild hypercalcemia and low urinary calcium excretion. However, the normal serum calcium value from 2 years ago, the patient's age, and the use of hydrochlorothiazide make this option a wrong choice. DXA (Answer B) is indicated once the diagnosis of primary hyperparathyroidism is unequivocal, but not at this stage. Measuring 1,25-dihydroxyvitamin D (Answer C) would not be informative or definitive. Finally, ordering a sestamibi parathyroid scan (Answer E) is premature until the diagnosis is determined and it is decided whether she meets surgical criteria.

Thiazide diuretics reduce urinary calcium excretion and can cause mild hypercalcemia. In addition, some patients with latent or preexisting undiagnosed hyperparathyroidism may be prescribed thiazides, resulting in further elevations of serum calcium and an unmasking of the disorder. Following discontinuation of the thiazide, these individuals remain hypercalcemic, although perhaps less so, and are found to have surgically proven hyperparathyroidism. Thus, if a patient taking a thiazide becomes hypercalcemic, the drug should be withdrawn, if possible, and calcium and PTH should be assessed approximately 3 months later. Persistent hypercalcemia (with elevated or high-normal PTH) after drug withdrawal suggests that the thiazide has unmasked true primary hyperparathyroidism.

In a population-based study of residents of Olmsted County, Minnesota, thiazide-associated hypercalcemia was identified on average 5.2 years after initiating thiazides, and it persisted in 71% of patients who discontinued the thiazide. Among all patients with thiazide-associated hypercalcemia, 24% were subsequently diagnosed with primary hyperparathyroidism. The mean maximum serum calcium concentration in these patients was 10.85 mg/dL (2.7 mmol/L).

Although the optimal management strategy in patients with thiazide-related primary hyperparathyroidism is unclear, asymptomatic patients with unequivocal biochemical evidence of hyperparathyroidism weeks or months after stopping thiazides are best managed like patients with asymptomatic primary hyperparathyroidism. Interestingly, in patients with primary hyperparathyroidism who are not surgical candidates, introduction of thiazides may reduce hypercalciuria and PTH levels without significantly increasing serum calcium.

Educational Objective
Evaluate hyperparathyroidism in patients taking thiazide diuretics.

Reference(s)
Griebeler ML, Kearns AE, Ryu E, et al. Thiazide-associated hypercalcemia: incidence and association with primary hyperparathyroidism over two decades. *J Clin Endocrinol Metab.* 2016; 101(3):1166-1172. PMID: 26751196

Tsvetov G, Hirsch D, Shimon I, et al. Thiazide treatment in primary hyperparathyroidism-a new indication for an old medication? *J Clin Endocrinol Metab.* 2017;102(4):1270-1276. PMID: 28388724

Riss P, Kammer M, Selberherr A, et al. The influence of thiazide intake on calcium and parathyroid hormone levels in patients with primary hyperparathyroidism. *Clin Endocrinol (Oxf).* 2016;85(2):196-201. PMID:

Wermers RA, Kearns AE, Jenkins GD, Melton LJ 3rd. Incidence and clinical spectrum of thiazide-associated hypercalcemia. *Am J Med.* 2007; 120(10):911.e9-e15. PMID: 17904464

25 ANSWER: B) Perform preoperative parathyroid imaging

This patient meets criteria for normocalcemic primary hyperparathyroidism. This is defined as persistently normal total and ionized serum calcium levels in the setting of persistently elevated serum intact PTH, along with normal 25-hydroxyvitamin D, serum creatinine, and 24-hour urinary calcium excretion levels. Such patients are often discovered during a workup for low bone mineral density or kidney stone disease.

Normocalcemic hyperparathyroidism (as opposed to hypercalcemic hyperparathyroidism) is defined as normal serum total and ionized calcium levels with concomitant elevated PTH levels on at least 2 separate occasions. It is a diagnosis of exclusion and cannot be made unless the following conditions are excluded:

- Chronic kidney disease (estimated glomerular filtration rate <60 mL/min per 1.73 m^2)
- Drugs: thiazides, lithium, bisphosphonates, denosumab
- Malabsorption (eg, celiac disease, if urinary calcium excretion is low, anemia is present, etc)
- Hypercalciuria
- Vitamin D deficiency (aim for 25-hydroxyvitamin D level of ≥30 ng/mL [≥74.9 nmol/L] or greater)

In general, the same criteria for surgical intervention are used for patients with normocalcemic primary hyperparathyroidism and patients with asymptomatic primary hyperparathyroidism (*see criteria for parathyroid surgery below*). Because this patient already meets surgical criteria by virtue of her osteoporosis, obtaining a DXA of the one-third distal radius (Answer A) is not necessary. Longitudinal studies indicate that parathyroidectomy improves bone mineral density in patients with both hypercalcemic and normocalcemic primary hyperparathyroidism. For patients who decline surgery or are not surgical candidates, alendronate has been shown to significantly improve bone mineral density. Cinacalcet, which is US FDA approved for treatment of primary hyperparathyroidism in non-surgical patients, has not been shown to improve bone mineral density, but a combination of cinacalcet and alendronate in such patients may be beneficial.

Preoperative parathyroid imaging (eg, ultrasonography and/or sestamibi scan) (Answer B) is the best next step for this patient. Imaging detects approximately 80% of abnormal parathyroid tissue, and there can be false-negative results. There is evidence that all imaging studies may be less sensitive in patients with normocalcemic hyperparathyroidism compared with hypercalcemic hyperparathyroidism. Additionally, some studies suggest that multiglandular disease is more common among patients with normocalcemic hyperparathyroidism.

Without a personal or family history of kidney stones or an abnormally high urinary calcium excretion, imaging for renal stones (Answer C) would not be the most appropriate next step in a woman of this age. She is already getting enough calcium, so doubling calcium supplementation (Answer D) is unlikely to affect her serum PTH level. Many patients with normocalcemic hyperparathyroidism eventually demonstrate elevated serum calcium levels, but measuring calcium and PTH in 6 months is not correct, as this patient meets surgical criteria. Most clinicians recommend retesting serum calcium and albumin every 6 to 12 months in patients with normocalcemic hyperparathyroidism who do not meet surgical criteria.

The recommendations for the evaluation of patients with asymptomatic primary hyperparathyroidism are outlined (*see table*).

Table 3. Recommendations for the Evaluation of Patients With Asymptomatic PHPT

Recommended
  Biochemistry panel (calcium, phosphate, alkaline
      phosphatase activity, BUN, creatinine), 25(OH)D
  PTH by second- or third-generation immunoassay
  BMD by DXA
      Lumbar spine, hip, and distal 1/3 radius
  Vertebral spine assessment
      X-ray or VFA by DXA
  24-h urine for:
      Calcium, creatinine, creatinine clearance
      Stone risk profile
  Abdominal imaging by x-ray, ultrasound, or CT scan
Optional
  HRpQCT
  TBS by DXA
  Bone turnover markers (bone-specific alkaline phosphatase
      activity, osteocalcin, P1NP [select one]; serum CTX,
      urinary NTX [select one])
  Fractional excretion of calcium on timed urine sample
  DNA testing if genetic basis for PHPT is suspected

Abbreviations: BUN, blood urea nitrogen; P1NP, procollagen type 1 N-propeptide; CTX, C-telopeptide cross-linked collagen type I; NTX, N-telopeptide of type I collagen. This evaluation is for PHPT, not to distinguish between PHPT and other causes of hypercalcemia.

Table reprinted from Bilezikian JP, Brandi ML, Eastell R, et al. Guidelines for the management of asymptomatic primary hyperparathyroidism: summary statement from the Fourth International Workshop. *J Clin Endocrinol Metab.* 2014;99(10):3561-3569.

Criteria for parathyroid surgery in an asymptomatic patient with primary hyperparathyroidism:

- Age <50 years
- Serum calcium >1 mg/dL above upper normal limit
- T-score less than –2.5 at any skeletal site on DXA or vertebral compression fracture identified on imaging
- Creatinine clearance <60 mL/min per 1.73 m^2
- Kidney stones on imaging or nephrocalcinosis
- Urinary calcium excretion >400 mg/24 h and increased stone risk by biochemical stone risk analysis

Educational Objective
Evaluate normocalcemic hyperparathyroidism.

Reference(s)
Cusano NE, Silverberg SJ, Bilezikian JP. Normocalcemic primary hyperparathyroidism. *J Clin Densitom.* 2013;16(1):33-39. PMID: 23374739

Rejnmark L, Amstrup AK, Mollerup CL, Heickendorff L, Mosekilde L. Further insights into the pathogenesis of primary hyperparathyroidism: a nested case-control study. *J Clin Endocrinol Metab.* 2013;98(1):87-96. PMID: 23150677

Lowe H, McMahon DJ, Rubin MR, Bilezikian JP, Silverberg SJ. Normocalcemic primary hyperparathyroidism: further characterization of a new clinical phenotype. *J Clin Endocrinol Metab.* 2007;92(8):3001-3005. PMID: 17536001

Bilezikian JP, Brandi ML, Eastell R, et al. Guidelines for the management of asymptomatic primary hyperparathyroidism: summary statement from the Fourth International Workshop. *J Clin Endocrinol Metab.* 2014;99(10):3561-3569. PMID: 25162665

26 ANSWER: C) Multiple endocrine neoplasia type 1

This young woman presents with multiple endocrine neoplasia (MEN) type 1 (Answer C). A number of red flags in this case should raise the possibility of hereditary primary hyperparathyroidism and particularly of MEN type 1. First, the patient is young, presenting about 3 decades earlier than the typical age for sporadic (nonfamilial) primary hyperparathyroidism. Second, she and her father had kidney stones, suggesting a possible familial syndrome. Third, she is on an oral contraceptive for secondary amenorrhea, raising the possibility of pituitary disease (eg, prolactinoma) and a multigland endocrine syndrome. Fourth, following bilateral neck exploration and removal of 2 abnormal-appearing parathyroid glands, she remained hypercalcemic.

Other characteristic features of primary hyperparathyroidism in MEN type 1 include:

- A 1:1 male-to-female ratio in contrast to the female predominance in sporadic hyperparathyroidism.
- Approximately 80% to 85% of patients with sporadic disease have single parathyroid adenomas. In contrast, primary hyperparathyroidism associated with MEN type 1 is characterized by multiglandular disease eventually affecting all 4 glands. There can be marked asymmetry in size among the parathyroids so that, upon initial neck exploration, some parathyroid glands in MEN type 1 may appear to be grossly normal. However, even the smaller glands generally exhibit hypercellularity on histologic examination.
- Even after apparently successful subtotal parathyroidectomy, there is a very high rate of recurrent hyperparathyroidism in MEN type 1, consistent with the genetic mutation affecting all of the glands. In contrast, sporadic primary hyperparathyroidism rarely recurs.

Indications to perform MEN type 1 genetic testing in patients with primary hyperparathyroidism are as follows:

- Parathyroid adenoma before age 30 to 35 years
- Atypical or multigland parathyroid adenomas at any age
- 2 or more types of endocrine tumors: parathyroid, pancreatic, pituitary
- First-degree relatives of a person with a known MEN type 1 pathogenic variant

Educational Objective
Diagnose multiple endocrine neoplasia type 1.

Reference(s)
Thakker RV, Newey PJ, Walls GV, et al; Endocrine Society. Clinical practice guidelines for multiple endocrine neoplasia type 1 (MEN1). *J Clin Endocrinol Metab.* 2012;97(9):2990-3011. PMID: 22723327

Lassen T, Friis-Hansen L, Rasmussen AK, Knigge U, Feldt-Rasmussen U. Primary hyperparathyroidism in young people. When should we perform genetic testing for multiple endocrine neoplasia 1 (MEN-1)? *J Clin Endocrinol Metab.* 2014;99(11):3983-3987. PMID: 24731012

27 ANSWER: B) Zoledronate, 5 mg intravenously (1 dose)

This patient has Paget disease of the pelvis with symptomatic extension into the left hip joint, and he therefore needs treatment. Historically known as "osteitis deformans," Paget disease is a localized disorder of bone remodeling that progresses slowly and leads to deformities of affected bones, as well as skeletal, joint, neurologic, and vascular complications. Microscopic studies show signs of excessive bone resorption and disorganized, dysregulated bone formation. This weakens the bone, leading to deformity, pain, fracture, neurologic impingement, and/or joint complications. In mild cases, there are no symptoms, and the disease is detected incidentally on radiographs or by an elevated alkaline phosphatase level.

In some parts of the world, Paget disease is the second most common bone disorder after osteoporosis, although in recent years, its prevalence and severity appear to be decreasing. The disease is easily diagnosed and effectively treated, but its pathogenesis remains incompletely understood. It can affect one (monostotic) or multiple (polyostotic) bones, most commonly the pelvis, femur, lumbar vertebrae, and skull, but it never affects the entire skeleton and does not spread from one bone to another. Rarely, Paget disease can transform into osteosarcoma.

Symptoms of Paget disease include bone pain, bone deformity, loss of hearing, tinnitus, cranial nerve dysfunction, osteoarthritis, high-output heart failure, fracture, and hypercalcemia. Some patients have no symptoms at all. The diagnosis is made by documenting an elevated serum alkaline phosphatase concentration, along with normal levels of calcium, phosphate, and liver transaminases. Characteristic radiographic findings on skeletal survey and bone scans can be helpful to diagnose the disease and determine the extent of the condition. Treatment includes oral or intravenous bisphosphonates.

The best recommendation for this patient is zoledronate, 5 mg intravenously (1 dose) (Answer B). The listed doses of alendronate (Answer A) and risedronate (Answer C) are not appropriate for Paget disease. Calcitonin nasal spray (Answer D) is considered to be a much less effective therapy for Paget disease compared with bisphosphonates. Physical therapy alone (Answer E) is not appropriate for a patient with active, symptomatic Paget disease and would not alleviate his bone pain.

The 2014 Endocrine Society clinical practice guideline recommends treatment with a bisphosphonate for "most patients with active Paget's disease who are at risk for future complications," but this has been challenged by others who contend that the only symptom proven to be ameliorated by bisphosphonate treatment is bone pain. Studies suggest that a single dose of zoledronate can control pain and sustain reductions in bone resorption for several years. The Endocrine Society guideline suggests that the definition of "remission" with any given treatment should include: (1) symptom control and (2) reduction of bone turnover to below the midpoint of the reference range.

Table 2. Recommended Bisphosphonate Dosing Regimens

Drug	Dosage
Zoledronate[a]	5 mg given as a single infusion over 15 min. Retreatment is seldom required within 5 y
Alendronate	40 mg/d for 6 mo. Retreatment may be required between 2 and 6 y
Risedronate	30 mg/d for 2 mo. Retreatment may be required between 1 and 5 y

Table reproduced with permissions from Singer FR, Bone HG 3rd, Hosking DJ, et al; Endocrine Society. Paget's disease of bone: an Endocrine Society clinical practice guideline. *J Clin Endocrinol Metab.* 2014;99(12):4408-4422.
Note: Image in the stem is reproduced from Genuth SM, Klein L. Hypoparathyroidism and Paget's disease: the effect of parathyroid hormone administration. *J Clin Endocrinol Metab.* 1972;35(5):693-699.

Educational Objective
Apply treatment guidelines for Paget disease.

Reference(s)
Reid IR, Miller P, Lyles K, et al. Comparison of a single infusion of zoledronic acid with risedronate for Paget's disease. *N Engl J Med.* 2005; 353(9):898-908. PMID: 16135834

Singer FR, Bone HG 3rd, Hosking DJ, et al; Endocrine Society. Paget's disease of bone: an Endocrine Society clinical practice guideline. *J Clin Endocrinol Metab.* 2014;99(12):4408-4422. PMID: 25406796

Ralston SH. Clinical practice. Paget's disease of bone. *N Engl J Med.* 2013;368(7):644-650. PMID: 23406029

Genuth SM, Klein L. Hypoparathyroidism and Paget's disease: the effect of parathyroid hormone administration. *J Clin Endocrinol Metab.* 1972;35(5):693-699. PMID: 4262771

28 ANSWER: B) Primary hyperparathyroidism with osteitis fibrosa cystica

In this patient, the development of hypercalcemia after partial treatment of vitamin D deficiency indicates that primary hyperparathyroidism was masked by profound vitamin D deficiency. Imaging revealed a 1.3-cm parathyroid adenoma that was successfully resected, resulting in gradual healing of bone lesions and normocalcemia. Osteitis fibrosa cystica or "brown tumors" are most commonly associated with hypercalcemic primary hyperparathyroidism but may occur with severe secondary hyperparathyroidism due to vitamin D deficiency or renal disease. Primary hyperparathyroidism with osteitis fibrosa cystica (Answer B) is this patient's most likely diagnosis. The bony lesions of osteitis fibrosa cystica generally affect fingers, facial bones, ribs, pelvis, and long bones. The histopathologic changes include osteoclast-lined cysts with areas of fibrosis, intratrabecular tunneling, and hemosiderin pigmentation resulting in brown tumors. Lesions can be mistaken for malignancies, but they generally heal with resolution of the hyperparathyroidism.

Parathyroid carcinoma (Answer A) accounts for less than 1% of cases of primary hyperparathyroidism and generally presents quite differently than benign primary hyperparathyroidism. The incidence of parathyroid cancer is equal between the 2 genders rather than being predominant in women. Moreover, patients with parathyroid carcinomas are much more likely to have symptoms, larger tumor sizes, bone and kidney disease, marked hypercalcemia, and serum PTH concentrations that are 5- to 10-fold higher than the upper normal limit. The combination of a neck mass, severe symptomatic hypercalcemia, and very elevated PTH levels should raise the possibility of parathyroid carcinoma. Although the primary treatment is wide surgical resection, it is important to avoid biopsy of the neck mass to avoid hemorrhage and seeding of the carcinoma. Cinacalcet can have an important adjuvant role in managing the hypercalcemia. In general, benign parathyroid adenomas do not progress or change to carcinomas, except in hyperparathyroidism–jaw tumor syndrome. The absence of a neck mass, the bone lesions, and the duration of symptoms make this diagnosis very unlikely.

Hyperparathyroidism–jaw tumor syndrome (Answer C) is a hereditary syndrome caused by inactivating germline pathogenic variants in the *CDC73* gene, resulting in autosomal dominant familial hyperparathyroidism. Patients with hyperparathyroidism–jaw tumor syndrome are predisposed to ossifying fibromas of the jaw, cystic and neoplastic renal lesions, uterine tumors, and parathyroid neoplasia with an increased risk of parathyroid cancer. Parathyroid carcinoma is reported to occur in approximately 15% of patients with hyperparathyroidism–jaw tumor syndrome. In these patients, all parathyroid glands are at risk for tumor development, but the tumors can occur asynchronously over many years. This patient's knee findings and the results of the mandibular mass biopsy essentially rule out this condition.

Giant-cell tumors (Answer D) have not been associated with ectopic PTH secretion.

Note: Images in the stem are reproduced from Hussain M, Hammam M. Management challenges with brown tumor of primary hyperparathyroidism masked by severe vitamin D deficiency: a case report. *J Med Case Rep*. 2016;10:166.

Educational Objective
Recognize masking of severe primary hyperparathyroidism by vitamin D deficiency complicated by osteitis fibrosa cystica.

Reference(s)

Hussain M, Hammam M. Management challenges with brown tumor of primary hyperparathyroidism masked by severe vitamin D deficiency: a case report. *J Med Case Rep*. 2016; 10:166. PMID: 27277007

Misiorowski W, Czajka-Oraniec I, Kochman M, Zgliczynski W, Bilezikian JP. Osteitis fibrosa cystica-a forgotten radiologic feature of primary hyperparathyroidism. *Endocrine*. 2017;58(2): 380-385. PMID: 28900835

29 ANSWER: E) Foreign-body granulomata

This 45-year-old patient presents with non-PTH–associated symptomatic hypercalcemia due to foreign-body granulomata from silicone implants (Answer E). The activated macrophages surrounding the silicone express the 1α-hydroxylase enzyme and convert 25-hydroxyvitamin D to 1,25-dihydroxyvitamin D. Chronically elevated calcitriol results in release of calcium and phosphate from bone, increased calcium and phosphate absorption from the gut, hypercalciuria, nephrocalcinosis, nephrolithiasis, and in some cases, renal failure. During this time, damage from hypercalciuria can be extensive. Polymethylmethacrylate and paraffin oil have also been associated with this syndrome. Cases have included body builders, transgender women, patients with HIV wasting syndrome, and patients wanting to improve cosmetic appearance using body sculpting and fillers.

In a recent review, typical patients were approximately 50 years old, female (including transgender), and used silicone followed by polymethylmethacrylate injections. The most common injection site was the buttocks followed by the breast. Hypercalcemia developed, on average, 8 years after the initial procedure and was close to 14 mg/dL (3.5 mmol/L) at presentation with elevated calcitriol. Management involves hydration, glucocorticoids, and bisphosphonates; surgery is rarely successful. Renal failure is the most common complication (~80%).

Systemic sarcoidosis (Answer A) could present similarly, but it would be associated with classic pulmonary, skin, bone, or ocular findings, which this patient does not have. B-cell lymphomas (Answer B) can produce calcitriol-induced hypercalcemia, but one would expect fever, night sweats, lymphadenopathy, and/or radiographic findings typical for lymphoma. Disseminated coccidioidomycosis (Answer C) or Valley fever, is a fungal disease common in the southwest United States and would present with more prominent pulmonary symptoms. Although associated with hypercalcemia, the mechanism is unknown, as calcitriol levels are not usually elevated. Leiomyosarcoma (Answer D) is not associated with this syndrome.

Educational Objective
Diagnose hypercalcemia associated with cosmetic injections.

Reference(s)
Tachamo N, Donato A, Timilsina B, et al. Hypercalcemia associated with cosmetic injections: a systematic review. *Eur J Endocrinol.* 2018;178(4):425-430. PMID: 29453291

Amiraian DE, Accurso JM, Jain MK. Severe hypercalcemia related to silicone granulomas as discovered by FDG-PET. *Indian J Nucl Med.* 2017;32(4):343-344. PMID: 29142355

Edwards BJ, Saraykar S, Sun M, et al. Resection of granulomatous tissue resolves silicone induced hypercalcemia. *Bone Rep.* 2015;5:163-167. PMID: 28589383

30 ANSWER: B) Inactivating pathogenic variant in the *GNAS* gene inherited from her mother

This young woman has classic signs of pseudohypoparathyroidism type 1A. Pseudohypoparathyroidism is a group of disorders defined by end-organ resistance to PTH that results in hypocalcemia, hyperphosphatemia, and elevated PTH levels. The syndrome is caused by pathogenic variants in the *GNAS* gene that encodes the α subunit of the G protein, which is linked to the PTH receptor. The pathogenic variants prevent generation of adenylyl cyclase when PTH binds to its receptor, and, therefore, failure of signal transduction by PTH. Interestingly, *GNAS* is imprinted in humans, so that expression of the allele for a specific tissue is dependent on whether the allele is inherited from the mother or father. Thus, pseudohypoparathyroidism type 1A is an autosomal dominant disease with a loss-of-function pathogenic variant in *GNAS* that only manifests when the mutation is inherited from the mother (Answer B). Affected patients have the biochemical abnormalities listed above, as well as a classic phenotypic appearance known as Albright hereditary osteodystrophy. Such patients have round facies, short stature, obesity, developmental delay, and short fourth metacarpal bones as shown in the x-ray in the vignette. Additionally, patients with pseudohypoparathyroidism type 1A have resistance to various other G-protein–coupled hormones, including TSH, LH, FSH, and GnRH.

In contrast, those with paternally transmitted pathogenic variants in the *GNAS* gene (Answer C) have the physical phenotype of Albright hereditary osteodystrophy but normal serum calcium, phosphate, and PTH concentrations. This is referred to as pseudopseudohypoparathyroidism.

DiGeorge syndrome (22q11.2 deletion syndrome) (Answer A) results from abnormal development of the third and fourth branchial pouches and is associated with parathyroid aplasia or hypoplasia, thymic aplasia or hypoplasia, cardiac abnormalities, developmental delay, and characteristic facial appearance. In this setting, PTH would be low, not high.

An activating pathogenic variant in the gene encoding the calcium-sensing receptor (*CASR*) (Answer D) is the usual cause of autosomal dominant hypocalcemia and manifests with hypocalcemia and inappropriately normal PTH concentrations. The very high PTH level seen in this case is not consistent with autosomal dominant hypocalcemia.

Autoimmune polyglandular syndrome type 1 results in immunologic destruction of the parathyroid glands and presents with hypoparathyroidism, primary adrenal insufficiency, and mucocutaneous candidiasis, none of which is present in this case. Autoimmune polyglandular syndrome type 1 is due to pathogenic variants in the autoimmune regulator gene (*AIRE*) (Answer E).

Note: Image in the stem is reprinted from Virágh K, Toke J, Sallai A, Jakab Z, Racz K, Toth M. Gradual development of brachydactyly in pseudohypoparathyroidism. *J Clin Endocrinol Metab.* 2014;99(6):1945-1946.

Educational Objective

Explain the genetics underlying pseudohypoparathyroidism type 1A (an inactivating pathogenic variant in the *GNAS* gene inherited from the mother).

Reference(s)

Virágh K, Toke J, Sallai A, Jakab Z, Racz K, Toth M. Gradual development of brachydactyly in pseudohypoparathyroidism. *J Clin Endocrinol Metab*. 2014;99(6):1945-1946. PMID: 24684469

Mantovani G. Clinical review: pseudohypoparathyroidism: diagnosis and treatment. *J Clin Endocrinol Metab*. 2011;96(10): 3020-3030. PMID: 21816789

Diabetes Mellitus Section 1 Board Review

Serge A. Jabbour, MD

1 ANSWER: A) Iron deficiency

Although the international standardization of the hemoglobin A_{1c} assay has decreased potential technical errors in interpreting results, a number of biologic and patient-specific factors can cause misleading results.

Hemoglobin A_{1c} values are influenced by red blood cell survival. Thus, falsely high values in relation to mean blood glucose values can be obtained when red blood cell turnover is low, resulting in a disproportionate number of older red cells. This problem can occur in patients with iron, vitamin B_{12}, or folate deficiency anemia (thus, Answer A is correct).

In contrast, rapid red blood cell turnover leads to a greater proportion of younger red cells and falsely low hemoglobin A_{1c} values. Examples include patients with hemolysis (Answer C); patients treated for iron, vitamin B_{12}, or folate deficiency; and patients treated with erythropoietin.

It should be noted that hemoglobin A_{1c} values tend to be lower in pregnancy (Answer D) because the average blood glucose concentration is about 20% lower in pregnant women than in nonpregnant women, and in the first half of pregnancy there is a rise in red cell mass and a slight increase in red blood cell turnover.

Laboratory error (Answer B) is unlikely to happen twice—both of the patient's hemoglobin A_{1c} values were high at 7.8% (62 mmol/mol) and 8.5% (69 mmol/mol).

High nighttime blood glucose values (Answer E) do not typically occur suddenly and without a rise in fasting blood glucose.

Educational Objective
Diagnose iron deficiency anemia as a cause of falsely high hemoglobin A_{1c} values.

Reference(s)

National Glycohemoglobin Standardization Program (NGSP) Web site. Factors that interfere with HbA1c test results. Available at: http://www.ngsp.org/factors.asp. Accessed for verification February 2019

Ahmad J, Rafat D. HbA1c and iron deficiency: a review. *Diabetes Metab Syndr.* 2013;7(2): 118-122. PMID: 23680254

Silva JF, Pimentel AL, Camargo JL. Effect of iron deficiency anaemia on HbA1c levels is dependent on the degree of anaemia. *Clin Biochem.* 2016; 49(1-2):117-120. PMID: 26365695

2 ANSWER: E) Proteinuria

The turnover of serum proteins, mainly albumin, is more rapid than that of hemoglobin; thus, serum fructosamine values (glycated proteins, mostly albumin) reflect mean blood glucose values over a much shorter period (1 to 2 weeks). There is generally a good correlation between serum fructosamine and hemoglobin A_{1c} values. Fructosamine responds more rapidly with changes in blood glucose control than does hemoglobin A_{1c}. Falsely low fructosamine values in relation to mean blood glucose values occur with rapid albumin turnover, for example, in patients with protein-losing enteropathy or nephrotic syndrome (Answer E).

Biotin (Answer B), hemolysis (Answer C), and hypothyroidism (Answer D) do not falsely lower fructosamine. Laboratory errors (Answer A) do rarely occur, but in this case, the heavy proteinuria explains the normal fructosamine value.

Educational Objective
Diagnose nephrotic syndrome as a cause of falsely low fructosamine values.

Reference(s)

Vetter SW. Glycated serum albumin and AGE receptors. *Adv Clin Chem.* 2015;72:205-275. PMID: 26471084

Koga M. Glycated albumin; clinical usefulness. *Clin Chim Acta.* 2014;433:96-104. PMID: 24631132

Parrinello CM, Selvin E. Beyond HbA1c and glucose: the role of nontraditional glycemic markers in diabetes diagnosis, prognosis, and management. *Curr Diab Rep.* 2014;14(11):548. PMID: 25249070

3 ANSWER: B) Diabetic ketoacidosis

SGLT-2 inhibitors are associated with euglycemic diabetic ketoacidosis and ketosis (Answer B) as a consequence of their noninsulin-dependent glucose clearance, hyperglucagonemia, and volume depletion. Patients with type 1 or type 2 diabetes who experience nausea, vomiting, or malaise or develop a metabolic acidosis in the setting of SGLT-2 inhibitor therapy should be promptly evaluated for the presence of urine and/or serum ketones. In the setting of type 1 diabetes, SGLT-2 inhibitors should only be used with great caution, extensive counseling, and close monitoring given that their use in such patients is off-label. The efficacy and safety of SGLT-2 inhibitors are being studied in patients with type 1 diabetes.

Four SGLT-2 inhibitors are approved in the United States for the treatment of type 2 diabetes: canagliflozin, dapagliflozin, empagliflozin, and ertugliflozin. Dapagliflozin, empagliflozin, and ertugliflozin are not associated with higher fracture rates (Answer A) or hyperkalemia (Answer E). Canagliflozin has been associated with hyperkalemia (in patients with moderate renal impairment and on drugs that can interfere with potassium excretion) and an increased risk of bone fractures (mainly upper extremities). Only canagliflozin and sertugliflozin have label warnings regarding lower-limb amputations (Answer D). Dapagliflozin is the only SGLT-2 inhibitor with a label warning about bladder tumors (Answer C).

Educational Objective

Counsel patients about SGLT-2 inhibitors and diabetic ketoacidosis in the setting of type 1 diabetes mellitus (off-label use).

Reference(s)

Peters AL, Buschur EO, Buse JB, Cohan P, Diner JC, Hirsch IB. Euglycemic diabetic ketoacidosis: a potential complication of treatment with sodium-glucose cotransporter 2 inhibition. *Diabetes Care.* 2015;38(9):1687-1693. PMID: 26078479

Erondu N, Desai M, Ways K, Meininger G. Diabetic ketoacidosis and related events in the canagliflozin type 2 diabetes clinical program. *Diabetes Care.* 2015;38(9):1680-1686. PMID: 26203064

US Food and Drug Administration. FDA Drug Safety Communication: FDA revises labels of SGLT2 inhibitors for diabetes to include warnings about too much acid in the blood and serious urinary tract infections. December 4, 2015. Available at: http://www.fda.gov/Drugs/DrugSafety/ucm475463.htm. Accessed for verification February 2019

4 ANSWER: D) Increase evening insulin detemir to 14 units

During pregnancy, normalization of blood glucose levels reduces the risk of congenital malformations during the first 8 to 10 weeks of pregnancy and the risk of macrosomia and related comorbidities over the course of the pregnancy. The American Diabetes Association recommends that the hemoglobin A_{1c} level be less than 6.0% to 6.5% (42-48 mmol/mol) during early pregnancy, with a lower target (<6.0% [<42 mmol/mol]) by the second and third trimesters. The American Diabetes Association also recommends maintaining fasting and preprandial glucose levels less than 95 mg/dL (<5.3 mmol/L) with either a peak (1-hour) postprandial level less than 140 mg/dL (<7.8 mmol/L) or a 2-hour postprandial level less than 120 mg/dL (<6.7 mmol/L). Because this patient's fasting blood glucose levels are higher than 90 mg/dL (>5.0 mmol/L), increasing the evening insulin detemir (Answer D) is the best course of action.

Continuing the same regimen (Answer A) would not improve her high fasting blood glucose. Given that her peak postprandial glucose measurements are within the target range, changing her insulin-to-carbohydrate ratio (Answer B) is not indicated. Changing the morning insulin detemir dose (Answer C) would affect her evening blood glucose values, which are within range.

Changing the sensitivity (or correction) factor (Answer E) would not affect her high fasting glucose levels.

Educational Objective
Make basic recommendations for management of glycemia during pregnancy.

Reference(s)
American Diabetes Association. 14. Management of diabetes in pregnancy: standards of medical care in diabetes-2019. *Diabetes Care.* 2019;42(Suppl 1):S165-172. PMID: 30559240

McCance DR. Pregnancy and diabetes. *Best Pract Res Clin Endocrinol Metab.* 2011;25(6):945-958. PMID: 22115168

Kitzmiller JL, Block JM, Brown FM, et al. Managing preexisting diabetes for pregnancy: summary of evidence and consensus recommendations for care. *Diabetes Care.* 2008;31(5):1060-1079. PMID: 18445730

5 ANSWER: D) Lower his hemoglobin A$_{1c}$ to <7.0% (<53 mmol/mol)

Glycemic control has clearly been shown to decrease the risk of onset or progression of diabetic nephropathy in patients with type 1 diabetes. Thus, lowering his hemoglobin A$_{1c}$ to less than 7.0% (<53 mmol/mol) (Answer D) is correct.

In patients with diabetes complicated by either albuminuria or hypertension, the use of either an ACE inhibitor or an angiotensin-receptor blocker as first-line therapy is recommended (in nonpregnant patients). Because this patient has neither albuminuria nor hypertension, there are no data to support the use of an ACE inhibitor (Answer A) or an angiotensin-receptor blocker (Answer B). Blood pressure control (<140/90 mm Hg), blood glucose control, and limiting protein intake to 0.8 g/kg per day (the recommended daily allowance) may be recommended. However, there is no additional benefit to lowering his blood pressure to less than 120/70 mm Hg (Answer E). Higher levels of protein intake (>1.3 g/kg per day) have been associated with increased albuminuria, more rapid kidney function loss, and cardiovascular disease mortality and therefore should be avoided. Reducing this patient's protein intake to less than 0.5 g/kg per day (Answer C) is not recommended because it would not alter glycemic measures, cardiovascular risk measures, or the course of glomerular filtration rate decline.

Educational Objective
Recommend interventions to decrease the risk of future diabetic nephropathy in a normoalbuminuric, normotensive patient with type 1 diabetes mellitus.

Reference(s)
American Diabetes Association. 4. Comprehensive medical evaluation and assessment of comorbidities: standards of medical care in diabetes-2019. *Diabetes Care.* 2019;41(Suppl 1): S34-S45. PMID: 30559230

Bilous R, Chaturvedi N, Sjølie AK, et al. Effect of candesartan on microalbuminuria and albumin excretion rate in diabetes: three randomized trials. *Ann Intern Med.* 2009;151(1):11-20. PMID: 19454554

Mauer M, Zinman B, Gardiner R, et al. Renal and retinal effects of enalapril and losartan in type 1 diabetes. *N Engl J Med.* 2009;361(1):40-51. PMID: 19571282

6 ANSWER: C) Discontinuation of insulin and initiation of glimepiride

Monogenic forms of diabetes comprise a heterogeneous group of disorders. They are caused by single gene mutations and are characterized by impaired insulin secretion. Up to 5% of all diabetes cases are monogenic and affected patients are often undiagnosed or are misclassified as having type 1 or type 2 diabetes.

Accurate diagnosis is important because of the special implications for treatment, prognosis, and familial risk. Monogenic diabetes includes MODY (maturity-onset diabetes of the young), mitochondrial diabetes, and neonatal diabetes. Many gene mutations have been identified that cause diabetes by disturbing the coupling of blood glucose concentration and insulin secretion.

The patient in this vignette has MODY, characterized by (1) young age at diagnosis, often under 25 years, (2) a marked family history of diabetes in every generation due to autosomal dominant inheritance, (3) absence of obesity and signs of insulin resistance, (4) commonly mild hyperglycemia without the need for insulin therapy, and (5) negative results for β-cell antibodies. The diagnosis can be confirmed by genetic testing where available. MODY 3 (due to an *HNF1A* pathogenic variant [hepatocyte nuclear factor-1-alpha gene on chromosome 12]), the most prevalent MODY form, presents with early glycosuria and hyperglycemia, which is often postprandial. Optimal treatment of MODY 3 is sulfonylureas (thus, Answer C is correct and Answer A is incorrect). One study documented a significantly greater drop in hemoglobin A_{1c} level with a sulfonylurea compared with metformin (Answer D). Almost 70% of patients previously treated with insulin are successfully switched to sulfonylureas once an *HNF1A* pathogenic variant is identified. Patients with MODY 3 are at risk for microvascular and macrovascular complications of type 1 and type 2 diabetes. In addition, patients with MODY 3 appear to have an increased risk of cardiovascular mortality compared with unaffected family members. There are no data on the use of SGLT-2 inhibitors (Answer B) in patients with MODY.

Educational Objective

Diagnose monogenic diabetes mellitus that was initially misdiagnosed as type 1 diabetes and assess the treatment implications.

Reference(s)

Henzen C. Monogenic diabetes mellitus due to defects in insulin secretion. *Swiss Med Wkly.* 2012;142:w13690. PMID: 23037711

Thanabalasingham G, Owen KR. Diagnosis and management of maturity onset diabetes of the young (MODY). *BMJ.* 2011;343:d6044. PMID: 22012810

Wherrett DK, Bundy B, Becker DJ, et al; Type 1 Diabetes TrialNet GAD Study Group. Antigen-based therapy with glutamic acid decarboxylase (GAD) vaccine in patients with recent-onset type 1 diabetes: a randomised double-blind trial. *Lancet.* 2011;378(9788):319-327. PMID: 21714999

Shepherd M, Shields B, Ellard S, Rubio-Cabezas O, Hattersley AT. A genetic diagnosis of HNF1A diabetes alters treatment and improves glycaemic control in the majority of insulin-treated patients. *Diabet Med.* 2009;26(4):437-441. PMID: 19388975

7 ANSWER: A) Start insulin

This patient presents with a form of type 1 diabetes that may be seen in adults—latent autoimmune diabetes in adults (LADA). Patients with LADA can progress to the need for insulin very slowly, over years, or more rapidly, as in this patient. LADA may be present in up to 30% of patients with a clinical diagnosis of type 2 diabetes. Compared with type 2 diabetes, LADA is generally associated with a lower BMI, lower triglycerides, higher HDL cholesterol, and lower prevalence of hypertension. The Immunology of Diabetes Society has proposed the following criteria for LADA: age at onset of at least 30 years, positive for at least one type 1 diabetes autoantibody, and not requiring insulin within the first 6 months after diagnosis. Many experts think the latter criterion is too subjective. This patient's continued symptomatic hyperglycemia and lack of response to metformin are clues to the correct diagnosis. Failure to recognize it can delay appropriate treatment. The diagnosis is confirmed by the seropositivity of the antibodies (glutamic acid decarboxylase antibodies being the most sensitive immune parameter), especially if the titer is high.

This patient requires insulin (Answer A) to control his hyperglycemia; no other intervention has been well studied or shown to be effective in treating LADA. Thus, adding a sulfonylurea (Answer D), an SGLT-2 (Answer B), or a GLP-1 receptor agonist (Answer C) is incorrect.

Educational Objective

Diagnose latent autoimmune diabetes in adults (LADA) in a patient misdiagnosed as having type 2 diabetes and review treatment implications.

Reference(s)

O'Neil KS, Johnson JL, Panak RL. Recognizing and appropriately treating latent autoimmune diabetes in adults. *Diabetes Spectr.* 2016;29(4):249-252. PMID: 27899877

Laugesen E, Ostergaard JA, Leslie RD; Danish Diabetes Academy Workshop and Workshop Speakers. Latent autoimmune diabetes of the adult: current knowledge and uncertainty. *Diabet Med.* 2015;32(7):843-852. PMID: 25601320

Liao Y, Xiang Y, Zhou Z. Diagnostic criteria of latent autoimmune diabetes in adults (LADA): a review and reflection. *Front Med.* 2012;6(3):243-247. PMID: 22843304

Naik RG, Brooks-Worrell BM, Palmer JP. Latent autoimmune diabetes in adults. *J Clin Endocrinol Metab.* 2009;94(12):4635-4644. PMID: 19837918

⑧ ANSWER: B) Decrease insulin degludec to 40 units at bedtime; discontinue nateglinide

Individuals with severely insulin-deficient type 2 diabetes mellitus can experience hypoglycemia unawareness or hypoglycemia-associated autonomic failure. Hypoglycemia unawareness is characterized by a reduction in the sympathoadrenal and autonomic responses and is more common in those with longer duration of type 2 diabetes and in older adults. This syndrome can lead to a prolonged exposure to hypoglycemia, resulting in loss of consciousness, seizures, or brain damage. However, it is possible to improve the control of glycemia and reduce the frequency of hypoglycemia with short-term relaxation of glycemic targets. This hypoglycemia avoidance includes reducing insulin therapy for several weeks to allow the patient's blood glucose levels to run a little higher, thereby increasing sensitivity to symptoms. In addition, the glycemic targets in older patients are more relaxed, with a hemoglobin A_{1c} goal between 7.0% and 8.0% (53-64 mmol/mol). Accordingly, this patient's insulin dosage should be decreased by 10% to 20% and insulin secretagogues should be discontinued (Answer B). Although approaches that discontinue the insulin secretagogue are preferred, replacing degludec with the same dose of insulin detemir (Answer C) or NPH (Answer D) would not resolve the issue. An approach that continues the use of an insulin secretagogue (Answer A) should be avoided.

Educational Objective
Manage hypoglycemia in type 2 diabetes mellitus.

Reference(s)
American Diabetes Association. 12. Older adults: standards of medical care in diabetes-2019. *Diabetes Care.* 2019;42(Suppl 1):S139-S147. PMID30559238

American Diabetes Association. 9. Pharmacologic approaches to glycemic treatment: standards of medical care in diabetes-2019. *Diabetes Care.* 2019;42(Suppl 1):S90-S102. PMID 30559235

Cryer PE. Diverse causes of hypoglycemia-associated autonomic failure in diabetes. *N Engl J Med.* 2004;350(22):2272-2279. PMID: 15163777

⑨ ANSWER: C) Convert the insulin regimen to regular U500 insulin

Insulin is the preferred therapeutic option for patients with persistent hyperglycemia that fails to respond to other agents. However, in patients requiring more than 200 units of insulin a day, the volume of insulin given becomes a problem, both in terms of patient comfort and pharmacokinetics. Large-volume insulin injections are poorly absorbed. In these cases, U500 insulin (Answer C) should be considered. There is increasing evidence of more reliable delivery of insulin and successful outcomes with the use of U500 insulin in patients such as the one presented. Although the formulation of U500 is similar to that of regular insulin, the duration of action is up to 13 to 24 hours, permitting adequate delivery with 2 or 3 injections per day. Fortunately, U500 pens are now available and patients with severe insulin resistance are good candidates for U500 insulin.

Given the severity of this patient's hyperglycemia, switching to insulin degludec, even at a higher dose (Answer D), or adding linagliptin (Answer A) is unlikely to achieve a target hemoglobin A_{1c} level less than 7.0% (<53 mmol/mol). Switching to an insulin pump (Answer B) is not desirable because large volumes of insulin, either by injection or pump, are poorly absorbed and are unlikely to achieve the target hemoglobin A_{1c} level.

Educational Objective
Treat extreme insulin resistance with U500 insulin.

Reference(s)
Hood RC, Arakaki RF, Wysham C, Li YG, Settles JA, Jackson JA. Two treatment approaches for human regular U-500 insulin in patients with type 2 diabetes not achieving adequate glycemic control on high-dose U-100 insulin therapy with or without oral agents: a randomized, titration-to-target clinical trial. *Endocr Pract.* 2015;21(7):782-793. PMID: 25813411

Quinn SL, Lansang MC, Mina D. Safety and effectiveness of U-500 insulin therapy in patients with insulin-resistant type 2 diabetes mellitus. *Pharmacotherapy.* 2011;31(7):695-702. PMID: 21923457

Lane WS, Cochran EK, Jackson JA, et al. High-dose insulin therapy: is it time for U-500 insulin? *Endocr Pract.* 2009;15(1):71-79. PMID: 19211405

Garg R, Johnston V, McNally PG, Davies MJ, Lawrence IG. U-500 insulin: why, when and how to use in clinical practice. *Diabetes Metab Res Rev.* 2007;23(4):265-268. PMID: 17109474

10 ANSWER: A) Now

Although the mainstay of diabetes prevention should always focus on lifestyle management, including diet and physical activity counseling, the screening guidelines vary. Current guidelines (American Diabetes Association, World Health Organization) suggest a BMI criterion of 23 kg/m^2 for type 2 diabetes screening in Asian Americans (decreased from 25 kg/m^2 in the general population) because data demonstrate that Asian Americans are at greater risk for diabetes at a lower BMI than non-Asian populations. Therefore, this patient should be screened for type 2 diabetes now (Answer A). Delaying screening (Answers B, C, and D) would not serve his best interests.

In asymptomatic adults, diabetes screening should be considered in patients who are overweight or obese who have 1 or more of the following risk factors: first-degree relative with diabetes, high-risk race/ethnicity, history of cardiovascular disease, hypertension, HDL-cholesterol level <35 mg/dL (<0.90 mmol/L) and/or triglyceride level >250 mg/dL (>2.82 mmol/L), polycystic ovary syndrome (in women), and physical inactivity. Patients with prediabetes should have annual testing, and women diagnosed with gestational diabetes should have testing at least every 3 years.

According to the American Diabetes Association guidelines, screening for diabetes should begin at age 45 years regardless of other factors such as ethnicity, family history, BMI, blood pressure, and dyslipidemia.

Educational Objective

Select the appropriate criteria for type 2 diabetes mellitus/prediabetes screening in patients of diverse racial/ethnic backgrounds.

Reference(s)

American Diabetes Association. 3. Prevention or delay of type 2 diabetes: standards of medical care in diabetes-2019. *Diabetes Care.* 2019; 42(Suppl 1):S34-S45. PMID: 30559229

Pottie K, Jaramillo A, Lewin G, et al; Canadian Task Force on Preventive Health Care. Recommendations on screening for type 2 diabetes in adults [published correction appears in *CMAJ.* 2012;184(16):1815]. *CMAJ.* 2012; 184(15):1687-1696. PMID: 23073674

Siu AI; US Preventive Services Task Force. Screening for abnormal blood glucose and type 2 diabetes mellitus: U.S. Preventive Services Task Force Recommendation Statement. *Ann Intern Med.* 2015;163(11):861-868. PMID: 26501513

11 ANSWER: B) Zinc transporter 8 (ZnT8) antibody testing

In first-degree relatives of individuals with type 1 diabetes, screening before overt clinical symptoms develop, as occurred in this patient, can detect the disease in a clinically silent phase. Multiple positive antibodies are highly predictive of future disease development, while positivity for only 1 autoantibody may not indicate high risk. Several serum antibodies can be detected before the manifestation of autoimmune hyperglycemia, including islet-cell antibodies, insulin autoantibodies, glutamic acid decarboxylase antibodies, and antibodies to tyrosine phosphatase-like proteins. Analysis of zinc transporter 8 (ZnT8) antibodies (Answer B) increases the diagnostic sensitivity of islet autoantibodies for type 1 diabetes, as 26% of patients with antibody-negative type 1 diabetes (negative for insulin, glutamic acid decarboxylase, tyrosine phosphatase-like proteins, and islet-cell antibodies) have ZnT8 autoantibodies.

Fructosamine measurement (Answer A) may uncover hyperglycemia, but it is not helpful in characterizing the type of diabetes. This patient is much more likely to have type 1 diabetes than maturity-onset diabetes of the young (MODY), both statistically and because of the family history, and testing for pathogenic variants in the *GCK* gene (Answer C) or the *HNF1A* gene (Answer D) would not confirm the diagnosis of type 1 diabetes.

Educational Objective

Select the best test to confirm the diagnosis of type 1 diabetes mellitus.

Reference(s)

Mrena S, Virtanen SM, Laippala P, et al. Models for predicting type 1 diabetes in siblings of affected children. *Diabetes Care*. 2006;29(3):662-667. PMID: 16505523

Greenbaum CJ, Cuthbertson D, Krischer JP; Disease Prevention Trial of Type 1 Diabetes Study Group. Type 1 diabetes manifested solely by 2-h oral glucose tolerance test criteria. *Diabetes*. 2001;50(2):470-476. PMID: 11272162

Andersson C, Vaziri-Sani F, Delli A, et al; BDD Study Group. Triple specificity of ZnT8 autoantibodies in relation to HLA and other islet autoantibodies in childhood and adolescent type 1 diabetes. *Pediatr Diabetes*. 2013;14(2):97-105. PMID: 22957668

Vaziri-Sani F, Delli AJ, Elding-Larsson H, et al. A novel triple mix radiobinding assay for the three ZnT8 (ZnT8-RWQ) autoantibody variants in children with newly diagnosed diabetes. *J Immunol Methods*. 2011;371(1-2):25-37. PMID: 21708156

Vermeulen I, Weets I, Asanghanwa M, et al; Belgian Diabetes Registry. Contribution of antibodies against IA-2β and zinc transporter 8 to classification of diabetes under 40 years of age. *Diabetes Care*. 2011;34(8):1760-1765. PMID: 21715527

Gorus FK, Balti EV, Vermeulen I, et al. Screening for insulinoma antigen 2 and zinc transporter 8 autoantibodies: a cost-effective and age-dependent strategy to identify rapid progressors to clinical onset among relatives of type 1 diabetic patients. *Clin Exp Immunol*. 2013; 171(1):82-90. PMID: 23199327

12 ANSWER: E) Refer to a nutritionist

The American College of Cardiology/American Heart Association and the National Lipid Association blood cholesterol guidelines recommend statin treatment for individuals with diabetes aged 40 to 75 years with LDL-cholesterol levels between 70 and 189 mg/dL (1.81-4.90 mmol/L) who do not have clinical atherosclerotic cardiovascular disease. Thus, starting atorvastatin (Answer B) is incorrect in this case because the patient is 32 years old. The exception is if the patient has had type 1 diabetes for at least 20 years and has complications such as nephropathy (albuminuria, stage 3 chronic kidney disease). Without clinical albuminuria, adding an ACE inhibitor (Answer C) would not be expected to result in a cardiovascular disease benefit in a normotensive, normoalbuminuric patient with type 1 diabetes. For patients with a triglyceride level less than 500 mg/dL (5.65 mmol/L), treatment with a fibrate (Answer D) or omega-3 fatty acids (Answer A) is not indicated. In addition, in the ASCEND trial, among patients with diabetes without evidence of cardiovascular disease, there was no significant difference in the risk of serious vascular events between those who were assigned to receive omega-3 fatty acid supplementation and those who were assigned to receive placebo.

Her BMI is elevated and her lipids are abnormal, suggesting a poor diet. She would greatly benefit from seeing a nutritionist (Answer E).

Educational Objective

Determine when statin use is appropriate as part of cardiovascular risk reduction in patients with type 1 diabetes mellitus.

Reference(s)

American Diabetes Association. 10. Cardiovascular disease and risk management: standards of medical care in diabetes-2019. *Diabetes Care*. 2019;42(Suppl 1):S103-S123. PMID: 30559236

Stone NJ, Robinson J, Lichtenstein AH, et al; American College of Cardiology/American Heart Association Task Force on Practice Guidelines. 2013 ACC/AHA guideline on the treatment of blood cholesterol to reduce atherosclerotic cardiovascular risk in adults: a report of the American College of Cardiology/American Heart Association Task Force on Practice Guidelines. *Circulation*. 2014;129(25 Suppl 2):S1-S45. PMID: 24222016

Jacobson TA, Ito MK, Maki KC, et al. National Lipid Association recommendations for patient-centered management of dyslipidemia: part 1 - executive summary. *J Clin Lipidol*. 2014;8(5): 473-488. PMID: 25234560

Nathan DM, Cleary PA, Backlund JY, et al; Diabetes Control and Complications Trial/Epidemiology of Diabetes Interventions and Complications (DCCT/EDIC) Study Research Group. Intensive diabetes treatment and cardiovascular disease in patients with type 1 diabetes. *N Engl J Med*. 2005; 353(25):2643-2653. PMID: 16371630

The ASCEND Study Colaborative Group, Bowman L, Mafham M, et al. Effects of n-3 fatty acid supplements in diabetes mellitus. *N Engl J Med.* 2018;379(16):1540-1550. PMID: 30146932

Grundy SM, Stone NJ, Bailey AL, et al. 2018 AHA/ACC/AACVPR/AAPA/ABC/ACPM/ADA/AGS/APhA/ ASPC/NLA/PCNA guideline on the management of blood cholesterol: a report of the American College of Cardiology Foundation/ American Heart Association Task Force on Clinical Practice Guidelines. *J Am Coll Cardiol.* 2019;73(24):e285-e350. PMID: 30423393

13 ANSWER: B) Total iron-binding capacity and serum ferritin measurements

When diabetes is diagnosed, the possibility of secondary diabetes should be considered. Secondary diabetes occurs when a separate condition leads to hyperglycemia; this is considered distinct from routine type 1 or type 2 diabetes, although clinical features are often shared.

Broad categories of secondary diabetes include medication-induced (eg, corticosteroids), other endocrinopathies (eg, acromegaly), pancreatic diseases (eg, pancreatitis), infections (eg, cytomegalovirus), and genetic conditions (eg, Rabson-Mendenhall syndrome). One relatively common condition that should be considered is hemochromatosis, or iron overload. Primary hemochromatosis is the most common genetic disorder in the United States, affecting approximately 1 in every 200 to 300 Americans. It is more common in persons of Western European heritage. It results from increased absorption of iron through the gastrointestinal tract, with excess iron deposition in many tissues (pancreas, liver, pituitary, etc). Traditional teaching has been that hyperglycemia results from iron deposition in the pancreas, leading to islet-cell dysfunction. However, recent data suggest that the pathogenesis involves primarily insulin resistance with secondary β-cell decompensation, as in routine cases of type 2 diabetes. Secondary hemochromatosis includes conditions characterized by increased red blood cell breakdown or a history of many blood transfusions (thalassemia, sideroblastic anemia, hemolytic anemia). The clues in this case include hypogonadism (due to hypogonadotropic hypogonadism from pituitary iron deposition) and hepatic dysfunction and enlargement. The initial approach to diagnosis is assessing markers of iron stores, which can be performed by measuring the total iron-binding capacity and serum ferritin (Answer B). These 2 tests are used to calculate the transferrin saturation, a more useful indication of iron stores than either measure alone.

Glutamic acid decarboxylase antibodies (Answer A) would be elevated if this were type 1 diabetes or latent autoimmune diabetes in adults, but these diagnoses seem unlikely. Although liver ultrasonography (Answer C) could reveal fatty liver, it would not diagnose hemochromatosis. Pituitary MRI (Answer D) is done after documenting secondary hypogonadism (after checking free testosterone, LH, and FSH).

Educational Objective
Diagnose hemochromatosis as a cause of secondary diabetes mellitus.

Reference(s)
Bacon BR, Adams PC, Kowdley KV, Powell LW, Tavill AS; American Association for the Study of Liver Diseases. Diagnosis and management of hemochromatosis: 2011 practice guideline by the American Association for the Study of Liver Diseases. *Hepatology.* 2011;54(1):328-343. PMID: 21452290

Hatunic M, Finucane FM, Brennan AM, Norris S, Pacini G, Nolan JJ. Effect of iron overload on glucose metabolism in patients with hereditary hemochromatosis. *Metabolism.* 2010;59(3):380-384. PMID: 19815242

14 ANSWER: D) Lifestyle intervention

Lifestyle intervention (Answer D) is preferred over metformin (Answer C) on the basis of findings from available studies, mainly the landmark Diabetes Prevention Program. In the Diabetes Prevention Program, 3234 obese patients (average BMI, 34 kg/m^2) aged 25 to 85 years (average age, 51 years) at high risk for diabetes (based on BMI ≥24 kg/m^2 and fasting and 2-hour plasma glucose concentrations of 96 to 125 mg/dL [5.3-6.9 mmol/L] and 140 to 199 mg/dL [7.8-11.1 mmol/L], respectively) were randomly assigned to one of the following groups:

- Intensive lifestyle changes with the aim of reducing weight by 7% through a behavioral modification program aimed at a low-fat diet and exercise for 150 minutes per week
- Treatment with metformin (850 mg twice daily) plus information on diet and exercise

- Placebo plus information on diet and exercise.

After an average follow-up of 3 years, fewer patients in the intensive lifestyle group developed diabetes, as diagnosed by fasting plasma glucose and 2-hour post-load glucose concentrations (14% vs 22% and 29% in the metformin and placebo groups, respectively). The intensive lifestyle and metformin interventions reduced the cumulative incidence of diabetes by 58% and 31%, respectively. Lifestyle intervention was effective in men and women in all age groups and in all ethnic groups.

In a follow-up observational study (the Diabetes Prevention Program Outcomes Study), the benefit of the lifestyle intervention was shown to persist more than 10 years. In this study, 85% of patients originally enrolled in the Diabetes Prevention Program joined the long-term follow-up and were offered group-implemented lifestyle intervention. Patients originally assigned to metformin continued receiving it (unblinded). During a cumulative 10 years of follow-up, the incidence of diabetes in the lifestyle and metformin groups was significantly reduced by 34% and 18%, respectively, compared with placebo.

The Actos Now for Prevention of Diabetes study assessed the ability of pioglitazone (Answer E) (30 to 45 mg daily) to reduce the risk of developing diabetes in 600 patients with impaired glucose tolerance and 1 or more components of the metabolic syndrome. After a median follow-up period of 2.4 years, fewer patients randomly assigned to pioglitazone developed diabetes (5.0% vs 16.7% with placebo; hazard ratio, 0.28; 95% confidence interval, 0.16-0.49). Weight gain was significantly greater with pioglitazone (3.9 vs 0.77 kg), and edema was more frequent (12.9% vs 6.4%). Pioglitazone should not be used for diabetes prevention in this patient because of potential adverse effects (fluid retention, weight gain, heart failure), especially since he already has 2+ edema on examination.

There are no studies on dapagliflozin (Answer B) or exenatide (Answer A) with respect to diabetes prevention.

Educational Objective

Identify prediabetes (impaired fasting glucose and impaired glucose tolerance) and recommend the best way to prevent progression to diabetes.

Reference(s)

Dunkley AJ, Bodicoat DH, Greaves CJ, et al. Diabetes prevention in the real world: effectiveness of pragmatic lifestyle interventions for the prevention of type 2 diabetes and of the impact of adherence to guideline recommendations: a systematic review and meta-analysis. *Diabetes Care.* 2014;37(4):922-933. PMID: 24652723

Knowler WC, Barrett-Connor E, Fowler SE, et al; Diabetes Prevention Program Research Group. Reduction in the incidence of type 2 diabetes with lifestyle intervention or metformin. *N Engl J Med.* 2002;346(6):393-403. PMID: 11832527

Diabetes Prevention Program Research Group, Knowler WC, Fowler SE, et al. 10-year follow-up of diabetes incidence and weight loss in the Diabetes Prevention Program Outcomes Study [published correction appears in *Lancet.* 2009; 374(9707):2054]. *Lancet.* 2009;374(9702):1677-1686. PMID: 19878986

DeFronzo RA, Tripathy D, Schwenke DC, et al; ACT NOW Study. Pioglitazone for diabetes prevention in impaired glucose tolerance [published corrections appear in *N Engl J Med.* 2011; 365(2):189 and *N Engl J Med.* 2011;365(9):869]. *N Engl J Med.* 2011;364(12):1104-1115. PMID: 21428766

15   ANSWER: C) Assessment for ketones

In patients with type 1 diabetes, the urine should be tested for ketones if the blood glucose concentration is above 300 mg/dL (>16.7 mmol/L) for unexplained reasons, especially if the person feels unwell at the time. Testing for ketonuria should also be performed during periods of illness or stress or if there are symptoms compatible with ketoacidosis such as nausea, vomiting, and abdominal pain. If ketonuria is present in the setting of hyperglycemia, diabetic ketoacidosis should be suspected and the patient should be ideally sent to the emergency department for more testing (serum ketones, electrolytes, bicarbonate, pH, etc) and treated accordingly with intravenous fluids and insulin drip if diabetic ketoacidosis is indeed present.

While basal rate testing (Answer A), diabetes education (Answer B), and a continuous glucose sensor (Answer D) are all needed to help this patient achieve a lower hemoglobin A_{1c}, none of these options is the best immediate step to take now. These steps can be done over weeks to months. Therapy for stress management (Answer E) is appropriate if she is willing to explore it, but again, this is not immediately necessary.

Educational Objective
Determine when checking urine ketones is appropriate in a patient with type 1 diabetes mellitus.

Reference(s)
Cao X, Zhang X, Xian Y, Wu J, et al. The diagnosis of diabetic acute complications using the glucose-ketone meter in outpatients at endocrinology department. *Int J Clin Exp Med*. 2014;7(12):5701-5705. PMID: 25664094

Weber C, Kocher S, Neeser K, Joshi SR. Prevention of diabetic ketoacidosis and self-monitoring of ketone bodies: an overview. *Curr Med Res Opin*. 2009;25(5):1197-1207. PMID: 19327102

Goldstein DE, Little RR, Lorenz RA, et al. Tests of glycemia in diabetes. *Diabetes Care*. 2004;27(7): 1761-1773. PMID: 15220264

16   ANSWER: A) 1.5 L of 0.9% NaCl over the first hour, and intravenous insulin bolus of 10 units then 10 units per hour

This patient meets the criteria for the hyperosmolar hyperglycemic state (also known as hyperosmotic hyperglycemic nonketotic state). The diagnostic criteria are a plasma glucose concentration greater than 600 mg/dL (>33.3 mmol/L), effective serum osmolality greater than 320 mOsm/kg (>320 mmol/kg), arterial pH greater than 7.30, serum bicarbonate greater than 18 mEq/L (>18 mmol/L), and severe dehydration with absence of or minimal ketoacidosis.

The most common precipitating factors for hyperosmolar hyperglycemic state are infection (often pneumonia or urinary tract infection) and discontinuation of or inadequate insulin therapy. Compromised water intake due to underlying medical conditions, particularly in older patients, can promote the development of severe dehydration and the hyperosmolar hyperglycemic state. Other conditions and factors associated with the hyperosmolar hyperglycemic state include acute major illnesses such as myocardial infarction, cerebrovascular accident, sepsis, or pancreatitis, etc.

The hyperosmolar hyperglycemic state is treated with fluids and insulin. Because of severe dehydration, isotonic 0.9% NaCl is initiated at a rate of 15 to 20 mL/kg over the first hour (thus, Answers C, D, and E are

incorrect). A decision is then made as to whether to continue the 0.9% NaCl or switch to 0.45% NaCl depending on volume status and corrected serum sodium. In fact, in this patient, the corrected serum sodium was 145 mEq/L (145 mmol/L) (serum sodium may be corrected by adding 1.6 mg/dL to the measured serum sodium for each 100 mg/dL of glucose above 100 mg/dL [>5.6 mmol/L]). Administration of hypertonic saline at 3.0% (Answer E) might worsen the hypernatremia and hyperosmolarity.

Intravenous insulin treatment can be initiated with an intravenous bolus of regular insulin (0.1 units/kg body weight) followed within 5 minutes by a continuous infusion of regular insulin of 0.1 units/kg per hour (bolus of 10 units and 10 units as a drip in this patient who weighs 220 lb [100 kg]) (thus, Answer B is incorrect). Alternatively, the bolus dose can be omitted if a higher dose of continuous intravenous regular insulin (0.14 units/kg per hour) is initiated.

The best approach for this patient is to administer 1.5 L of 0.9% NaCl over the first hour, and then an intravenous insulin bolus of 10 units followed by 10 units per hour (Answer A).

Educational Objective
Manage the hyperosmolar hyperglycemic state.

Reference(s)
Dhatariya KK, Vellanki P. Treatment of diabetic ketoacidosis (DKA)/hyperglycemic hyperosmolar state (HHS): novel advances in the management of hyperglycemic crises (UK versus USA). *Curr Diab Rep*. 2017;17(5):33. PMID: 28364357

Kitabchi AE, Umpierrez GE, Miles JM, Fisher JN. Hyperglycemic crises in adult patients with diabetes. *Diabetes Care*. 2009;32(7):1335-1343. PMID: 19564476

Nyenwe EA, Kitabchi AE. Evidence-based management of hyperglycemic emergencies in diabetes mellitus. *Diabetes Res Clin Pract*. 2011; 94(3):340-351. PMID: 21978840

17 ANSWER: D) Polysomnography

In both men and women, the strongest risk factor for obstructive sleep apnea is obesity. The prevalence of obstructive sleep apnea progressively increases as BMI and associated markers increase (eg, neck circumference, waist-to-hip ratio). In a prospective study of nearly 700 adults with 4-year longitudinal follow-up, a 10% increase in weight was associated with a 6-fold increase in the risk of incident obstructive sleep apnea. In a population-based study of more than 1000 adults who underwent polysomnography, moderate-to-severe obstructive sleep apnea (apnea-hypopnea index ≥15 events/h) was present in 11% of patients who were normal weight, 21% of those who were overweight (BMI, 25-30 kg/m^2), and 63% of those who were obese (BMI >30 kg/m^2).

Most patients with obstructive sleep apnea first come to the attention of a clinician because of fatigue, daytime sleepiness, or report by the patient's bed partner of loud snoring, gasping, snorting, or interruptions in breathing while sleeping. Diagnostic testing for obstructive sleep apnea should be performed in any patient with unexplained excessive daytime sleepiness, which is the clinically relevant symptom of obstructive sleep apnea that is most responsive to treatment. In the absence of excessive daytime sleepiness, diagnostic testing is pursued if the patient snores and either works in a mission-critical profession (eg, airline pilots, bus drivers, and truck drivers) or has 2 or more additional clinical features of obstructive sleep apnea.

Full-night, attended, in-laboratory polysomnography (Answer D) is considered the gold-standard diagnostic test for obstructive sleep apnea. It involves monitoring the patient during a full night's sleep. Patients in whom obstructive sleep apnea is diagnosed and who choose positive airway pressure therapy are subsequently brought back for another study, during which their positive airway pressure device is titrated. Split-night, attended, in-laboratory polysomnography is similar, except the diagnostic portion of the study is performed during the first part of the night only. Those patients in whom obstructive sleep apnea is diagnosed during the first part of the night and who choose positive airway pressure therapy can have their positive airway pressure device titrated during the second part of the night.

There is no role for a cosyntropin-stimulation test (Answer A). This patient has no other symptoms suggestive of adrenal insufficiency, and he has normal blood pressure and electrolytes.

Total testosterone can be lower than normal because of obesity. Obesity decreases the serum concentration of SHBG, thereby decreasing the serum total testosterone concentration, usually without lowering the free testosterone concentration. The binding abnormality is proportional to the degree of obesity and is corrected by weight loss. Therefore, before diagnosing hypogonadism, serum free testosterone should be measured by equilibrium dialysis. If it is normal, pituitary MRI (Answer B) and prolactin measurement (Answer C) are not necessary. This patient also has normal libido, which is consistent with a normal gonadal axis; the erectile dysfunction is most likely due to his diabetes and other comorbidities.

Free T$_4$ measurement (Answer E) is incorrect because the normal TSH level excludes primary hypothyroidism unless he has central hypothyroidism. However, there is no indication that he has hypothyroidism (no history of pituitary surgery, no radiation, and no obvious pituitary hormone abnormalities).

Educational Objective

Identify sleep apnea in obese patients with type 2 diabetes mellitus.

Reference(s)

Peppard PE, Young T, Barnet JH, Palta M, Hagen EW, Hla KM. Increased prevalence of sleep-disordered breathing in adults. *Am J Epidemiol.* 2013;177(9):1006-1014. PMID: 23589584

Qaseem A, Dallas P, Owens DK, Starkey M, Holty JE, Shekelle P; Clinical Guidelines Committee of the American College of Physicians. Diagnosis of obstructive sleep apnea in adults: a clinical practice guideline from the American College of Physicians. *Ann Intern Med.* 2014;161(3):210-220. PMID: 25089864

Cooper LA, Page ST, Amory JK, Anawalt BD, Matsumoto AM. The association of obesity with sex hormone-binding globulin is stronger than the association with ageing--implications for the interpretation of total testosterone measurements. *Clin Endocrinol (Oxf).* 2015; 83(6):828-833. PMID: 25777143

18 ANSWER: E) Pioglitazone

Nonalcoholic fatty liver disease (NAFLD) is observed worldwide and is the most common liver disorder in Western industrialized countries, where the major risk factors are common (central obesity, type 2 diabetes mellitus, dyslipidemia, and metabolic syndrome). One of the management options for NAFLD includes optimization of blood glucose control in those with diabetes. In addition, certain antidiabetes agents have been shown to improve liver histology such as steatosis, lobular inflammation, hepatocellular ballooning, and fibrosis.

The effect of thiazolidinediones on histologic parameters in nonalcoholic steatohepatitis (NASH) was examined in a meta-analysis of 4 randomized trials that compared thiazolidinediones with placebo in 334 patients with NASH. The analysis found that compared with placebo, thiazolidinediones were more likely to improve hepatic histologic parameters such as ballooning degeneration, lobular inflammation, and steatosis. Improvement in fibrosis was not seen when all thiazolidinediones were examined, but when the analysis was limited to 3 studies that used pioglitazone (Answer E), there was a significant improvement in fibrosis among patients treated with pioglitazone compared with placebo.

The effectiveness of metformin (Answer A) for the treatment of NASH was evaluated in a meta-analysis that included 3 randomized trials of metformin with histologic data available both before and after treatment. There was no difference between the patients who received metformin and the control patients with regard to histologic response (steatosis, ballooning, inflammation, or fibrosis) or changes in alanine aminotransferase levels.

There are no available data on changes in liver histology in patients with NASH and type 2 diabetes regarding dulaglutide (Answer C), dapagliflozin (Answer B), or sitagliptin (Answer D).

Another option to treat NASH is liraglutide. In a randomized trial, 52 patients with NASH (one-third had type 2 diabetes) were assigned to either receive liraglutide or placebo for 48 weeks. An end-of-treatment biopsy was performed in 23 patients in the liraglutide arm and in 22 patients in the placebo arm. NASH resolved in 9 patients (39%) who received liraglutide and in 2 patients (9%) who received placebo. With regard to fibrosis progression, patients who received liraglutide were less likely to have progression of fibrosis.

Educational Objective
Explain the effect of various antidiabetes agents on nonalcoholic steatohepatitis.

Reference(s)

Portillo-Sanchez P, Cusi K. Treatment of nonalcoholic fatty liver disease (NAFLD) in patients with type 2 diabetes mellitus. *Clin Diabetes Endocrinol.* 2016;2(9):1-9. PMID: 28702244

Rakoski MO, Singal AG, Rogers MA, Conjeevaram H. Meta-analysis: insulin sensitizers for the treatment of non-alcoholic steatohepatitis. *Aliment Pharmacol Ther.* 2010;32(10):1211-1221. PMID: 20955440

Armstrong MJ, Gaunt P, Aithal GP, et al. Liraglutide safety and efficacy in patients with non-alcoholic steatohepatitis (LEAN): a multicentre, double-blind, randomised, placebo-controlled phase 2 study. *Lancet.* 2016;387(10019):679-690. PMID: 26608256

19 ANSWER: A) 2-Hour oral glucose tolerance test

A 2-hour oral glucose tolerance test (Answer A) (with measurement of fasting and 2-hour glucose) is recommended for all women with polycystic ovary syndrome at initial diagnosis. If this is not feasible, fasting glucose should be measured together with glycated hemoglobin (hemoglobin A_{1c}). This approach is consistent with a number of professional organizations' guidelines (eg, the American College of Obstetricians and Gynecologists, American Association of Clinical Endocrinologists, the Endocrine Society, the Androgen Excess Society) and with a consensus panel representing the European Society of Human Reproduction and Embryology and the American Society of Reproductive Medicine.

The rationale for an oral glucose tolerance test is that a standard fasting glucose measurement (Answer D) lacks the sensitivity to detect impaired glucose tolerance or early type 2 diabetes that could be identified by an oral glucose tolerance test in a substantial number of women with polycystic ovary syndrome.

Limited studies have shown poor sensitivity of hemoglobin A_{1c} (Answer C) measurement for detecting impaired glucose tolerance.

In a retrospective observational study at an academic tertiary-care medical center, 208 premenopausal women with polycystic ovary syndrome underwent clinical evaluation (Ferriman-Gallwey score, BMI, waist circumference, blood pressure), hormone analyses (testosterone, SHBG, fasting lipids, insulin, glucose, hemoglobin A_{1c}), transvaginal ultrasonography, and 2-hour oral glucose tolerance tests measuring capillary blood glucose at 0 minutes and 120 minutes, insulin, and C-peptide. The main outcome measures were the results of the oral glucose tolerance test and hemoglobin A_{1c} values. Type 2 diabetes was diagnosed in 20 patients based on results of oral glucose tolerance testing. The sensitivity and specificity of a hemoglobin A_{1c} value of 6.5% or greater ($\geq$48 mmol/mol) for the diagnosis of diabetes were 35% and 99%, respectively, compared with the diagnosis established by oral glucose tolerance testing.

Patients with polycystic ovary syndrome and normal glucose tolerance should be rescreened at least once every 2 years or more frequently if additional risk factors are identified. Patients with impaired glucose tolerance should be screened annually for development of type 2 diabetes.

No tests of insulin resistance are necessary to diagnose polycystic ovary syndrome, nor are they needed to select treatments. There is currently no validated test for measuring insulin resistance in a clinical setting, including insulin levels (Answer B) or glucose-to-insulin ratios (Answer E).

Educational Objective

Guide the screening for prediabetes and type 2 diabetes in women with polycystic ovary syndrome.

Reference(s)

Velling Magnussen L, Mumm H, Andersen M, Glintborg D. Hemoglobin A1c as a tool for the diagnosis of type 2 diabetes in 208 premenopausal women with polycystic ovary syndrome. *Fertil Steril.* 2011;96(5):1275-1280. PMID: 21982282

Salley KE, Wickham EP, Cheang KI, Essah PA, Karjane NW, Nestler JE. Glucose intolerance in polycystic ovary syndrome--a position statement of the Androgen Excess Society. *J Clin Endocrinol Metab.* 2007;92(12):4546-4556. PMID: 18056778

American Association of Clinical Endocrinologists Polycystic Ovary Syndrome Writing Committee. American Association of Clinical Endocrinologists position statement on metabolic and cardiovascular consequences of polycystic ovary syndrome. *Endocr Pract.* 2005; 11(2):126-134. PMID: 15915567

Legro RS, Arslanian SA, Ehrmann DA, et al; Endocrine Society. Diagnosis and treatment of polycystic ovary syndrome: an Endocrine Society clinical practice guideline. *J Clin Endocrinol Metab.* 2013;98(12):4565-4592. PMID: 24151290

20 ANSWER: E) TPO antibodies

Up to 20% of patients with type 1 diabetes mellitus have positive antithyroid antibodies (TPO and/or thyroglobulin antibodies) (Answer E). Patients with circulating antibodies may be euthyroid, or they may develop autoimmune hypothyroidism, with a prevalence of about 2% to 5% in patients with type 1 diabetes. Rarely, children and adolescents with type 1 diabetes are hyperthyroid, with a reported prevalence of about 1%, with circulating thyroid-stimulating immunoglobulins (Answer B).

About 5% of patients with type 1 diabetes mellitus develop celiac disease (gluten-sensitive enteropathy diagnosed by a positive small-bowel biopsy sample), and 7% to 10% have tissue transglutaminase antibodies (Answer A).

Less than 1% to 2% of children and adolescents with type 1 diabetes have autoimmune adrenalitis with circulating antibodies to steroid 21-hydroxylase (Answer C).

Autoimmune polyglandular syndrome type 1, also referred to as the autoimmune polyendocrinopathy-candidiasis-ectodermal dystrophy (APECED) syndrome, is a rare autosomal recessive disorder. Hypoparathyroidism or chronic mucocutaneous candidiasis is usually the first manifestation, characteristically appearing during childhood or early adolescence, and always by the early 20s. Adrenal insufficiency usually develops later, at age 10 to 15 years. Hypoparathyroidism may or may not occur in association with parathyroid gland antibodies (Answer D) that are directed against the calcium-sensing receptor.

Educational Objective

List the prevalence of various autoimmune conditions (mostly Hashimoto thyroiditis) in patients with type 1 diabetes mellitus.

Reference(s)

Warncke K, Fröhlich-Reiterer EE, Thon A, et al; DPV Initiative of the German Working Group for Pediatric Diabetology; German BMBF Competence Network for Diabetes Mellitus. Polyendocrinopathy in children, adolescents, and young adults with type 1 diabetes: a multicenter analysis of 28,671 patients from the German/Austrian DPV-Wiss database. *Diabetes Care.* 2010;33(9):2010-2012. PMID: 20551013

Dost A, Rohrer TR, Fröhlich-Reiterer E, et al; DPV Initiative and the German Competence Network Diabetes Mellitus. Hyperthyroidism in 276 children and adolescents with type 1 diabetes from Germany and Austria. *Horm Res Paediatr.* 2015;84(3):190-198. PMID: 26202175

Likhari T, Magzoub S, Griffiths MJ, Buch HN, Gama R. Screening for Addison's disease in patients with type 1 diabetes mellitus and recurrent hypoglycaemia. *Postgrad Med J.* 2007; 83(980):420-421. PMID: 17551075

21 ANSWER: D) Refer for psychological evaluation

Eating disorders are relatively common in patients with diabetes, especially in female adolescents and young adults with type 1 diabetes. Eating disorders have a deleterious effect on glycemic control and on long-term outcome in these patients. One study evaluated 91 female patients with type 1 diabetes (mean age, 15 years) at baseline and at follow-up 4 to 5 years later. The following findings were noted:

Twenty-six (29%) had a self-reported eating disorder at baseline, which persisted in 16 (18%) at follow-up.

Among the patients with normal eating patterns at baseline, 15% had disordered eating at follow-up.

Dieting or omission of insulin for weight loss and bulimia nervosa were the most common eating disorders. Bulimia nervosa is characterized by recurrent episodes of binge eating and inappropriate compensatory

behaviors (such as self-induced vomiting), as well as frequent comorbid psychopathology. Insulin omission leading to weight loss is a unique purging behavior available to patients with type 1 diabetes, observed mainly in females.

Eating disorders are suspected in a patient with type 1 diabetes when there is poor glycemic control associated with recurrent episodes of diabetic ketoacidosis (due to omission of insulin) and recurrent hypoglycemia (deliberately inducing hypoglycemia through intentional insulin overdosing to justify eating sweets and high-carbohydrate meals, often followed by self-induced vomiting), frequently missed medical appointments, refusal to be weighed, and preoccupation with appearance. It is important to evaluate patients with diabetes, especially young women, for an eating disorder (or misreporting of insulin administration) and arrange appropriate psychological counseling and support when indicated (Answer D). Pharmacotherapy (Answer E) can be used at a later stage; first-line treatment is a selective serotonin reuptake inhibitor.

Switching to insulin pump therapy (Answer A) would not help, as her eating disorder must be addressed first. Her ACTH level, electrolytes, and blood pressure are normal, making Addison disease an extremely unlikely diagnosis. Thus, a cosyntropin-stimulation test (Answer B) is unnecessary. Biotin can lead to falsely low TSH in certain assays. Because this patient's TSH is normal, she is not hyperthyroid and there is no need to measure TSH again after the patient has stopped biotin (Answer C).

Educational Objective

Screen for eating disorders in patients with type 1 diabetes mellitus.

Reference(s)

Pinhas-Hamiel O, Hamiel U, Levy-Shraga Y. Eating disorders in adolescents with type 1 diabetes: challenges in diagnosis and treatment. *World J Diabetes.* 2015;6(3):517-526. PMID: 25897361

Mannucci E, Rotella F, Ricca V, Moretti S, Placidi GF, Rotella CM. Eating disorders in patients with type 1 diabetes: a meta-analysis. *J Endocrinol Invest.* 2005;28(5):417-419. PMID: 16075924

Ardabilygazir A, Afshariyamchlou S, Mir D, Sachmechi I. Effect of high-dose biotin on thyroid function tests: case report and literature review. *Cureus.* 2018;10(6):e2845. PMID: 30140596

22 ANSWER: E) Hepatic glucose output and β-cell dysfunction

GLP-1 is an incretin produced from the proglucagon gene in L cells of the small intestine and is secreted in response to nutrients. GLP-1 is deficient in patients with type 2 diabetes. DPP-4 inhibitors are a class of oral diabetes drugs that inhibit the enzyme DPP-4. This is a ubiquitous enzyme expressed on the surface of most cell types that deactivates GLP-1; therefore, its inhibition could potentially affect glucose regulation through multiple effects.

Incretin-based therapies include DPP-4 inhibitors and GLP-1 receptor agonists. DPP-4 inhibitors, through increasing endogenous GLP-1, can stimulate glucose-dependent insulin secretion from the β cells and can lower glucagon secretion, thereby lowering hepatic glucose output (Answer E). GLP-1 receptor agonists exert the same effects and, in addition, slow gastric emptying and decrease food intake.

DPP-4 inhibitors have no effect on insulin action (Answers A and D) or satiety (Answers B and C).

Educational Objective
Summarize the pathogenesis of type 2 diabetes mellitus and the mechanism of action of incretin therapies.

Reference(s)
DeFronzo RA, Eldor R, Abdul-Ghani M. Pathophysiologic approach to therapy in patients with newly diagnosed type 2 diabetes. *Diabetes Care.* 2013;36(Suppl 2):S127-S138. PMID: 23882037

Demuth HU, McIntosh CH, Pederson RA. Type 2 diabetes--therapy with dipeptidyl peptidase IV inhibitors. *Biochim Biophys Acta.* 2005;1751(1): 33-44. PMID: 15978877

Koliaki C, Doupis J. Incretin-based therapy: a powerful and promising weapon in the treatment of type 2 diabetes mellitus. *Diabetes Ther.* 2011; 2(2):101-121. PMID: 22127804

23 ANSWER: D) Diazepam

This patient has stiff-person syndrome (SPS), formerly called stiff-man syndrome. This disorder is characterized by progressive muscle stiffness, rigidity, and spasm involving the axial muscles, resulting in severely impaired ambulation. It is caused by increased muscle activity due to decreased inhibition of the CNS that results from the blockade of glutamic acid decarboxylase, an enzyme critical for maintaining inhibitory pathways in the CNS. The subsequent decline in the levels of gamma amino butyric acid (GABA) in the CNS due to glutamic acid decarboxylase antibodies causes a loss of neural inhibition. SPS is often associated with type 1 diabetes mellitus (type 1 diabetes is observed in about 30% of patients with SPS), which may be a reflection of shared pathogenetic features, as well as other autoimmune disorders. It may rarely occur as a paraneoplastic syndrome.

Establishing the diagnosis of SPS requires a high index of suspicion. The presence of the following features is generally considered necessary for making the diagnosis, although there are no formally accepted criteria:

Stiffness in the axial and limb muscles resulting in impairment of ambulation

Presence of superimposed episodic spasms that are precipitated by sudden movement, noise, or emotional upset

A positive therapeutic response to oral diazepam or findings of continuous motor-unit activity on electromyography that are abolished by intravenous diazepam (Answer D)

Absence of other neurologic disorders that may explain the clinical features

Prednisone (Answer A), gabapentin (Answer B), amitriptyline (Answer C), and potassium (Answer E) are not effective in treating SPS. Long-term, high-dosage glucocorticoid therapy might work, but glucocorticoids are avoided because of the resultant associated adverse effects in patients with diabetes.

Educational Objective
Diagnose stiff-person syndrome in a patient with type 1 diabetes mellitus.

Reference(s)

Sarva H, Deik A, Ullah A, Severt WL. Clinical spectrum of stiff person syndrome: a review of fecent reports. *Tremor Other Hyperkinet Mov (N Y)*. 2016;6:340. PMID: 26989571

Baizabal-Carvallo JF, Jankovic J. Stiff-person syndrome: insights into a complex autoimmune disorder. *J Neurol Neurosurg Psychiatry*. 2015; 86(8):840-848. PMID: 25511790

McKeon A, Robinson MT, McEvoy KM, et al. Stiff-man syndrome and variants: clinical course, treatments, and outcomes. *Arch Neurol*. 2012; 69(2):230-238. PMID: 22332190

24 ANSWER: B) Split the insulin bolus into standard/extended for high-fat meals

Food contains 3 different fuels (carbohydrate, fat, and proteins) that affect glycemia through different mechanisms. The fat in certain foods such as ice cream may delay the absorption of carbohydrates from the gastrointestinal tract and reduce the expected rise in blood glucose, leading to early hypoglycemia from the insulin bolus. Certain high-fat meals such as pizza create a rapid temporary insulin resistance (high free fatty acids from high-fat meals cause insulin resistance) for up to 6 to 12 hours after a meal, making blood glucose rise later after the insulin bolus effect is gone. Also, excess free fatty acids contribute to gluconeogenesis.

In addition, large quantities of protein, such as a 12-ounce steak, can cause a rise in blood glucose. Almost 50% of protein calories are slowly converted to glucose (amino acids contribute to gluconeogenesis) over a period of several hours (4-12 hours). Excessive amino acid availability can interfere with insulin action.

In this case of a high-fat meal, the only solution is to split the bolus into standard/extended bolus where the percentage of each component varies depending on the meal and the patient (Answer B). It could start with 50%/50% split where the extended bolus is given over 2 hours. Then, depending on results, the percentage and duration of the extended bolus could be changed accordingly.

Changing his insulin-to-carbohydrate ratio to 1 unit per 12 g for high-fat meals (Answer A) is incorrect because less insulin would make the late hyperglycemia worse. Aspart-niacinamide (Answer D) is faster acting than aspart and would exacerbate the early hypoglycemia. Eating more carbohydrates (Answer C) would lead to more weight gain and his BMI is already higher than normal. Metoclopramide (Answer E) is used to treat gastroparesis, which the patient does not have.

Educational Objective

Explain the benefit of extended insulin bolus with high-fat meals.

Reference(s)

Lopez PE, Smart CE, McElduff P, et al. Optimizing the combination insulin bolus split for a high-fat, high-protein meal in children and adolescents using insulin pump therapy. *Diabet Med*. 2017; 34(10):1380-1384. PMID: 28574182

Van der Hoogt M, van Dyk JC, Doman RC, Pieters M. Protein and fat meal content increase insulin requirement in children with type 1 diabetes – role of duration of diabetes. *J Clin Transl Endocrinol*. 2017;10:15-21. PMID: 29204367

Bell KJ, Toschi E, Steil GM, Wolpert HA. Optimized mealtime insulin dosing for fat and protein in type 1 diabetes: application of a model-based approach to derive insulin doses for open-loop diabetes management. *Diabetes Care*. 2016;39(9):1631-1634. PMID: 27388474

25 ANSWER: A) Eat breakfast, take insulin glargine (14 units) and insulin lispro with an insulin-to-carbohydrate ratio of 1:20

With an adequate concentration of insulin on board, aerobic activities are associated with reductions in blood glucose concentrations. By contrast, anaerobic activities usually do not reduce blood glucose concentrations, and may be associated with elevations in glycemia in certain circumstances. Aerobic exercise is associated with a more modest rise (2- to 4-fold) in catecholamines, while anaerobic exercise is associated with a much higher increase in catecholamine release (14- to 18-fold rise). It is also well established that exercise increases muscle glucose uptake through insulin-dependent and insulin-independent mechanisms. Glycemia during exercise is also affected by substrate availability, as well as insulin concentrations. The net balance effect varies between individuals. However, in general, assuming insulin is present and the blood glucose level is within the normal range, aerobic activity can lead to hypoglycemia, usually during or immediately after exercise, although in some patients, delayed hypoglycemia hours after exercise can be seen.

In the presented scenario, the best way to prevent hypoglycemia is to cut back on the mealtime bolus by 50%, just an hour before playing tennis (Answer A). Skipping insulin glargine (Answers B and D) would lead to late hyperglycemia and possibly diabetic ketoacidosis, as skipping basal insulin could cause ketone formation in this setting. Taking the full bolus at breakfast could lead to hypoglycemia during exercise and lowering the insulin glargine dose (Answer C) could lead to late hyperglycemia.

Educational Objective

Manage insulin therapy during exercise.

Reference(s)

Colberg SR, Laan R, Dassau E, Kerr D. Physical activity and type 1 diabetes: time for a rewire? *J Diabetes Sci Technol.* 2015;9(3):609-618. PMID: 25567144

Thabit H, Leelarathna L. Basal insulin delivery reduction for exercise in type 1 diabetes: finding the sweet spot. *Diabetologia.* 2016;59(8):1628-1631. PMID: 27287376

Basu R, Johnson ML, Kudva YC, Basu A. Exercise, hypoglycemia, and type 1 diabetes. *Diabetes Technol Ther.* 2014;16(6):331-337. PMID: 24811269

26 **ANSWER: C) Aspart-niacinamide**

Faster-acting insulin aspart injection is a rapid-acting insulin analogue for subcutaneous administration used to lower blood glucose. Aspart is homologous with regular human insulin with the exception of a single substitution of the amino acid proline by aspartic acid in position B28. Addition of niacinamide (vitamin B_3) to aspart (Answer C) promotes formation of insulin aspart monomers after subcutaneous injection, leading to more rapid absorption of faster aspart into the bloodstream than conventional insulin aspart. In a pooled analysis of 6 randomized controlled trials in participants with type 1 diabetes, onset of appearance was twice as fast and early insulin exposure was 2-fold greater, leading to a 74%

greater early glucose-lowering effect with faster-acting insulin aspart than with conventional insulin aspart.

In the Onset trials, the primary endpoint was change in hemoglobin A_{1c} concentrations from baseline to the end of the trial. There were no significant differences in most of the trials between faster-acting insulin aspart and conventional insulin aspart in terms of hemoglobin A_{1c} reduction. However, postprandial plasma glucose control was better with faster-acting insulin aspart, at least in the first 30 to 60 minutes after a meal. Safety (hypoglycemia) and tolerability of both insulins was similar in most trials.

Glulisine-fatty acid (Answer A), aspart-arginine (Answer B), and glulisine-glutamic acid (Answer D) do not exist.

Note: Image in stem is reprinted from the prescribing information for FIASP [package insert]. Plainsboro, NJ: Novo Nordisk Inc; September 2018. (used with permission of Novo Nordisk Inc.; © 2018 Novo Nordisk, all rights reserved)

Educational Objective

Determine when fast-acting insulin aspart is an option to treat diabetes mellitus.

Reference(s)

Davis A, Kuriakose J, Clements JN. Faster insulin aspart: a new bolus option for diabetes mellitus. *Clin Pharmacokinet.* 2019;58(4):421-430. PMID: 29978361

Russell-Jones D, Bode BW, De Block C, et al. Fast-acting insulin aspart improves glycemic control in basal-bolus treatment for type 1 diabetes: results of a 26-week multicenter, active-controlled, treat-to-target, randomized, parallel-group trial (onset 1). *Diabetes Care.* 2017;40(7): 943-950. PMID: 28356319

Bowering K, Case C, Harvey J, et al. Faster aspart versus insulin aspart as part of a basal-bolus regimen in inadequately controlled type 2 diabetes: the onset 2 trial. *Diabetes Care.* 2017; 40(7):951-957. PMID: 28483786

FIASP [package insert]. Plainsboro, NJ: Novo Nordisk Inc; September 2018.

27 ANSWER: E) Stop vitamin C, as it can interfere with sensor glucose readings

The flash glucose monitoring system was approved by the US FDA in October 2017 and became available by prescription in the United States by the end of 2017. Calibration free, it is a disk worn on the arm for 10 to 14 days, which is designed to largely replace the recommended 4 to 10 painful fingerstick blood glucose readings required each day for the self-management of diabetes. The initial device was designed for 10 days, but in August 2018 the US FDA approved the 14-day version.

In randomized controlled trials, use of the flash glucose monitoring system is associated with reduced hypoglycemia and, in observational studies, with improved hemoglobin A_{1c} levels. User satisfaction is high and adverse events are low. Accuracy of this system in adults, children, and in women during pregnancy is comparable to that of currently available real-time continuous glucose monitors. The cost of the flash glucose monitoring system is lower than that of real-time continuous glucose monitors.

Glucose data can be visualized in multiple devices and platforms and summarized in an ambulatory glucose profile to aid pattern recognition and adjustment of insulin doses. Both users and health care professionals must be appropriately educated to harness the full benefits. Further randomized controlled trials to assess the long-term impact on hemoglobin A_{1c}, particularly in patients with high baseline hemoglobin A_{1c} values and in specific age groups (eg, such as adolescents and young adults), are warranted. The potential effect on diabetes-related complications is yet to be realized.

The manufacturer has undertaken tests to evaluate the flash glucose monitoring system with 16 potentially interfering substances. Testing confirmed no clinically significant interference for the substances tested, with the exception of ascorbic acid and salicylic acid. Taking ascorbic acid may falsely raise glucose readings and salicylic acid may slightly lower glucose readings. The level of inaccuracy depends on the amount of interfering substance.

In this patient, high doses of vitamin C led to falsely high sensor glucose readings. Therefore, vitamin C should be stopped (Answer E). Cinnamon (Answer C) and acetaminophen (Answer D) do not interfere with sensor readings. The patient's diabetes is well-controlled and her normal blood glucose values determined by fingerstick are consistent with her hemoglobin A_{1c} value. Therefore, it would be incorrect to adjust her insulin based on the sensor data (Answer A). Changing the site of the sensor from the arm to the abdomen (Answer B) is incorrect because the arm is the FDA-approved site. One study showed that the accuracy and precision of the flash glucose monitoring system placed on the upper thigh are similar to those when it is worn on the upper arm, but the abdomen performed unacceptably poorly.

The table summarizes the main features of the flash glucose monitoring system (*see table*).

Table 1. Overview of Features in the FreeStyle Libre Systems Approved in the United States

This overview is representative of the FreeStyle Libre systems approved in the United States at time of publication.* The FreeStyle Libre system is approved in the European Union (EU) as of September 2014 and in the United States as of November 2017. The FreeStyle Libre 14 day system is approved in the United States as of July 2018. EU and US systems have differences in patient indication and interface options. Refer to the table for features of US approved systems only.	
Minimum use age:	≥18 years
Sensor placement:	Back of arm; placement is not approved for other sites
Sensor warm-up period:	▶ FreeStyle Libre system: 12 hours after insertion before able to retrieve glucose data ▶ FreeStyle Libre 14 day system: 1 hour after insertion before able to retrieve glucose data
Sensor wear time:	▶ FreeStyle Libre system: 10 days ▶ FreeStyle Libre 14 day system: 14 days
Calibration:	Factory calibrated; does not require daily calibration
Insulin dosing:	Individuals are able to use sensor glucose reading for treatment decisions without confirmatory fingerstick monitoring. Under the following conditions, sensor glucose readings may not be accurate, and you should conduct a fingerstick: ▶ If inaccurate reading is suspected ▶ If experiencing symptoms that may be due to low or high blood glucose ▶ If experiencing symptoms that do not match sensor glucose readings ▶ During times of rapidly changing glucose of more than 2 mg/dL per minute (i.e., straight up or down trend arrow) ▶ When the sensor glucose reading does not include a current glucose number or trend arrow ▶ To confirm hypoglycemia or impending hypoglycemia as reported by the sensor ▶ When "Check Blood Glucose" symbol appears in the reader ▶ During the first 12 hours of wearing a FreeStyle Libre 14 day Sensor
Cautions and Contraindications:	▶ The system is not approved for use in pregnant women or persons on dialysis and has not been evaluated in these populations. ▶ The system has not been evaluated for use in patients with hypoglycemia unawareness and will not automatically alert to current or impending hypoglycemic event without scanning the sensor. The system will not automatically notify the user when experiencing hypoglycemia or hyperglycemia unless the sensor is scanned.
Potential Interferents:	▶ Salicylic acid (used in aspirin and other pain relievers) at doses ≥650 mg may cause falsely lower glucose values ▶ Ascorbic acid (vitamin C) at doses ≥500 mg may cause falsely higher readings. ▶ At lower doses, salicylic acid and ascorbic acid are known to have minimal effect on sensor glucose readings in the FreeStyle Libre systems.

* For full indications for use and safety information, seek out product information from the manufacturer.

Table reproduced with permissions from Kudva YC, Ahmann AJ, Bergenstal RM, et al. Approach to using trend arrows in the FreeStyle Libre Flash Glucose Monitoring Systems in adults. *J Endoc Soc.* 2018;2(12):1320-1337. PMID: 20474069

Educational Objective
List the substances known to interfere with glucose readings derived from the flash glucose monitoring system.

Reference(s)
Leelarathna L, Wilmot EG. Flash forward: a review of flash glucose monitoring. *Diabetic Med.* 2018; 35(4):472-482. PMID: 29356072

Chen C, Zhao XL, Li ZH, Zhu ZG, Qian SH, Flewitt AJ. Current and emerging technology for continuous glucose monitoring. *Sensors (Basel)*. 2017;17(1):pii: E182. PMID: 28106820

Charleer S, Mathieu C, Nobels F, Gillard P. Accuracy and precision of flash glucose monitoring sensors inserted into the abdomen and upper thigh compared with the upper arm. *Diabetes Obes Metab*. 2018;20(6):1503-1507. PMID: 29381253

Kudva YC, Ahmann AJ, Bergenstal RM, et al. Approach to using trend arrows in the FreeStyle Libre Flash Glucose Monitoring Systems in adults. *J Endoc Soc*. 2018;2(12):1320-1337. PMID: 20474069

28 ANSWER: C) Aspirin

The 2018 American Diabetes Association guidelines recommend the following:

- Use aspirin therapy (75-162 mg daily) as a secondary prevention strategy in those with diabetes and a history of atherosclerotic cardiovascular disease (level of evidence: A)
- For patients with atherosclerotic cardiovascular disease and documented aspirin allergy, clopidogrel (75 mg daily) should be used (level of evidence: B)
- Dual antiplatelet therapy (with low-dosage aspirin and a P2Y12 inhibitor) is reasonable for a year after an acute coronary syndrome (level of evidence: A) and may have benefits beyond this period (level of evidence: B)
- Aspirin therapy (75-162 mg daily) may be considered as a primary prevention strategy in those with type 1 or type 2 diabetes who are at increased cardiovascular risk. This includes most men and women with diabetes aged 50 years or older who have at least 1 additional major risk factor (family history of premature atherosclerotic cardiovascular disease, hypertension, dyslipidemia, smoking, or albuminuria) and are not at increased risk of bleeding (level of evidence: C)

Recently, a large randomized controlled trial compared aspirin, 100 mg daily, vs placebo in patients with diabetes but no evident cardiovascular disease. The primary efficacy outcome was the first serious vascular event (ie, myocardial infarction, stroke, or transient ischemic attack, or death from any vascular cause, excluding any confirmed intracranial hemorrhage). The primary safety outcome was the first major bleeding event (ie, intracranial hemorrhage, sight-threatening bleeding event in the eye, gastrointestinal bleeding, or other serious bleeding). Secondary outcomes included gastrointestinal tract cancer. A total of 15,480 participants were included. During a mean follow-up of 7.4 years, serious vascular events occurred in a significantly lower percentage of participants in the aspirin group than in the placebo group (658 participants [8.5%] vs 743 [9.6%]; rate ratio, 0.88; 95% confidence interval, 0.79-0.97; *P* = .01). In contrast, major bleeding events occurred in 314 participants (4.1%) in the aspirin group, compared with 245 (3.2%) in the placebo group (rate ratio, 1.29; 95% confidence interval, 1.09-1.52; *P* = .003), with most of the excess being gastrointestinal bleeding and other extracranial bleeding. There was no significant difference between the aspirin group and the placebo group in the incidence of gastrointestinal tract cancer (157 [2.0%] and 158 [2.0%] participants, respectively) or all cancers (897 [11.6%] and 887 [11.5%] participants, respectively). Long-term follow-up of these outcomes is planned. Aspirin use prevented serious vascular events in persons who had diabetes and no evident cardiovascular disease at trial entry, but it also caused major bleeding events. The absolute benefits were largely counterbalanced by the bleeding hazard.

Neither lixisenatide (Answer B) nor sitagliptin (Answer D) has been shown to significantly lower the 3-point major adverse cardiovascular events in their respective cardiovascular outcomes trials, ELIXA (Evaluation of Lixisenatide in Acute Coronary Syndrome) and TECOS (Trial Evaluating Cardiovascular Outcomes with Sitagliptin). Empagliflozin (Answer A) did significantly lower major adverse cardiovascular events, but more than 99% of patients had established cardiovascular disease (secondary prevention) as opposed to the patient in this vignette who is not known to have cardiovascular disease (primary prevention).

Educational Objective
Determine when low-dosage aspirin is indicated in patients with diabetes mellitus as a primary prevention strategy for cardiovascular disease.

Reference(s)

American Diabetes Association. 10. Cardiovascular disease and risk management: standards of medical care in diabetes-2019. *Diabetes Care.* 2019;41(Suppl 1):S103-S123. PMID: 30559236

The ASCEND Study Collaborative Group, Bowman L, Mafham M, et al. Effects of aspirin for primary prevention in persons with diabetes mellitus. *N Engl J Med.* 2018;379(16):1529-1539. PMID: 30146931

Cefalu WT, Kaul S, Gerstein HC, et al. Cardiovascular outcomes trials in type 2 diabetes: where do we go from here? Reflections from a Diabetes Care Editors' Expert Forum. *Diabetes Care.* 2018; 41(1):14-31. PMID: 29263194

29 ANSWER: D) Add insulin glargine, 10 units at bedtime

This patient has chronic kidney disease and symptoms and signs of heart failure. Saxagliptin (Answer A) should not be used. Among the recent cardiovascular safety outcomes trials testing DPP-4 inhibitors, the SAVORTIMI53 study (Saxagliptin Assessment of Vascular Outcomes Recorded in Patients with Diabetes Mellitus–Thrombolysis in Myocardial Infarction 53) demonstrated a 3.5% risk of hospitalization for heart failure with saxagliptin vs 2.8% with placebo (hazard ratio, 1.27; 95% confidence interval, 1.07-1.51; *P* = .007). The new American Diabetes Association/European Association for the Study of Diabetes guidelines also warn against the use of saxagliptin in the setting of heart failure (the drug has a warning on its label). In addition, when the estimated glomerular filtration rate is less than 50 mL/min per 1.73 m^2, saxagliptin should be used at a dosage of 2.5 mg daily.

Glimepiride, 4 mg daily (half-maximum dosage) is the maximal effective dosage. Going up to 8 mg daily (Answer B) will not result in any significant decrease in hemoglobin A$_{1c}$.

Metformin (Answer C) should not be used in patients with an estimated glomerular filtration rate less than 30 mL/min per 1.73 m^2, and a dosage reduction (to 1000 mg daily or less) should be considered when the estimated glomerular filtration rate is less than 45 mL/min per 1.73 m^2. In addition, metformin should not be used in the setting of acute heart failure because of the potential for lactic acidosis. In this patient, the metformin dosage should certainly not be increased (Answer C), and an argument could be made that metformin should be stopped until he undergoes cardiac evaluation.

Although empagliflozin (Answer E) would be beneficial in a patient with type 2 diabetes who has heart failure, it is not indicated in patients with an estimated glomerular filtration rate less than 45 mL/min per 1.73 m^2.

The only correct option is adding insulin glargine (Answer D), as this is the only safe way to decrease the hemoglobin A$_{1c}$ to goal in a patient with possible heart failure, as well as kidney disease.

Educational Objective

Recommend insulin therapy in a patient with uncontrolled type 2 diabetes mellitus who has a decreased glomerular filtration rate and possible heart failure.

Reference(s)

Davies MJ, D'Alessio DA, Fradkin J, et al. Management of hyperglycemia in type 2 diabetes, 2018. A consensus report by the American Diabetes Association (ADA) and the European Association for the Study of Diabetes (EASD). *Diabetes Care.* 2018;41(12):2669-2701. PMID: 30291106

Scirica BM, Bhatt DL, Braunwald E, et al; SAVOR-TIMI 53 Steering Committee and Investigators. Saxagliptin and cardiovascular outcomes in patients with type 2 diabetes mellitus. *N Engl J Med.* 2013;369(14):1317-1326. PMID: 23992601

30 ANSWER: D) Liraglutide

Overall, cardiovascular outcome trials of DPP-4 inhibitors have demonstrated safety (ie, noninferiority relative to placebo for the primary major adverse cardiovascular events endpoint, but not cardiovascular benefit). The TECOS trial (Trial Evaluating Cardiovascular Outcomes with Sitagliptin) comparing sitagliptin with placebo showed no cardiovascular benefit with sitagliptin (Answer A).

In the SUSTAIN 6 trial (Trial to Evaluate Cardiovascular and Other Long-term Outcomes with Semaglutide in Subjects with Type 2 Diabetes), semaglutide (Answer A) compared with placebo demonstrated an absolute risk reduction of 2.3% with a hazard ratio of 0.74 for major adverse cardiovascular events (95% confidence interval, 0.58-0.95; *P* = .02 for superiority) over 2.1 years. However, the reduction in events appeared to be driven by the rate of stroke rather than death due to cardiovascular disease. The EXSCEL trial (Exenatide Study of Cardiovascular Event Lowering) compared exenatide extended-release with placebo over 3.2 years in 14,752 participants with type 2 diabetes. While the medication was safe (noninferior), the hazard ratio for major adverse cardiovascular events in the entire trial was 0.91 (95% confidence interval, 0.83-1.0; $P = .06$), which did not reach the threshold for demonstrated superiority vs placebo; absolute risk reduction was 0.8%. All-cause death was lower in the exenatide arm (absolute risk reduction, 1%; hazard ratio, 0.86; 95% confidence interval, 0.77-0.97), but it was not considered to be significant in the hierarchical testing procedure applied.

Liraglutide (Answer D), studied in the LEADER trial (Liraglutide Effect and Action in Diabetes: Evaluation of Cardiovascular Outcome Results) demonstrated an absolute risk reduction of 1.9% with a hazard ratio of 0.87 (95% confidence interval, 0.78-0.97; $P = .01$ for superiority) for the primary composite outcome of cardiovascular death, nonfatal myocardial infarction, and nonfatal stroke (major adverse cardiac events) compared with placebo over 3.8 years. Each component of the composite contributed to the benefit, and the hazard ratio for cardiovascular death was 0.78 (95% confidence interval, 0.66-0.93; $P = .007$; absolute risk reduction, 1.7%). The LEADER trial also demonstrated a hazard ratio of 0.85 (95% confidence interval, 0.74-0.97; $P = .02$; absolute risk reduction, 1.4%) for all-cause mortality.

Canagliflozin compared with placebo was studied in the CANVAS Program (Canagliflozin Cardiovascular Assessment Study), composed of 2 similar trials—CANVAS and CANVAS Renal) in participants with type 2 diabetes, 66% of whom had a history of cardiovascular disease. Participants were followed for a median of 3.6 years. In the combined analysis of the 2 trials, the primary composite endpoint of myocardial infarction, stroke, or cardiovascular death was reduced with canagliflozin (26.9 vs 31.5 participants per patient-year with placebo; hazard ratio, 0.86; 95% confidence interval, 0.75-0.97; $P = .02$) for superiority in the pooled analysis. Findings were consistent in the component studies. Although there was a trend toward benefit regarding cardiovascular death, the difference compared with placebo was not significant in the CANVAS Program.

Educational Objective

Compare and contrast the cardiovascular outcome trials in diabetes mellitus.

Reference(s)

Davies MJ, D'Alessio DA, Fradkin J, et al. Management of hyperglycemia in type 2 diabetes, 2018. A consensus report by the American Diabetes Association (ADA) and the European Association for the Study of Diabetes (EASD). *Diabetes Care*. 2018;41(12):2669-2701. PMID: 30291106

Green JB, Bethel MA, Armstrong PW, et al; TECOS Study Group. Effect of sitagliptin on cardiovascular outcomes in type 2 diabetes. *N Engl J Med*. 2015;373(3):232-242. PMID: 26052984

Neal B, Perkovic V, Matthews DR. Canagliflozin and cardiovascular and renal events in type 2 diabetes. *N Engl J Med*. 2017;377(21):2099. PMID: 29166232

Marso SP, Bain SC, Consoli A, et al; SUSTAIN-6 Investigators. Semaglutide and cardiovascular outcomes in patients with type 2 diabetes. *N Engl J Med*. 2016;375(19):1834-1844. PMID: 27633186

Marso SP, Daniels GH, Brown-Frandsen K, et al; LEADER Steering Committee; LEADER Trial Investigators. Liraglutide and cardiovascular outcomes in type 2 diabetes. *N Engl J Med*. 2016; 375(4):311-322. PMID: 27295427

Holman RR, Bethel MA, Mentz RJ, et al; EXSCEL Study Group. Effects of once-weekly exenatide on cardiovascular outcomes in type 2 diabetes. *N Engl J Med*. 2017;377(13):1228-1239. PMID: 28910237

Diabetes Mellitus Section 2 Board Review

Michelle F. Magee, MD

31 **ANSWER: C) Administer insulin lispro, 10 units with meals; discontinue insulin drip 2 to 3 hours after the first dose of glargine is administered**

Transition from intravenous to subcutaneous insulin therapy is frequently accompanied by rebound hyperglycemia. Patients with type 1 diabetes on intravenous infusions who are transferring from the intensive care unit to a medical-surgical ward require transition to subcutaneous insulin management to meet basal, nutritional, and corrective (supplemental) insulin requirements. Subcutaneous insulin requirements can be calculated from the estimated total daily insulin dose while on stable intravenous insulin therapy, may be weight-based, or may be based on the preadmission insulin regimen if it was providing adequate glycemic control.

The first consideration in making this transition from intravenous to subcutaneous insulin is determination of appropriate dosing of basal insulin. When the insulin drip rate is used as the basis for the determination of the total daily insulin requirement at the time of transition to subcutaneous insulin, several studies recommend starting at a daily insulin dose that is approximately 60% to 80% of the total number of units of intravenous insulin used in the preceding 12 to 24 hours. In this case, this represents the patient's basal insulin requirement, as he was not eating while in the intensive care unit, so it is 40 units of insulin glargine. This may be given once daily or split into 2 doses.

The second consideration in this case is determining an appropriate mealtime insulin dose. The meal dose of 10 units of insulin in this case is calculated as 0.1 units/kg with each meal, and when it is administered as a rapid-acting insulin analogue (lispro), it can be given with or even directly at the end of the meal.

Finally, the timing of when the insulin drip is to be stopped must be considered. It is important to allow time to the onset of action of the first injection of subcutaneous insulin before stopping the drip to prevent rebound hyperglycemia. In the presented scenario, it is 9 AM and the patient will most likely not eat until after transfer from the intensive care unit, so the first dose of basal insulin may be given now and the drip should be stopped 2 hours later to allow time for the onset of action of the long-acting insulin (Answer C). This will help avoid rebound hyperglycemia.

A mealtime dose of 15 units of insulin lispro (Answer A) is high for this man. It would lead to a skewed distribution of prandial to basal insulin, with more than 50% of his total daily dose being prandial, which would increase the risk for hypoglycemia. It is considered prudent to underestimate, rather than overestimate, the amount of insulin given with meals, especially when the patient is just beginning to eat. It is generally considered safe to limit the allocation of daily insulin given with meals or enteral feedings to 40% of the total daily insulin dose.

When regular insulin is given with meals (Answer B), it must be administered 30 to 45 minutes before the meal to allow time for the onset of action to enable coverage of the postprandial blood glucose rise. However, 3 units of regular insulin, while given with sufficient time to allow for its onset of action before meals (Answer D), will most likely be too little to control his postprandial blood glucose. If the drip were being stopped at a meal, the first dose of mealtime insulin could be given and the insulin drip could be stopped concurrent with the first dose of a rapid-acting insulin analogue (lispro in this case) or 30 minutes after administration of regular insulin.

Finally, an additional strategy that can help to avoid posttransition rebound hyperglycemia is to begin subcutaneous insulin as once-daily basal insulin therapy at a dosage of 0.25 units/kg per day starting within 12 hours of initiating intravenous insulin therapy.

Educational Objective
Devise a rational plan for transitioning from intravenous insulin to a subcutaneous insulin regimen in hospitalized patients.

Reference(s)

Handelsman Y, Blomgarden ZT, Grunberger G, et al. American Association of Clinical Endocrinologists and American College of Endocrinology - clinical practice guidelines for developing a diabetes mellitus comprehensive care plan - 2015. *Endocr Pract.* 2015;21(Suppl 1):1-87. PMID: 25869408

American Diabetes Association. 14. Diabetes care in the hospital: standards of medical care in diabetes-2018. *Diabetes Care.* 2018;41(Suppl 1):S144-S151. PMID: 29222385

Umpierrez GE, Hellman R, Korytkowski MT, et al; Endocrine Society. Management of hyperglycemia in hospitalized patients in non-critical care setting: an Endocrine Society clinical practice guideline. *J Clin Endocrinol Metab.* 2012;97(1):16-38. PMID: 22223765

Hsia E, Seggelke S, Gibbs J, et al. Subcutaneous administration of glargine to diabetic patients receiving insulin infusion prevents rebound hyperglycemia. *J Clin Endocrinol Metab.* 2012;97(9):3132-3137. PMID: 22685233

32 ANSWER: D) Basal insulin daily plus regular insulin every 6 hours when his blood glucose is greater than 180 mg/dL (>10.0 mmol/L) to achieve most blood glucose values between 140 and 180 mg/dL (7.8-10.0 mmol/L)

It is now widely accepted that proper attention to glycemic management both in the intensive care unit and in the general medical-surgical wards is an important aspect of high-quality, safe inpatient care. A 2009 American Association of Clinical Endocrinologists–American Diabetes Association consensus statement endorsed the use of intravenous insulin in the intensive care unit setting, targeting blood glucose values between 140 and 180 mg/dL (7.8-10.0 mmol/L). In this vignette, the postoperative blood glucose is clearly uncontrolled, placing the patient at increased risk of infection, among other potential complications.

Scheduled basal insulin given once daily combined with supplemental scale regular insulin given every 6 hours when blood glucose is above the upper limit of his target range (Answer D) is an appropriate regimen for this man while he remains on nothing-by-mouth status. The dose of basal insulin could also be appropriately split into a twice-daily regimen. If a rapid-acting insulin analogue is to be used for correction dosing, it would be dosed every 4 hours, rather than every 6 hours based on the known physiologic duration of action of regular and rapid-acting insulin analogues, respectively.

A regular insulin sliding-scale regimen (Answer A) would reduce glucose levels to some degree, but it has been associated with increased rates of both hyperglycemia and hypoglycemia when compared with regimens that include some basal insulin. Aspart premixed insulin such as 70/30 (Answer B) has little role in the hospital setting because it is an inflexible product and does not allow for adjustments in the dose of the intermediate insulin separate from the rapid-acting insulin analogue (and vice versa). GLP-1 receptor agonists such as liraglutide (Answer C) should be used only in outpatients and they have no current role in the hospital setting. Intravenous insulin infusion (Answer E) could be used, but many hospitals are not equipped to manage insulin infusions outside of the intensive care unit, and the titration target should be 140 to 180 mg/dL, not 80 to 110 mg/dL.

Educational Objective
Manage preexisting diabetes mellitus in hospitalized patients.

Reference(s)

Moghissi ES, Korytkowski MT, DiNardo M, et al; American Association of Clinical Endocrinologists; American Diabetes Association. American Association of Clinical Endocrinologists and American Diabetes Association consensus statement on inpatient glycemic control. *Diabetes Care.* 2009;32(6):1119-1131. PMID: 19429873

Lleva RR, Inzucchi SE. Hospital management of hyperglycemia. *Curr Opin Endocrinol Diabetes Obes.* 2011;18(2):110-118. PMID: 21358407

33 ANSWER: D) Reduced albuminuria

Five to ten years after successful pancreas transplant, mesangial volume and mesangial matrix volume are significantly decreased compared with the same measurements at 0 and 5 years. In some patients, the width of the glomerular and tubular basement membranes and the mesangial volumes return to normal, and nodular glomerular lesions disappear. Tubular atrophy appears improved, possibly due to reabsorption of diseased nephrons. In all patients, urine albumin excretion improves significantly. Thus, reduced albuminuria (Answer D) can be expected within 5 years after a successful pancreas transplant.

After successful pancreas transplant, the velocity of motor and sensory nerve conduction, as well as clinical neuropathy, stabilizes but does not regress (Answer B). Abnormalities of gastric motility do not improve (Answer C). Quality-of-life studies consistently demonstrate benefits, such as return to work and successful pregnancies. Although initial reports indicated that established retinopathy does not improve, one study has shown that retinopathy was more likely to be arrested in patients who were successful pancreas recipients, when compared with those who lost the allograft. However, retinopathy does not regress (Answer A).

Educational Objective
Describe the potential benefits of pancreas transplant observed 5 to 10 years after successful transplant.

Reference(s)
de Sá JR, Monteagudo PT, Rangel EB, et al. The evolution of diabetic chronic complications after pancreas transplantation. *Diabetol Metab Syndr.* 2009;1(1):11. PMID: 19825148

Boggi U, Rosati CM, Marchetti P. Follow-up of secondary diabetic complications after pancreas transplantation. *Curr Opin Organ Transplant.* 2013;18(1):102-110. PMID: 23283247

34 ANSWER: B) Temporarily relax tight glucose targets

Up to 30% of patients with type 1 or longstanding type 2 diabetes mellitus have impaired or absent awareness of hypoglycemia. As plasma glucose levels fall, compromised physiologic counterregulatory defenses include failure of an increase in glucagon secretion and attenuated epinephrine secretion. This, together with inability to reduce circulating insulin levels, results in the clinical syndrome of defective counterregulation, which markedly increases the risk of recurrent severe hypoglycemia. Hypoglycemia-attenuating defense against subsequent hypoglycemia is a concept referred to as hypoglycemia-associated autonomic failure. The mainstay of treatment for this condition is the scrupulous avoidance of hypoglycemia. Patients with hypoglycemia unawareness and/or severe hypoglycemia and tight control should be advised to relax their glucose targets (Answer B) for a period to allow awareness to potentially return with adrenergic symptoms.

This patient should continue his usual dietary regimen (consistent carbohydrate or matching insulin to carbohydrates). Frequent small meals (Answer A) would not address the root of his problem. Switching to insulin pump therapy (Answer C) would not address the underlying cause of the hypoglycemia unawareness (repetitive hypoglycemic episodes) or guarantee its avoidance. A pump with a closed-loop suspend or autosuspend for hypoglycemia function might be considered in his long-term management plan; however, he has had tight glycemic control on a multiple daily injection regimen as evidenced by his hemoglobin A_{1c} level and again, the urgent need here is to address the blunted glycemic awareness. There would also be a delay in initiating pump therapy and a learning curve regarding its use. While a number of educational programs focusing on hypoglycemia detection and avoidance (Dose Adjustment for Normal Eating [DAFNE], Blood Glucose Awareness Training [BGAT], Hypoglycemia Awareness and Avoidance [HAAT]) have demonstrated effectiveness in reducing the occurrence of hypoglycemia, such an education program (Answer D) is not the most immediate fix for this patient, nor would it address the cause.

Educational Objective
Recommend management for severe hypoglycemia and hypoglycemia unawareness in type 1 diabetes mellitus.

Reference(s)

Alsahli M, Gerich JE. Hypoglycemia. *Endocrinol Metab Clin North Am.* 2013;42(4):657-676. PMID: 24286945

Little SA, Leelarathna L, Barendse SM, et al. Severe hypoglycaemia in type 1 diabetes mellitus: underlying drivers and potential strategies for successful prevention. *Diabetes Metab Res Rev.* 2014;30(3):175-190. PMID: 24185859

Choudhary P, Amiel SA. Hypoglycaemia: current management and controversies. *Postgrad Med J.* 2011;87(1026):298-306. PMID: 21296797

Oyer DS. The science of hypoglycemia in patients with diabetes. *Curr Diabetes Rev.* 2013;9(3):195-208. PMID: 23506375

Cryer PE. Mechanisms of hypoglycemia-associated autonomic failure in diabetes. *N Engl J Med.* 2013;369(4):362-372. PMID: 23883381

Awoniyi O, Rehman R, Dagogo-Jack S. Hypoglycemia in patients with type 1 diabetes: epidemiology, pathogenesis, and prevention. *Curr Diab Rep.* 2013;13(5):669-678. PMID: 23912765

Morales J, Schneider D. Hypoglycemia. *Am J Med.* 2014;127(Suppl 10):S17-S24. PMID: 25282009

35 ANSWER: B) Recommend assessment of her coronary artery calcium score

The 2013 American College of Cardiology/American Heart Association blood cholesterol guideline recommends that patients such as the one described in this vignette initiate moderate-intensity statin treatment (ie, individuals with diabetes aged 40 to 75 years with LDL-cholesterol levels between 70 and 189 mg/dL [1.81-4.90 mmol/L] and without clinical atherosclerotic cardiovascular disease). However, particularly when a patient resists starting statin therapy, consideration of determining the coronary calcium score (Answer B) may increasingly be factored into this kind of decision. A coronary artery calcium score of 0 results in a downward shift in estimated cardiovascular disease risk and may be used to help guide discussions regarding the likely benefit of preventive pharmacotherapy. Conversely, a high score would strongly support the recommendation that she start statin therapy and discussion as to whether evaluation for the presence of coronary artery disease is also warranted.

A minor reduction in hemoglobin A_{1c} from 7.2% (55 mmol/mol) to less than 7.0% (<53 mmol/mol) (Answer A) is unlikely to have any impact on this patient's cardiovascular disease risk. Her earlier levels of glycemic control are more likely to correlate with risk for cardiovascular disease. Without clinical albuminuria, which would also be an indication for statin use, adding an ACE inhibitor (Answer C) to the regimen of a normotensive, normoalbuminuric patient with type 1 diabetes would not be expected to result in a cardiovascular disease benefit according to the American Diabetes Association 2018 Standards of Medical Care. With a BMI of 24.5 kg/m^2, there is no need to recommend weight loss (Answer D). Because the potential adverse effects from bleeding most likely offset the potential benefits, aspirin (Answer E) is not routinely recommended for cardiovascular disease prevention in adults with diabetes who have a low risk of cardiovascular disease (10-year risk <5%, such as in men younger than 50 years and women younger than 60 years with no major additional cardiovascular disease risk factors).

Educational Objective

Incorporate the use of the coronary artery calcium score in the assessment of cardiovascular disease risk.

Reference(s)

Greenland P, Blaha MJ, Budoff MJ, Erbel R, Watson KE. Coronary calcium risk score and cardiovascular risk. *J Am Coll Cardiol.* 2018;72(4):434-447. PMID: 30025580

Blaha MJ, Cainzos-Achirica M, Greenland P, et al. Role of coronary artery calcium score of zero and other negative risk markers for cardiovascular disease: the multi-ethnic study of atherosclerosis (MESA). *Circulation.* 2016;133(9):849-858. PMID: 26801055

American Diabetes Association. 9. Cardiovascular disease and risk management: standards of medical care in diabetes-2018. *Diabetes Care.* 2018;41(Suppl 1):S86-S104. PMID: 29222380

Stone NJ, Robinson JG, Lichtenstein AH, et al; American College of Cardiology/American Heart Association Task Force on Practice Guidelines. 2013 ACC/AHA guideline on the treatment of blood cholesterol to reduce atherosclerotic cardiovascular risk in adults: a report of the American College of Cardiology/American Heart Association Task Force on Practice Guidelines [published correction appears in *Circulation*. 2014;129(25 Suppl 2): S46-S48]. *Circulation*. 2013;129(25 Suppl 2): S1-S45. PMID: 24222016

Nathan DM, Cleary PA, Backlund JY, et al; Diabetes Control and Complications Trial/Epidemiology of Diabetes Interventions and Complications (DCCT/EDIC) Study Research Group. Intensive diabetes treatment and cardiovascular disease in patients with type 1 diabetes. *N Engl J Med*. 2005; 353(25):2643-2653. PMID: 16371630

Randomised placebo-controlled trial of lisinopril in normotensive patients with insulin-dependent diabetes and normoalbuminuria or microalbuminuria. The EUCLID Study Group. *Lancet*. 1997;349(9068):1787-1792. PMID: 9269212

36 ANSWER: D) Standard supervised 72-hour fast

This patient's history is consistent with progressive hypoglycemic episodes over the past year that are now markedly worsening. Although his symptoms only occur during the day with an apparent relationship to meals, his glucose while fasting is lower than would be expected for a man of this age and body weight. A glucose concentration of 57 mg/dL (3.2 mmol/L) is not low enough to enable interpretation of the insulin and C-peptide results, as his blood glucose was not less than 54 mg/dL (<3.0 mmol/L) (the cut point at which insulin counterregulatory hormones will be triggered and insulin secretion will be suppressed). He should undergo a standard evaluation for hypoglycemia, so the next step is a supervised 72-hour fast (Answer D). This will determine whether his hypoglycemia is associated with inappropriate insulin secretion and assess the possibility that he has an insulinoma.

Localization studies, such as CT (Answer A) or MRI, are useful subsequent steps in localizing an insulinoma if this is suspected after a supervised fast, but they are potentially misleading in the absence of clear biochemical evidence of hyperinsulinemic hypoglycemia. Surreptitious use of sulfonylureas has been described in patients with lab values suggesting insulinoma, but such patients typically have access to these drugs at work or through family members. Therefore, a sulfonylurea screen (Answer B) is not the best next step. Heavy alcohol drinking is associated with hypoglycemia, but this is usually in the context of malnutrition or insulin use, neither of which is present

in this case. Thus, measurement of blood alcohol and γ-glutamyl transpeptidase (Answer C) is incorrect. Reactive hypoglycemia, of the type that might occur with a meal tolerance test (Answer E), is very rare except in individuals with previous gastric surgery.

Educational Objective

Guide the appropriate evaluation of hypoglycemia.

Reference(s)

FJ Service. Diagnostic approach to adults with hypoglycemic disorders. *Endocrinol Metab Clin North Am*. 1999;28(3):519-532. PMID: 10500929

37 ANSWER: A) Adrenal insufficiency

This patient with type 1 diabetes and possibly hypothyroidism (as evidenced by her elevated TSH) most likely has adrenal insufficiency (Answer A) with an autoimmune basis. In a patient with type 1 diabetes who experiences progressive decline in total daily insulin requirements with no obvious precipitating factors, it is important to consider a diagnosis of adrenal insufficiency. This woman has a classic presentation, namely persistent hypoglycemia and a falling insulin requirement. She also has orthostatic hypotension, defined as a decrease in systolic blood pressure greater than 20 mm Hg and a reflex increase in heart rate upon standing, which may or may not be present at the time the diagnosis is considered. Biochemical features of adrenal insufficiency such as mild hyperkalemia or hypernatremia, which are seen with acute adrenal insufficiency, are often not present in these patients.

Orthostatic hypotension can also result from cardiovascular autonomic neuropathy (Answer B), but one would not expect a reflex increase in heart rate if this were present. In the setting of cardiovascular autonomic neuropathy, signs of advanced peripheral neuropathy (Answer D) are often present (they are mild this case). Although this patient with longstanding type 1 diabetes may also have hypothyroidism (Answer C), it would not cause orthostatic hypotension. Because the patient's serum sodium concentration is normal, there is no evidence to suspect a salt-wasting nephropathy (Answer E).

Educational Objective

Identify the clinical signs and symptoms suggestive of adrenal insufficiency in the setting of type 1 diabetes mellitus.

Reference(s)

Barker JM. Clinical review: type 1 diabetes-associated autoimmunity: natural history, genetic associations, and screening. *J Clin Endocrinol Metab.* 2006;91(4):1210-1217. PMID: 16403820

Cutolo M. Autoimmune polyendocrine syndromes. *Autoimmun Rev.* 2014;13(2):85-89. PMID: 24055063

Pop-Busui R. Cardiac autonomic neuropathy in diabetes: a clinical perspective. *Diabetes Care.* 2010;33(2):434-441. PMID: 20103559

Vinik AI, Ziegler D. Diabetic cardiovascular autonomic neuropathy. *Circulation.* 2007;115(3):387-397. PMID: 17242296

38 ANSWER: C) Reduce basal insulin to 20 units in the morning, stop the mealtime insulin, and start linagliptin

Patients with inadequately controlled type 2 diabetes may be prescribed multiple daily insulin injections. It is increasingly recognized that this can impose a self-care burden, particularly among older patients. Measuring blood glucose and injecting insulin multiple times daily and, where appropriate, problem solving to adjust insulin doses and/or take correction doses requires complex self-care decision-making skills. The use of rapid-acting or short-acting insulin also increases hypoglycemia risk, which is of concern in older patients, such as the one presented in this vignette.

Hypoglycemia in elderly patients with diabetes increases the risk of cardiovascular and cerebrovascular events, progression of dementia, injurious falls, emergency department visits, and hospitalization. Hypoglycemic episodes are often difficult to diagnose in this population and are easily missed by intermittent fingerstick blood glucose measurements, as has been shown using continuous glucose monitoring. Munshi et al used continuous glucose monitoring to evaluate hypoglycemia in older patients with type 2 diabetes who had a hemoglobin A_{1c} level greater than 8.0% (>64 mmol/mol). Community-living older patients seen at a diabetes center with a hemoglobin A_{1c} level greater than 8.0% were evaluated with blinded continuous glucose monitoring for a 3-day period while they continued their usual daily activities. Patients checked their blood glucose concentration 4 times daily while wearing the continuous glucose monitor and recorded symptoms suggestive of hypoglycemia. Forty adults aged 75 ± 5 years were evaluated. The mean hemoglobin A_{1c} level was 9.3% ± 1.3%. Most patients (58%) were taking insulin alone. Twenty-six of 40 patients (65%) had at least 1 episode of hypoglycemia (median glucose value of 63 mg/dL (3.5 mmol/L) (range, 42-69 mg/dL [2.3-3.8 mmol/L]) over the 3-day period. Among those with a hemoglobin A_{1c} value between 8.0% and 9.0% (64 to 75 mmol/mol) and greater than 9.0% (>75 mmol/mol), the hypoglycemia rate was 54% and 46%, respectively.

In addition, large studies have shown lack of benefit and higher risk of morbidity and mortality with tight glycemic control. The American Diabetes Association recommends relaxing glycemic control for vulnerable patients, with a goal of less than 7.5% (<58 mmol/mol) in otherwise healthy older adults with few coexisting chronic conditions and intact cognitive and functional status. Among those with multiple coexisting conditions, cognitive impairment or functional dependence goals that are less stringent (eg, <8.0% [<64 mmol/mol] or <8.5% [<69 mmol/mol]), would be considered appropriate.

This patient's basal insulin dose should clearly be reduced, as she becomes hypoglycemic when lunch is late. Her erratic morning blood glucose values suggest that she is also having nocturnal hypoglycemia. Her multiple daily insulin injection regimen requires problem solving, as she must determine when and how to take correction insulin doses. Her C-peptide level indicates that she is still making insulin. She is taking fewer than 10 units of rapid-acting analogue before meals, so it is reasonable to discontinue her mealtime insulin and to add an oral agent that does not independently cause hypoglycemia, such as linagliptin, per national guidelines (Answer C).

Referring her to a diabetes educator (Answer A) is a reasonable adjunctive measure, but it will not lower her risk for hypoglycemia without a concurrent adjustment in her antihyperglycemic medication regimen. Reducing her insulin doses and continuing the multiple daily injection regimen (Answer B) may reduce the frequency of hypoglycemia, but this would still require her to do problem solving, which seems to be challenging for her. Finally, stopping both of her insulins is likely to result in hyperglycemia, as her total daily dose is currently 52 units. The Simplify regimen recommends reducing insulin doses sequentially and replacing mealtime insulin first with an oral agent. Repaglinide with meals (Answer D) might be a reasonable oral agent for this patient, as we know she is still able to secrete C-peptide; however, it would still require her to take it 3 times daily, so a once-daily agent such as a DPP-4 inhibitor makes more sense for her now.

Educational Objective
Simplify the antihyperglycemic regimen in older adults with type 2 diabetes mellitus to prevent hypoglycemia.

Reference(s)
Kirkman MS, Briscoe VJ, Clark N, et al. Diabetes in older adults. *Diabetes Care*. 2012;35(12):2650-2664. PMID: 23100048

Munshi MN, Segal AR, Suhl E, et al. Frequent hypoglycemia among elderly with poor glycemic control. *Arch Intern Med*. 2011;171(4):362-364. PMID: 21357814

Munshi MN, Slyne C, Segal AR, Saul N, Lyons C, Weinger K. Simplification of insulin regimen in older adults and risk of hypoglycemia. *JAMA Intern Med*. 2016;176(7):1023-1025. PMID: 27273335

39 ANSWER: B) Tissue transglutaminase antibody assessment

The incidence of celiac disease in individuals with type 1 diabetes mellitus is 5% to 7%. Affected patients may report typical symptoms of celiac sprue (bloating, diarrhea, abdominal pain, weight loss) or be relatively asymptomatic. Sometimes a chronic inflammatory rash (dermatitis herpetiformis) develops suddenly, lasts for weeks to months, and may also be associated with other gastrointestinal diseases. The best initial test is measurement of tissue transglutaminase antibodies (Answer B).

Colonoscopy (Answer A) would not be diagnostic. An upper gastrointestinal series with small-bowel follow-through (Answer D) would probably show nonspecific small-bowel findings but would also not be diagnostic. TPO antibody measurement (Answer C) is irrelevant to this case. A skin biopsy (Answer E) should diagnose the rash as dermatitis herpetiformis, but it would not identify the specific associated gastrointestinal condition—in this case, celiac disease.

Educational Objective
Recognize the signs and symptoms of celiac disease and initiate appropriate evaluation.

Reference(s)
Vermeersch P, Geboes K, Marien G, Hoffman I, Hiele M, Bossuyt X. Serological diagnosis of celiac disease: comparative analysis of different strategies. *Clin Chim Acta*. 2012;413(21-22):1761-1767. PMID: 22771970

Barker JM. Clinical review: type 1 diabetes-associated autoimmunity: natural history, genetic associations, and screening. *J Clin Endocrinol Metab*. 2006;91(4):1210-1217. PMID: 16403820

Acerini CL, Ahmed ML, Ross KM, Sullivan PB, Bird G, Dunger DB. Coeliac disease in children and adolescents with IDDM: clinical characteristics and response to gluten-free diet. *Diabetic Med*. 1998;15(1):38-44. PMID: 9472862

40 ANSWER: D) A benign course

Isolated glucosuria in the absence of diabetes or other renal dysfunction is diagnostic of familial renal glucosuria. The incidence of this autosomal co-dominant condition is 3 in 1000 persons, and it is due to pathogenic variants in the sodium-glucose transporter 2 (*SLC5A2* gene) that impair glucose transport in the proximal tubule of the kidney. Familial renal glucosuria has variable penetrance, but affected patients have lifelong excretion of abnormal amounts of glucose in the urine (1 to 150 g/24 h). In the limited case reports and animal models of familial renal glycosuria, glycosuria has not caused renal dysfunction. The otherwise benign course of this condition (Answer D) has been used to justify the development of SGLT-2 inhibitors to treat diabetes.

Glycosuria is sometimes present in patients with chronic kidney disease who do not have diabetes. Whether glycosuria in chronic kidney disease implies a channelopathy or proximal tubulopathy is not known. In persons with chronic kidney disease, glucosuria is associated with a decreased risk for end-stage renal disease (adjusted hazard ratio, 0.77; confidence interval, 0.62-0.97; $P = .024$) and for rapid renal function decline (adjusted odds ratio, 0.63; confidence interval, 0.43-0.95; $P = .032$) (thus, Answer B is incorrect). It is not associated with all-cause mortality (Answer A) or cardiovascular events (Answer C).

Educational Objective
Describe the long-term health implications of glucosuria in persons who do not have diabetes.

Reference(s)

Lee H, Han KH, Park HW, et al. Familial renal glucosuria: a clinicogenetic study of 23 additional cases. *Pediatr Nephrol.* 2012;27(7):1091-1095. PMID: 22314875

Santer R, Calado J. Familial renal glucosuria and SGLT2: from a mendelian trait to a therapeutic target. *Clin J Am Soc Nephrol.* 2010;5(1):133-141. PMID: 19965550

Hung CC, Lin HY, Lee JJ, et al. Glycosuria and renal outcomes in patients with nondiabetic advanced chronic kidney disease. *Sci Rep.* 2016;6:39372. PMID: 28008953

41 ANSWER: B) Diuretic effect of glucose reabsorption and consequent reduction in plasma volume

Glucose reabsorption is handled by proximal tubular proteins called sodium-glucose cotransporters 1 and 2 (SGLT-1 and SGLT-2). SGLT-2 inhibitors increase the excretion of glucose by inhibiting the action of these SGLT-2 proteins, thereby preventing glucose reabsorption in the proximal convoluted tubule of the kidneys. The most prominent explanation for cardioprotection by the SGLT-2 inhibitors is thought to be their diuretic effect and the consequent reduction in plasma volume (Answer B).

Although conventional diuretics and thiazides show no or moderate reduction in risk of heart failure, the diuretic action of SGLT-2 inhibitors does not induce reflex activation of the sympathetic nervous system and its consequent neurohormonal cardiac dysregulation (Answer A). The proximal inhibition of glucose and sodium reabsorption has beneficial consequences on renal function, as opposed to distal inhibition (Answer C). Other cardioprotective mechanisms include metabolic processes, including increased plasma glucagon and ketones (not decreased ketones [Answer D]), which are thought to confer protection against increases in blood pressure and vascular damage.

The kidneys may increase blood glucose levels by promoting renal gluconeogenesis, renal glycogenolysis, or glucose reabsorption in the proximal convoluted tubule. The mechanism of action of SGLT-2 inhibitors is primarily dependent on blood glucose levels and is independent of insulin's actions. SGLT-2 inhibitors do not inhibit sodium and chloride or glucagon excretion.

Educational Objective

Explain the purported mechanisms whereby SGLT-2 inhibitors affect cardiovascular disease outcomes.

Reference(s)

Schwarz PEH, Timpel P, Harst L, et al. Blood sugar regulation for cardiovascular health promotion and disease prevention. *J Am Coll Cardiol.* 2018; 72(15):1829-1844. PMID: 30286928

Jung CH, Jang JE, Park JY. A novel therapeutic agent for type 2 diabetes mellitus: SGLT2 inhibitor. *Diabetes Metab J.* 2014;38(4):261-273. PMID: 25215272

42 ANSWER: D) Insulin

Patients with cystic fibrosis–related diabetes (CFRD) produce an insufficient amount of insulin; therefore, insulin is recommended by the American Diabetes Association as the optimal therapeutic option for glycemic control. Evidence in the literature demonstrates that when insulin is used to achieve glycemic control, there is demonstrable improvement in weight, protein anabolism, pulmonary function, and survival. There is not, however, adequate evidence to support the superiority of one specific insulin regimen over another in CFRD.

Data from several randomized controlled studies suggest that oral agents (those studied include glyburide [Answer B], metformin [Answer A], repaglinide, and thiazolidinediones [Answer C]) are not as effective as insulin in improving nutritional status or blood glucose control in patients with CFRD.

In addition, it should be noted that mortality has not been evaluated as an outcome in CFRD studies to date.

Educational Objective

Manage hyperglycemia in patients with cystic fibrosis–related diabetes.

Reference(s)

Moran A, Pekow P, Grover P, et al; Cystic Fibrosis Related Diabetes Therapy Study Group. Insulin therapy to improve BMI in cystic fibrosis-related diabetes without fasting hyperglycemia: results of the cystic fibrosis related diabetes therapy trial. *Diabetes Care.* 2009;32(10):1783-1788. PMID: 19592632

Onady GM, Stolfi A. Insulin and oral agents for managing cystic fibrosis-related diabetes. *Cochrane Database Syst Rev*. 2013;7:CD004730. PMID: 23893261

Moran A, Brunzell C, Cohen RC, et al; CFRD Guidelines Committee. Clinical care guidelines for cystic fibrosis-related diabetes: a position statement of the American Diabetes Association and a clinical practice guideline of the Cystic Fibrosis Foundation, endorsed by the Pediatric Endocrine Society. *Diabetes Care*. 2010;33(12): 2697-2708. PMID: 21115772

43 ANSWER: C) Reduced peripheral glucose disposal

In a healthy state, glucose enters the circulation from food ingestion, and endogenous glucose production (predominantly hepatic) is evenly matched by glucose disposal into peripheral tissues, mainly skeletal muscle and fat.

The pathogenesis of hyperglycemia in patients with type 2 diabetes is multifactorial and complex. Primary defects are evident in skeletal muscle and adipocytes, where decreased insulin action (referred to as insulin resistance) is demonstrated early in the disease course—in fact, before any elevation in blood glucose concentrations. This results in decreased glucose disposal (Answer C) under experimental conditions. Metformin and thiazolidinediones increase peripheral glucose disposal.

Initially, the pancreatic β cell compensates for the insulin resistance by augmenting its secretion of insulin, resulting in the maintenance of normal blood glucose concentrations. In those individuals who develop diabetes, pancreatic compensation falters, and insulin secretion is no longer able to surmount the decreased insulin action in peripheral tissues. Defects are initially demonstrated in the postprandial setting, when major augmentation of insulin secretion is necessary for glucose disposal. The most marked deficit is in first-phase insulin secretion, with a sluggish initial β-cell response to early increases in blood glucose concentrations from carbohydrate ingestion. Ultimately, insulin secretion is inadequate to maintain normal glucose levels even in the postabsorptive phase, and fasting hyperglycemia develops. Insulin secretagogues, thiazolidinediones, and incretins can augment pancreatic insulin secretion (Answer A). However, this is not the primary defect in type 2 diabetes.

Increased hepatic glucose production is a third well-documented pathophysiologic defect in type 2 diabetes, reflecting hepatic insulin resistance in combination with insufficient insulin levels and unsuppressed glucagon levels in the portal vein.

Inappropriate reabsorption of glucose from the proximal convoluted tubule in type 2 diabetes also has a role in the pathogenesis of hyperglycemia. In those without diabetes, about 180 g of glucose is filtered daily by the glomeruli, and this is then reabsorbed in the proximal convoluted tubule. This is achieved by passive transporters, namely, facilitated glucose transporters, and active cotransporters, namely, SGLT-2. SGLT-2 inhibitors work by inhibiting SGLT-2 in the proximal convoluted tubule to prevent reabsorption of glucose and facilitate its excretion in urine. As glucose is excreted, its plasma levels fall, which leads to an improvement in all glycemic parameters. This mechanism of action is dependent on blood glucose levels and, unlike the actions of thiazolidinediones (mediated through glucose transporters), is independent of the actions of insulin. Thus, there is minimal potential for hypoglycemia, and no risk of overstimulation or fatigue of the β cells. Because their mode of action relies on normal renal glomerular-tubular function, the efficacy of SGLT-2 inhibitors is reduced in persons with renal impairment. The inappropriate absorption of glucose is not a primary defect in the pathogenesis of type 2 diabetes. In addition, the SGLT-2 inhibitors reduce, rather than increase (Answer B), expression of the receptor.

Unless autonomic neuropathy is present, there are no abnormalities of gastric emptying (Answer D) in type 2 diabetes. The endogenous secretion of incretins is impaired in type 2 diabetes. The defects in incretin secretion are most likely a secondary defect in type 2 diabetes. When incretin agents are used to treat type 2 diabetes, one of their mechanisms of action is reduced gastric emptying. This helps to attenuate the magnitude of postprandial glucose excursions and may contribute to a feeling of fullness or bloating.

In summary, the pathogenesis of type 2 diabetes is complex and involves lesions in multiple organ systems that are responsible for maintaining normal glucose homeostasis.

Educational Objective

Examine the pathophysiology of type 2 diabetes mellitus.

Reference(s)

Defronzo RA. Banting lecture. From the triumvirate to the ominous octet: a new paradigm for the treatment of type 2 diabetes mellitus. *Diabetes*. 2009;58(4):773-795. PMID: 19336687

Rizza RA. Pathogenesis of fasting and postprandial hyperglycemia in type 2 diabetes: implications for therapy. *Diabetes*. 2010;59(11):2697-2707. PMID: 20705776

Samuel VT, Shulman GI. Mechanisms for insulin resistance: common threads and missing links. *Cell*. 2012;148(5):852-871. PMID: 22385956

44 ANSWER: D) Begin treatment with a phosphodiesterase inhibitor

Erectile dysfunction is very common and affects at least 50% of men with diabetes mellitus. Diabetes mellitus can cause erectile dysfunction through a number of pathophysiologic pathways, including neuropathy, endothelial dysfunction, cavernosal smooth muscle structural/functional changes, and hormonal changes.

Testosterone levels gradually decline in men—typically about 1% per year after age 30 or 40. This man's testosterone level is normal for his age. Phosphodiesterase inhibitors (Answer D) are the mainstay of therapy for erectile dysfunction when testosterone deficiency is not present. They enhance blood flow into the corpora cavernosa and thereby improve erectile quality. As he does not have testosterone deficiency, treatment with testosterone (Answer B) is not indicated.

While improving his glucose control and hemoglobin A_{1c} level (Answer A) may delay progression of neuropathy and vascular features of erectile dysfunction in the long term, it will not improve his erectile function.

Many drugs are associated with erectile dysfunction, including blood pressure medications, such as β-adrenergic blockers and calcium-channel blockers, but not ACE inhibitors. Thus, stopping his ACE inhibitor (Answer C) is incorrect.

Educational Objective

Recommend treatment of erectile dysfunction in a man with type 1 diabetes mellitus.

Reference(s)

Hatzimouratidis K, Hatzichristou D. How to treat erectile dysfunction in men with diabetes: from pathophysiology to treatment. *Curr Diab Rep*. 2014;14(11):545. PMID: 25193347

Mobley DF, Khera M, Baum N. Recent advances in treatment of erectile dysfunction. *Postgrad Med J*. 2017;93(1105):679-685. PMID: 28751439

Araujo AB, Mohr BA, McKinlay JB, et al. Changes in sexual function in middle-aged and older men: longitudinal data from the Massachusetts Male Aging Study. *J Am Geriatr Soc*. 2004;52(9):1502-1509. PMID: 15341552

McVary KT. Clinical practice. Erectile dysfunction. *N Engl J Med*. 2007;357(24):2472-2481. PMID: 18077811

45 ANSWER: B) Begin taking semaglutide and continue his current lifestyle regimen

Altering the macronutrient distribution of the diet is a very common strategy for commercial diet plans. Several randomized controlled studies of low-carbohydrate diets address this issue. In persons with obesity, intake of low-carbohydrate, ketogenic diets seems to cause greater weight loss and loss of body fat than calorie-restricted, low-fat diets, at least for periods of 3 to 6 months. In inpatient studies, isocaloric diets lead to the same degree of weight reduction as ketogenic diets, regardless of the proportions of fat and carbohydrate, and there are no major thermogenic advantages to lowering the percentage of carbohydrate and increasing the percentage of fat and protein in the diet. Studies in free-living participants have confirmed that diets based on such regimens do not increase the metabolic rate. While diuresis due to increased salt excretion occurs with caloric restriction in general, persons following low-carbohydrate diets lose fat mass comparably to those with equivalent weight loss from other regimens. The best explanation for the short-term effectiveness of low-carbohydrate regimens is that they are more satiating, or that they reduce caloric consumption by limiting food choices.

Based on evidence in the literature, there is no need to recommend that this patient change from his current diet (Answer A). It is important to monitor the usual markers of diabetes management—hemoglobin A_{1c}, blood pressure, and lipids—to ensure that he does not have a response to the low-carbohydrate diet that differs from that of participants in published clinical trials. However, as long as he continues to lose weight, or maintain a reduced body weight, he will most likely to have a positive response in clinical parameters.

Relative to pharmacotherapy that will help both his glycemic control and his weight, addition of semaglutide, a GLP-1 receptor agonist, to his treatment regimen (Answer B) will most likely enable attainment of both goals. Linagliptin would have a mild-to-moderate impact on his glycemic control, but use of DPP-4 inhibitors is not associated with weight loss. No studies have been conducted on the safety of SGLT-2 inhibitors in persons following a ketogenic diet (Answer D).

Increasing the frequency or intensity of his exercise regimen (Answer C) is unlikely to help him lose further weight. Exercise has been shown to be key to maintaining weight loss; however, in most cases it does not cause weight loss, as it is difficult to expend enough calories through exercise to create a net negative daily caloric balance.

It will be important for this patient to have a strategy for maintaining weight loss, including on-going regular exercise, when he stops following this diet. As with all diets that are successful in the short term, it is important to appreciate the difficulty that patients have with long-term adherence and to anticipate the sometimes dramatic changes in lipids and glycemic control that can ensue if there is rapid weight regain.

Educational Objective
Differentiate among options for medical nutrition therapy in patients with type 2 diabetes mellitus.

Reference(s)
Brehm BJ, Lattin BL, Summer SS, et al. One-year comparison of a high-monounsaturated fat diet with a high-carbohydrate diet in type 2 diabetes. *Diabetes Care.* 2009;32(2):215-220. PMID: 18957534

Samaha FF, Iqbal N, Seshadri P, et al. A low-carbohydrate as compared with a low-fat diet in severe obesity. *N Engl J Med.* 2003;348(21):2074-2081. PMID: 12761364

46 ANSWER: E) Institute dietary sodium restriction

This patient has had progression of her albuminuria despite blood pressure and glycemic measures that are near goal and use of an angiotensin-receptor blocker. There is now abundant evidence that inhibitors of the renin-angiotensin-aldosterone system effectively reduce excess albumin excretion and decrease the renal and cardiovascular end points associated with proteinuria. However, the effectiveness of angiotensin-receptor blockers and ACE inhibitors are blunted by high sodium intake and can be significantly improved by dietary sodium restriction (Answer E) or diuretics. This woman has been eating out (which has increased her sodium intake), she has signs of volume overload on examination (ankle edema), and her 24-hour urinary sodium excretion indicates that she is consuming the typical American high-salt diet. Restricting her to 4 to 6 g of sodium daily would most likely improve the effectiveness of her angiotensin-receptor blocker treatment. If this is not possible, starting either a loop diuretic or a thiazide would produce a similar effect.

Combination therapy with an angiotensin-receptor blocker and an ACE inhibitor (Answer A) has not been effective in changing the course of diabetic nephropathy and is less effective than either drug combined with sodium restriction. Notably, some agents in the SGLT-2 inhibitor class have been shown to have a renoprotective effect. In studies including the Empagliflozin, Cardiovascular Outcomes, and Mortality in Type 2 Diabetes (EMPA-REG OUTCOME) trial, these drugs have been shown to confer renoprotection. EMPA-REG randomly assigned 7020 patients with type 2 diabetes and cardiovascular disease to the SGLT-2 receptor empagliflozin at 2 doses vs placebo. At baseline, 26% of patients had an estimated glomerular filtration rate less than 60 mL/min per 1.73 m^2 and 40% had microalbuminuria or macroalbuminuria, as does this patient. After a median of 3.1 years of follow-up, not only was empagliflozin use linked to fewer cardiovascular and death events, but it also improved kidney-related outcomes. Specifically, it was associated with a significantly lower rate of incident macroalbuminuria (38%), doubling of serum creatinine, and estimated glomerular filtration rate of 45 mL/min per 1.73 m^2 or less (44%). Therefore, one consideration could be to replace one of her current glycemic medications with an SGLT-2 inhibitor. Because she has ankle edema, the pioglitazone could be stopped and/or the linagliptin could be replaced, as DPP-4 inhibitors have not been shown to be renoprotective.

The use of aldosterone antagonists such as spironolactone (Answer B) shows promise in improving short-term measures of nephropathy, but this combination has not been established in large outcomes trials.

Good glycemic control reduces the onset of nephropathy, but has shown less benefit in secondary prevention of end-stage renal disease. Addition of insulin glargine (Answer C) to reduce her hemoglobin A_{1c} level to less than 7.0% (<53 mmol/mol) is not likely to be of much benefit.

Protein restriction (Answer D) has been studied extensively in renal disease, but it is currently not recommended for patients such as the one presented because it does not affect the course of diabetic nephropathy.

Educational Objective

Manage nephropathy in the setting of type 2 diabetes mellitus.

Reference(s)

Doshi SM, Friedman AN. Diagnosis and management of type 2 diabetic kidney disease. *Clin J Am Soc Nephrol.* 2017;12(8):1366-1373. PMID: 28280116

Slagman MC, Waanders F, Hemmelder MH, et al; Holland Nephrology Study Group. Moderate dietary sodium restriction added to angiotensin converting enzyme inhibition compared with dual blockade in lowering proteinuria and blood pressure: randomised controlled trial. *BMJ.* 2011; 343:d4366. PMID: 21791491

Lambers Heerspink HJ, Holtkamp FA, Parving HH, et al. Moderation of dietary sodium potentiates the renal and cardiovascular protective effects of angiotensin receptor blockers. *Kidney Int.* 2012;82(3):330-337. PMID: 22437412

47 ANSWER: D) Decrease the evening dose of NPH insulin to 20 units and give it at bedtime

NPH insulin is the least expensive basal insulin available and is still the tier 1 basal insulin on some formularies. Therefore, it remains important to understand its pharmacokinetics and how to appropriately adjust dosages. This patient has poor glycemic control. Her fasting blood glucose values vary widely, which is a pattern that often indicates nocturnal lows. She clearly has overnight hypoglycemia periodically. These findings are due to the pharmacokinetics of NPH as a basal insulin. When given with the evening meal, the peak effect is in the early morning, and if only a small evening meal is consumed, hypoglycemia overnight can occur. However, because the effect of NPH insulin does not last 12 hours in all patients, glucose control is lost in some by the time of waking. She is experiencing both these effects. A good solution is to move her insulin to bedtime administration and to lower the dose. Importantly, shifting her evening NPH dose to bedtime will lower her risk for nocturnal hypoglycemia because the insulin effect will be most marked at breakfast. Thus, decreasing the evening dose of NPH insulin to 20 units and giving it at bedtime (Answer D) is the best course of action.

Despite her high hemoglobin A_{1c} level, increasing her NPH insulin dose to 28 units (Answers A and B) would exacerbate the tendency for overnight lows. No data in the vignette indicated whether she needs prandial insulin, so adding 6 units of regular insulin before meals and stopping glipizide (Answer C) is also incorrect. Further fingerstick blood glucose testing after meals would be required to determine whether she needs mealtime insulin.

Educational Objective

Manage insulin dosing using NPH insulin in a patient with type 2 diabetes mellitus.

Reference(s)

Leahy JL. Insulin treatment in type 2 diabetes mellitus. *Endocrinol Metab Clin North Am.* 2012; 41(1):119-144. PMID: 22575410

McCall AL. Insulin therapy and hypoglycemia. *Endocrinol Metab Clin North Am.* 2012;41(1): 57-87. PMID: 22575407

48 ANSWER: C) Stop insulin therapy; perform an oral glucose tolerance test in 1 month

Women with gestational diabetes often do not need to continue glucose-lowering medications post partum. They may revert to the level of glucose tolerance they had before becoming pregnant. Thus, continuing current therapy without reassessing this patient's status (Answer A) is incorrect. Home glucose monitoring is not recommended in these women because of the cost, inconvenience, and lack of evidence supporting the practice. However, a 75-g, 2-hour oral glucose tolerance test 6 to 12 weeks after delivery (Answer C) is recommended because of the increased prevalence of prediabetes and mild diabetes in women with gestational diabetes. After this test, metformin treatment may be indicated, but it should not be started empirically (Answer B).

Although hemoglobin A_{1c} (Answer D) is now used to diagnose diabetes in the general population, this measure has not been standardized for the evaluation of postgestational diabetes, and oral glucose tolerance testing is still preferred.

Even with normal results on postpartum oral glucose tolerance testing, women with a history of gestational diabetes should have periodic evaluation for diabetes, particularly before another planned pregnancy and after conception.

Educational Objective
Follow-up gestational diabetes mellitus in the postpartum period.

Reference(s)
Blumer I, Hadar E, Hadden DR, et al. Diabetes and pregnancy: an Endocrine Society clinical practice guideline. *J Clin Endocrinol Metab*. 2013;98(11): 4227-4249. PMID: 24194617

49 ANSWER: A) Start NPH insulin, 12 units with breakfast

Glucocorticoid therapy is a frequent cause of hyperglycemia or new-onset diabetes. The risk varies depending on other predispositions for diabetes and the steroid dosage. The mechanism of steroid-induced diabetes is a combination of insulin resistance and impaired proinsulin processing that leads to decreased insulin action.

The current recommendation for the treatment of hyperglycemia precipitated by steroids is to move straight to insulin therapy. A hallmark of steroid-induced diabetes is a disproportionate impact on prandial glucose levels such that hyperglycemia is much worse, and difficult to treat, during the day and is relatively better in the basal, overnight period. Therefore, insulin treatment should be focused during the periods when patients are eating, especially with relatively short-acting steroids given in the morning. Starting NPH insulin at a moderate dosage (Answer A) is the best course of action for this man. This regimen will provide insulin action over the course of the day while his blood glucose levels are running high.

At supraphysiologic steroid dosages, the resulting hyperglycemia is frequently refractory to oral agents. Thus, increasing the metformin dosage (Answers B, C, and D) is incorrect. Sitagliptin (Answer C) has a modest impact on blood glucose and is unlikely to adequately counter the hyperglycemic effect of the prednisone. He may also eventually need basal insulin (Answer D), but treating with basal insulin alone is less likely to be effective than use of an insulin that targets reduction in postprandial blood glucose.

It is important to note that as his steroid dosage is reduced, his insulin requirements will also decrease in parallel and reductions in the insulin dosage will be necessary to prevent hypoglycemia.

Educational Objective
Treat steroid-induced diabetes.

Reference(s)
Spanakis EK, Shah N, Malhotra K, Kemmerer T, Yeh HC, Golden SH. Insulin requirements in non-critically ill hospitalized patients with diabetes and steroid-induced hyperglycemia. *Hosp Pract*. 2014;42(2):23-30. PMID: 24769781

Baldwin D, Apel J. Management of hyperglycemia in hospitalized patients with renal insufficiency or steroid-induced diabetes. *Curr Diab Rep*. 2013;13(1):114-120. PMID: 23090580

50 ANSWER: A) Advise him to take his insulin bolus 10 to 15 minutes before meals

The time to onset of action of rapid-acting insulin lispro is 10 to 15 minutes. This patient is taking the dose with his meal, which does not allow enough time for it to be physiologically active to prevent the clear postprandial hyperglycemia peaks, as shown in the continuous glucose monitoring report. Moving the timing of insulin lispro administration to before the meal with a sufficient window to allow onset of its action (Answer A) would be expected to attenuate the postmeal glucose peaks.

This patient is already on a low-carbohydrate meal plan, so further restricting his carbohydrates with meals (Answer B) would not be expected to have a significant impact on his postmeal glucose excursions, nor would it be advisable from a nutrition standpoint.

In the absence of food and exercise, basal insulin should hold the blood glucose level steady. His premeal glucose values are within target range, which demonstrates that the basal insulin dose during this 12-hour window is appropriate. Therefore, performing a basal rate test (Answer C) is incorrect. Basal insulin rate testing can be conducted to help determine the appropriateness of basal dosing in cases where it is not clear if they are optimal. It is set up around the usual framework of mealtimes and sleep patterns and is initiated after the action of the most recently taken meal insulin bolus has dissipated for the period to be tested. If blood glucose drops during the test period, the basal rate is too high, and if it goes up, the basal rate may be too low. The basal rate can then be adjusted to move the glucose to the target value.

As automated closed-loop insulin pump and sensor systems are increasingly being used, the need for patients to conduct basal insulin testing will eventually be superseded by automated technology.

Finally, adjusting his insulin-to-carbohydrate ratio from 1:20 to 1:6 (Answer D) would lead to more than doubling his meal boluses, which would predispose him to hypoglycemia. A more modest adjustment in his insulin-to-carbohydrate ratio (eg, to 1:15) would also be expected to improve his postprandial blood glucose levels.

Educational Objective
Manage insulin based on blood glucose patterns.

Reference(s)
Walsh J, Roberts R. *Pumping Insulin.* 6th edition. San Diego, CA; Torrey Pines Press; 2017.

Gary Scheiner. Getting Down to Basals. Diabetes Self-Management. 2006. Available at: https://www.diabetesselfmanagement.com/managing-diabetes/treatment-approaches/getting-down-to-basals/ Accessed for verification May 2019.

51 ANSWER: A) Glutamic acid decarboxylase antibodies

This obese woman has diabetes that has been unresponsive to a variety of medications typically used to treat type 2 diabetes. Glutamic acid decarboxylase antibodies (Answer A) were measured based on her clinical presentation to assess for the presence of autoantibody-associated diabetes of the adult, and the result confirmed the diagnosis.

Latent autoimmune diabetes in adults (LADA) is an autoimmune form of diabetes defined by age at onset of more than 30 years, presence of diabetes-associated autoantibodies, and no insulin treatment requirement for a period after diagnosis (as has been the case in this patient). The 3 criteria conventionally used to define LADA are nonspecific; namely, age at diagnosis, autoantibody positivity, and need for insulin treatment. Metabolic changes at diagnosis of LADA reflect a broad clinical phenotype ranging from diabetic ketoacidosis to mild non–insulin-requiring diabetes. The latter phenotype is the most prevalent form of adult-onset autoimmune diabetes and is probably the most prevalent form of autoimmune diabetes in general. Patients with adult-onset autoimmune diabetes have less HLA-associated genetic risk and fewer diabetes-associated autoantibodies compared with patients with childhood-onset type 1 diabetes. Although LADA is associated with the same genetic and immunologic features as classic autoimmune type 1 diabetes, it also shares some genetic features with type 2 diabetes, which raises the question of genetic heterogeneity predisposing to this form of the disease.

The potential value of screening patients with adult-onset diabetes for diabetes-associated autoantibodies to identify those with LADA is emphasized by their lack of clinically distinct features, their different natural history compared with type 2 diabetes, and their potential need for a dedicated management strategy. Diabetes-associated autoantibodies include autoantibodies to glutamic acid decarboxylase, insulinoma-associated antigen IA-2, islet cells, and zinc transporter 8 (ZnT8A). The definition of autoantibody positivity is not unequivocal, and different cut-off points have been applied in different studies. Longitudinal studies observe changing autoantibody status over time, and even though most patients are positive for only one type of autoantibody, existing autoantibodies may be lost and other autoantibodies may develop.

This woman's blood glucose values are consistent with her hemoglobin A_{1c} level, so there is no reason to do alternative testing to confirm her current level of glycemic control. Fructosamine measurement (Answer B) will therefore not contribute to her management. Fasting insulin levels (Answer C) are used to assess the degree of insulin resistance, which is not a consideration in this patient right now. Finally, adult patients with LADA are more likely to have lower C-peptide levels than those without diabetes-associated autoantibodies, but because both cohorts may still make C-peptide, its measurement (Answer D) is not useful in distinguishing between the 2 conditions.

This patient's glutamic acid decarboxylase antibody level was 9832 IU/mL (<5.0 IU/mL is normal), which confirms a diagnosis of LADA. Islet-cell antibodies were undetectable (which was somewhat unanticipated). She is now taking basal-bolus insulin therapy and is learning about carbohydrate counting, insulin-to-carbohydrate ratios, and sick day rules for insulin management to prevent diabetic ketoacidosis in the event of an intercurrent illness. She is no longer taking dulaglutide, and her glycemic control is markedly improved.

Educational Objective
Diagnose latent autoimmune diabetes in adults.

Reference(s)
Laugesen E, Østergaard JA, Leslie RD; Danish Diabetes Academy Workshop and Workshop Speakers. Latent autoimmune diabetes of the adult: current knowledge and uncertainty. *Diabet Med.* 2015;32(7):843-852. PMID: 25601320

52 ANSWER: D) Switch to U500 regular insulin

This patient has markedly uncontrolled, symptomatic hyperglycemia. You have ascertained that her self-injection technique is good. She has insulin resistance as evidenced by her lack of responsiveness to a total daily dose of 230 units of U100 insulin lispro. She also has established congestive heart failure and chronic kidney disease.

There is a need for insulins that reduce the frequency of hyperglycemia and hypoglycemia and can reduce the burden of daily therapy (fewer injections, better delivery systems), especially in insulin-resistant patients taking high insulin dosages. Several concentrated insulin preparations are available in the United States. U500 regular insulin (Answer D) is 5 times more concentrated than U100 regular insulin and has a delayed onset and longer duration of action than U100 insulin. U500 regular insulin has both prandial and basal properties and is available in both prefilled pens and vials. Use of a prefilled pen would be expected to minimize the risk of dosing errors. Switching to U500 regular insulin is the best next step.

U300 insulin glargine and U200 insulin degludec are 3 and 2 times more concentrated, respectively, than the corresponding U100 preparations. They allow for higher doses of basal insulin administration per dose taken. They are basal insulins and do not provide any prandial insulin coverage. Pharmacy pricing for U500 regular insulin is relatively lower than for the other concentrated insulins, with a median national acquisition drug-associated cost (NADAC) being reported as $143 for vials and $184 for pens in 2017, compared with $285 for U200 insulin degludec and $239 for U300 insulin glargine.

Among patients with type 2 diabetes who have established cardiovascular disease, including congestive heart failure, and/or chronic kidney disease, the American Diabetes Association, the European Association for the Study of Diabetes, and the American College of Cardiology now recommend use of SGLT-2 inhibitors or GLP-1 receptor agonists as part of glycemic management. This recommendation is based on evidence that these agents improve cardiovascular outcomes, as well as secondary outcomes such as heart failure and progression of renal disease. A GLP-1 receptor agonist will be added to this patient's regimen. There are no data to support incremental cardiovascular benefit from combination of a GLP-1 receptor agonist with an SGLT-2 inhibitor. As the glycosuric effects of SGLT-2 inhibitors are dependent on glomerular filtration, these effects are attenuated in the presence of a reduced glomerular filtration rate. Because this patient will clearly need insulin treatment, adding an SGLT-2 inhibitor (Answer C) would only make her regimen more complex. Also, because of her chronic kidney disease, the glucose-lowering effect of an SGLT-2 inhibitor may be attenuated.

Increasing her insulin doses by 20% (Answer B) is unlikely to sufficiently overcome insulin resistance to improve her glycemic control, and it would not address the challenge of multiple daily insulin injections (5+ in this case).

Finally, there are challenges with insulin pump therapy (Answer A) in persons who have insulin resistance. High insulin doses required for management of insulin resistance necessitate frequent refills of the pump insulin reservoir. Concentrated basal insulins are not currently approved for use in insulin pumps.

Educational Objective
Determine when to prescribe a concentrated insulin.

Reference(s)
Heinemann L, Beals JM, Malone J, Anderson J, Jacobson JG, Sinha V, Corrigan SM. Concentrated insulins: History and critical reappraisal. *J Diabetes*. 2018;11(4):292-300. PMID: 30264527

Davies MJ, D'Alessio DA, Fradkin J, et al. Management of hyperglycemia in type 2 diabetes, 2018. A consensus report by the American Diabetes Association (ADA) and the European Association for the Study of Diabetes (EASD). *Diabetes Care*. 2018;41(12):2669-2701. PMID: 30291106

American Diabetes Association. 8. Pharmacologic approaches to glycemic treatment: standards of medical care in diabetes-2018. *Diabetes Care*. 2018;41 (Suppl 1):S73-S85. PMID: 29222379

53 ANSWER: A) Bradycardia

Severe hypoglycemia is strongly associated with increased all-cause and cardiovascular mortality in persons with type 2 diabetes mellitus. This has been demonstrated in landmark trials evaluating tight glycemic control and cardiac outcomes in type 2 diabetes, including the Action to Control Cardiovascular Risk in Diabetes (ACCORD), the Action in Diabetes and Vascular Disease trial (ADVANCE), and the Veterans Affairs Diabetes Trial (VADT).

The hemodynamic changes associated with hypoglycemia include an increase in heart rate and peripheral systolic blood pressure; a fall in central blood pressure; reduced peripheral arterial resistance (causing a widening of pulse pressure); and increased myocardial contractility, stroke volume, and cardiac output.

Hypoglycemia is hypothesized to cause arrhythmias through effects on cardiac repolarization and changes in cardiac autonomic activity. A study of spontaneous hypoglycemia in patients with type 2 diabetes and a history of cardiovascular disease or 2 or more risk factors treated with insulin found an increased risk for nocturnal bradycardia (Answer A), atrial ectopy, ventricular premature beats, and prolongation of the Q-T interval (not shortening [Answer D]). However, it did not show increased risk for complex ventricular premature beats (Answer C). Abnormal T-wave morphology was also observed. It has been suggested that excessive compensatory vagal activation after the counterregulatory phase may account for bradycardia and associated arrhythmias. Among supraventricular arrhythmias, transient atrial fibrillation is most frequently reported (not atrial flutter [Answer B]). Reports of ventricular arrhythmias associated with hypoglycemia are rare, perhaps because events are generally fatal if uncorrected.

Additionally, in view of his advanced age and his established cardiovascular disease, it is important to establish a less stringent target for hemoglobin A_{1c} and to adjust his insulin dose downward to ensure liberalization of glycemic control and to reduce further risk for severe hypoglycemic events. His patient characteristics/health status would be considered complex/intermediate in view of his hypoglycemia vulnerability, so a hemoglobin A_{1c} of 8.0% (64 mmol/mol) would be a reasonable target for this man.

Educational Objective

Explain the cardiac implications of severe hypoglycemia.

Reference(s)

Chow E, Bernjak A, Williams S, et al. Risk of cardiac arrhythmias during hypoglycemia in patients with type 2 diabetes and cardiovascular risk. *Diabetes Care.* 2013;63(5):1738-1747. PMID: 24757202

Frier BM, Schernthaner G, Heller SR. Hypoglycemia and cardiovascular risks. *Diabetes Care.* 2011;34(Suppl 2):S132-S137. PMID: 21525444

Kirkman MS, Briscoe VJ, Clark N, et al. Diabetes in older adults. *Diabetes Care.* 2012;35(12):2650-2664. PMID: 23100048

54 ANSWER: C) Rationing his insulin

Euglycemic diabetic ketoacidosis (DKA) is diagnosed when a patient presents with acidosis and ketosis but has a glucose level of 200 mg/dL or less (≤11.1 mmol/L). This condition has become an emerging concern. Causes of euglycemic DKA can include recent insulin administration, decreased caloric intake, substantial alcohol consumption, chronic liver disease, or rarely, glycogen storage issues. In addition, SGLT-2 inhibitors can cause euglycemic DKA. In May 2015, the US FDA added a warning about the risk of DKA with use of this class of drugs. One study suggested that the risk of DKA for patients using SGLT-2 inhibitors was twice as high as those prescribed a DPP-4 inhibitor, after controlling for other risk factors, although the risk of hospitalization was low. The exact cause of this relationship is unknown, but several theories include reduced insulin doses when the SGLT-2 inhibitor is initiated, an increase in glucagon, or decreased excretion of ketone bodies. Other related factors may be mild infection, increased activity, reduced food intake, or insulin reduction or omission. Case reports of euglycemic DKA occurring in patients taking SGLT-2 inhibitors have been documented in patients with both type 1 diabetes and type 2 diabetes. Many patients with euglycemic DKA present with nausea and vomiting but are misdiagnosed because of the lack of clear glucose elevation.

Insulin is lifesaving for persons with diabetes and is included on the Model List of Essential Medicines formulated by the World Health Organization. This means it should be available at all times at a price the individual and the community can afford. However, over the past decade, insulin prices have tripled in the United States, while out-of-pocket costs per prescription doubled. High costs of medications can contribute to nonadherence, but the prevalence of cost-related insulin underuse is unknown. The price of insulin tripled between 2002 and 2013, and since 2008, 3 of the makers have raised the list price of insulin at least 10 times. The FDA commissioner Scott Gottlieb has said that the FDA is going to be changing the way that they regulate insulin moving forward and there is much discussion and some early movement to address insulin pricing at the state and national levels. Compassionate and/or rebate programs for prescription drugs sometimes can be used as a bridge to obtain insulin as an enduring solution for individual patients is identified and put into place.

These issues may apply to any insulin-requiring diabetes patient without insurance, with Medicare Part D, and/or anyone who is underinsured. It is extremely important to discuss access to and affordability of insulin with individuals with diabetes, particularly those with type 1, who are prescribed insulin. Some insulins are less expensive than others for use as basal and bolus choices. These include U100 human regular insulin, U100 human NPH insulin, and premixed 70/30 insulin (NPH/regular). The vial and syringe option is less expensive than prefilled pens.

Educational Objective

Recall precipitating factors for euglycemic diabetic ketoacidosis.

Reference(s)

Herkert D, Vijayakumar P, Luo J, et al. Cost-related insulin underuse among patients with diabetes. *JAMA Intern Med.* 2019;179(1):112-114. PMID: 30508012

Rosenthal E. When high prices mean needless death. *JAMA Intern Med.* 2019;179(1):114-115. PMID: 30508014

Fralick M, Schneeweiss S, Patorno E. Risk of diabetic ketoacidosis after initiation of an SGLT2 inhibitor. *N Engl J Med.* 2017;376(23):2300-2302. PMID: 28591538

55 ANSWER: B) Ask her to show you how she self-administers a correction insulin dose using her pen

This patient was observed giving herself an insulin injection (Answer B). It was determined that she was correctly dialing the insulin dose into the pen and inserting the needle into the subcutaneous tissue space. However, she was then dialing the dose back down instead of pushing the button to inject the insulin. Therefore, she was not actually getting any insulin with her injections. Upon further questioning, she reported that she had changed her technique several months earlier because the insulin injections were causing discomfort, and she found when she changed from pushing the button to "dialing back," it did not hurt anymore.

She was instructed in proper technique for self-injection using a prefilled insulin pen. Her insulin doses were recalculated based on a weight-based formula, as it was not clear how much, if any insulin she had been injecting.

In accordance with the national standards for diabetes self-management education and support, all persons with diabetes should participate in diabetes self-management education and support. There are 4 critical times to evaluate the need for diabetes self-management education and support:

1. At diagnosis
2. Annually
3. When complicating factors arise (as is the case in this patient)
4. When transitions in care occur

If she has not already had diabetes self-management education and support (Answer A), including medical nutrition therapy, this would certainly be appropriate as an adjunctive strategy. However, she has already largely cut out simple carbohydrates from her diet and a change in meal plan would not have a big impact on her blood glucose levels until she is taking her insulin properly. While regular physical activity is recommended in conjunction with medical nutrition therapy as the cornerstone of type 2 diabetes management, initiating vigorous exercise (Answer C) while in a catabolic state, as is the case when marked symptomatic hyperglycemia is present, is not recommended. Finally, this patient has consistently elevated blood glucose and a markedly elevated hemoglobin A_{1c}

level, and it is highly unlikely that she is experiencing hypoglycemia or fluctuations in blood glucose patterns that data generated from continuous glucose monitoring (Answer D) would provide additional information about.

Educational Objective
Identify the need for insulin self-injection skills education.

Reference(s)
Powers MA, Bardsley J, Cypress M, et al. Diabetes self-management education and support in type 2 diabetes: a joint statement of the American Diabetes Association, the American Association of Diabetes Educators, and the Academy of Nutrition and Dietetics. *Diabetes Care.* 2015; 38(7):1372-1382. PMID: 26048904

56 ANSWER: A) Metformin

Despite this man's modest increase in risk for cardiovascular disease, metformin (Answer A) remains the first-line therapy agent of choice in international guidelines for diabetes management, including the recent 2018 American Diabetes Association and European Association for the Study of Diabetes Consensus Report on management of hyperglycemia in type 2 diabetes. Metformin should be combined with comprehensive lifestyle changes (including weight management and physical activity) if hemoglobin A_{1c} is above target, as is the case in this patient.

The major change in the new guidelines is based on accumulating evidence that specific SGLT-2 inhibitors and GLP-1 receptor agonists improve cardiovascular outcomes, as well as secondary outcomes such as heart failure and progression of renal disease, in patients with established cardiovascular disease or chronic kidney disease. Therefore, subsequent guidance in this overall approach when another drug is required is based on the presence or absence of established atherosclerotic cardiovascular disease or chronic kidney disease. As this patient has newly diagnosed diabetes, a modestly elevated hemoglobin A_{1c}, and no evidence of established cardiovascular disease or nephropathy, incorporation of an SGLT-2 inhibitor (Answer B) or a GLP-1 receptor agonist (Answer C) into his anti-hyperglycemic medication regimen is not indicated. The DPP-4 inhibitors (Answer D) do not confer advantages in terms of cardiovascular disease or renal outcome.

This man's calculated 10-year risk of heart disease or stroke is 14.1%. In patients with diabetes mellitus at higher risk, especially those with multiple risk factors or those 50 to 75 years of age, it is reasonable to recommend a high-intensity statin to reduce the LDL-cholesterol level by 50% or more. The American College of Cardiology/American Heart Association guidelines therefore suggest treatment with a high-intensity statin. This patient is taking atorvastatin, 40 mg daily. High-intensity dosing for atorvastatin is 80 mg daily, unless down-titration is required if the patient is unable to tolerate this dosage. He should be advised to increase his atorvastatin dosage to 80 mg daily. In addition, based on his age and calculated cardiovascular disease risk greater than 10%, he should be advised to start taking aspirin, 81 mg daily, as long as he is not at increased risk for bleeding and is willing to take it daily for at least 10 years.

Educational Objective

Explain how atherosclerotic cardiovascular disease risk is incorporated into selection of medications used to treat type 2 diabetes mellitus.

Reference(s)

http://www.cvriskcalculator.com/

Davies MJ, D'Alessio DA, Fradkin J, et al. Management of hyperglycemia in type 2 diabetes, 2018. A consensus report by the American Diabetes Association (ADA) and the European Association for the Study of Diabetes (EASD). *Diabetes Care*. 2018;41(12):2669-2701. PMID: 30291106

Grundy SM, Stone NJ, Bailey AL, et al. 2018 AHA/ACC/AACVPR/AAPA/ABC/ACPM/ADA/AGS/AphA/ASPC/NLA/PCNA guideline on the management of blood cholesterol: a report of the American College of Cardiology/American Heart Association Task Force on Clinical Practice Guidelines. *J Am Coll Cardiol*. 2019; 73(24):e285-e350. PMID: 20423393

57 ANSWER: A) Sitagliptin

In general, in the hospital setting for non-critically ill patients, a basal-bolus insulin regimen correction dose when blood glucose is high is preferred for glycemic management for individuals with good nutritional intake. In contrast, a single dose of long-acting insulin plus correction insulin is preferred for patients with poor or no oral intake. When a patient with type 2 diabetes has mild to moderate hyperglycemia and is otherwise clinically stable, the addition of an oral agent to the regimen—to prepare for discharge—may be considered. The Sita-Hospital Study was conducted in 5 US hospitals among 18- to 80-year-old adults with type 2 diabetes who had random blood glucose concentrations ranging from 140 to 400 mg/dL (7.8-22.2 mmol/L). For inclusion, patients needed to be eating and taking less than 0.6 units/kg per day of insulin. They were randomly assigned to sitagliptin (Answer A) plus basal insulin (n = 138) or a basal-bolus insulin regimen (n = 139).

Glycemic control between the groups assessed as the mean percentage of blood glucose values ranging from 70 to 180 mg/dL (3.9-10 mmol/L) did not differ at 57% for the sitagliptin plus basal insulin group and 59.6% for the basal-bolus group ($P = .58$). A relatively small percentage from each group experienced treatment failure (16% vs 19%, $P = .54$), which was recognized 2 to 3 days following randomization. There was no severe hypoglycemia (blood glucose <40 mg/dL [<2.2 mmol/L]). The only significant difference between groups was in the total daily insulin dose requirement (units/kg), which was lower at 0.2 (±0.1) for patients receiving sitagliptin compared with 0.3 (±0.2) for basal-bolus alone ($P < .0001$).

The researchers concluded that treatment with sitagliptin plus basal insulin is as effective and safe as (and a convenient alternative to) a labor-intensive basal-bolus insulin regimen for the management of hyperglycemia in patients with type 2 diabetes admitted to nonintensive care unit general medicine and surgery services.

Metformin (Answer B) in this patient is contraindicated because he has advanced heart failure. Pioglitazone (Answer C) could lead to fluid retention and exacerbation of congestive heart failure. Also, as its time to onset of action is in the range of 2 to 3 weeks, pioglitazone would not lead to short-term improvement in glycemic control during the current hospital stay. Use of an SGLT-2 inhibitor (Answer D) is associated with risk for ketoacidosis, urosepsis, urinary tract infections, and renal injury. Thus, SGLT-2 inhibitors cannot be recommended in the hospital setting, as their safety and effectiveness have not been established.

Educational Objective

Manage type 2 diabetes mellitus in the hospital on general medicine and surgery units.

Reference(s)

Lansang MC, Umpierrez GE. Inpatient hyperglycemia management: a practical review for primary medical and surgical teams. *Cleve Clin J Med.* 2016;83(Suppl 1):S34-S43. PMID: 27176681

Pasquel FJ, Gianchandani R, Rubin DJ, et al. Efficacy of sitagliptin for the hospital management of general medicine and surgery patients with type 2 diabetes (Sita-Hospital): a multicentre, prospective, open-label, non-inferiority randomised trial. *Lancet Diabetes Endocrinol.* 2017;5(2):125-133. PMID: 27964837

58 ANSWER: C) An SGLT-2 inhibitor

Heart failure is highly prevalent in patients with diabetes, occurring in more than 1 in 5 patients with diabetes who are older than 65 years. Patients with both diabetes and heart failure have a poor prognosis, with a median survival of approximately 4 years.

This patient has American Heart Association Class II Congestive Heart Failure, which is characterized by slight limitation in physical activity. Cardiovascular outcome trials of SGLT-2 inhibitors (Answer C) among persons with type 2 diabetes have demonstrated significant impact on cardiovascular outcomes, including risk for hospitalizations for heart failure, as shown in the table.

Trial	Outcomes	
EMPA-REG (n = 7020 with established cardiovascular disease) - empagliflozin		
	Study Drug	**Placebo**
Risk for heart failure admissions	2.7% (hazard ratio, 0.65; confidence interval, 0.50-0.85)	4.1%
CANVAS (n = 10,142 with high cardiovascular risk) - canagliflozin		
	Study Drug	**Placebo**
Risk for heart failure hospitalization	5.5/1000 patient-years (hazard ratio, 0.67; confidence interval, 0.52-0.87)	8.7/1000 patient-years
CVD-REAL (n = 309,045) observational comparison SGLT-2 inhibitors vs other antihyperglycemic drugs		
Risk for heart failure hospitalization	39% lower risk of heart failure with SGLT-2 inhibitors	
DECLARE-TIMI 58 (n = 17,160 with or at risk for CVD) - dapagliflozin		
Hospitalization rate for heart failure	Hazard ratio, 0.73 for study Rx; 95% confidence interval, (0.61-0.88)	

Empagliflozin reduced the primary major adverse cardiovascular event (MACE) endpoint compared with placebo treatment (10.5% vs 12.5%; hazard ratio, 0.86; 95% confidence interval, 0.74-0.99). Canagliflozin demonstrated significant reduction in the risk of cardiovascular death, nonfatal myocardial infarction, or nonfatal stroke (26.9 vs 31.5, respectively, per 1000 patient-years; hazard ratio, 0.86; 95% confidence interval, 0.75-0.97). Dapagliflozin did not reduce the primary MACE endpoint (8.8% in the dapagliflozin group and 9.4% for placebo; hazard ratio, 0.93; 95% confidence interval, 0.84-1.03; $P = .17$), but it did result in a lower rate of cardiovascular death or hospitalization for heart failure (4.9% vs 5.8%; hazard ratio, 0.83; 95% confidence interval, 0.73-0.95; $P = .005$). This reflects a reduced rate of hospitalizations for heart failure as shown in the table.

The ability of SGLT-2 inhibitors to optimize volume status through glycosuria and also to inhibit the sodium-hydrogen exchanger in the kidneys and heart is hypothesized to result in this impact on heart failure outcomes via a cascade of responses including increasing natriuresis, decreasing myocardial fibrosis, and increasing cardiac contractility. The results of these studies serve as the basis for positioning SGLT-2 inhibitors as second-line agents in the 2018 American Diabetes Association and European Association for the Study of Diabetes Consensus Report on the management of hyperglycemia in type 2 diabetes.

GLP-1 receptor agonists (Answer A) have not been shown to significantly reduce risk for hospitalizations due to heart failure, but it is important to note that liraglutide (LEADER trial) did reduce risk for the primary MACE outcome of cardiovascular death, nonfatal myocardial infarction, and nonfatal stroke. No prospective randomized controlled trial has evaluated whether metformin (Answer B) is the optimal first-line agent in patients with diabetes and heart failure. Finally, several studies have suggested that increased heart failure risk is seen with thiazolidinedione use (Answer D).

Educational Objective
Manage antihyperglycemic agents in a patient with type 2 diabetes mellitus and congestive heart failure.

Reference(s)
Sharma A, Cooper LB, Fiuzat M, et al. Anti-hyperglycemic therapies to treat patients with heart failure and diabetes mellitus. *JACC Heart Fail.* 2018;6(10):813-822. PMID: 30098964

Wiviott SD, Raz I. Dapagliflozin and cardiovascular outcomes in type 2 diabetes. *N Engl J Med.* 2019; 380(4):347-357. PMID: 30415602

Zinman B, Wanner C, Lachin JM, et al; EMPA-REG OUTCOME Investigators. Empagliflozin, cardiovascular otucomes, and mortality in type 2 diabetes. *N Engl J Med.* 2015;373(22):2117-2128. PMID: 26378978

Neal B, Perkovic V, Mahaffey KW, et al; CANVAS Program Collaborative Group. Canagliflozin and cardiovascular and renal events in type 2 diabetes. *N Engl J Med.* 2017;377(7):644-657. PMID: 28605608

Davies MJ, D'Alessio DA, Fradkin J, et al. Management of hyperglycemia in type 2 diabetes, 2018. A consensus report by the American Diabetes Association (ADA) and the European Association for the Study of Diabetes (EASD). *Diabetes Care.* 2018;41(12):2669-2701. PMID: 30291106

Kosiborod M, Cavender MA, Fu AZ, et al; CVD-REAL Investigators and Study Group. Lower risk of heart failure and death in patients initiated on sodium-glucose cotransporter-2 inhibitors versus other glucose-lowering drugs: the CVD-REAL Study (Comparative Effectiveness of Cardiovascular Outcomes in New Users of Sodium-Glucose Cotransporters-2 Inhibitors). *Circulation.* 2017;136(3):249-259. PMID: 28522450

59 ANSWER: C) Perforating collagenosis
The association of specific skin disorders with diabetes mellitus has been well established. Current literature suggests that approximately 30% to 91% of patients with diabetes experience at least one cutaneous manifestation of a systemic disease in their lifetime.

In this case, skin biopsy revealed an ulcer with a fibrin base and focal collagen fibers perforating through the hyperplastic epithelium adjacent to the ulcer. There was a mixed inflammatory infiltrate composed of neutrophils and lymphocytes. These findings are consistent with acquired or reactive perforating collagenosis (Answer C). It may also be referred to as perforating folliculitis or Kyrle disease. It is characterized by hyperkeratotic papules with transepidermal elimination of degenerated material, including collagen or elastic fibers. This is a distinct entity seen most commonly in persons with diabetes or chronic kidney disease. It has also been associated with hyperparathyroidism, hypothyroidism, and liver disease. It may be difficult to treat, but often responds to light therapy. This patient started a course of twice-weekly light therapy.

Hypersensitivity to insect bites (Answer A) is also a consideration in the differential diagnosis of scattered pruritic lesions, but this would not specifically be associated with diabetes. Necrobiosis lipoidica diabeticorum (Answer B) is a rare chronic and granulomatous skin disorder that affects 0.3% of patients with diabetes. The skin lesions are characterized by thinning of the skin, dilated capillaries, and lipid deposits. This appearance is quite different from the lesions seen in this case. While the etiology and pathogenesis of necrobiosis lipoidica diabeticorum is still controversial, it is thought that microangiopathy has an important role. The legs are the most common site for necrobiosis lipoidica diabeticorum, but involvement of other areas such as the abdomen, upper extremities, and scalp has been reported. Benefit has been reported from different treatment regimens such as corticosteroid therapy (topical, intralesional and systemic), enhancers of wound healing, surgery, and immunomodulating therapies (including photochemotherapy).

Before the introduction of recombinant human insulin to the market in the early 1980s, insulin allergy (Answer D) was a common occurrence. Allergy to human insulin preparations, although rare, can still occur. When insulin allergy is suspected, it is important to rule out causes such as allergies to inactive ingredients in the insulin formulation (eg, protamine sulfate, zinc, and metacresol) and allergies to latex or alcohol swabs that are used in the insulin preparation and injection process. Allergies to inactive ingredients in the insulin formulation can often be resolved by switching to a different type of insulin that does not contain the responsible inactive ingredient. In rare cases, an individual can be allergic to the insulin molecule itself. Insulin allergy may present as a localized reaction at the injection site or a more severe, generalized reaction that can range from urticaria to anaphylaxis. The lesions exhibited by the patient in this vignette are not true urticaria.

Educational Objective

Differentiate among specific skin disorders associated with diabetes mellitus.

Reference(s)

Rapini RP, Hebert AA, Drucker CR. Acquired perforating dermatosis. *Arch Dermatol.* 1989; 125(8):1074-1078. PMID: 2757403

Kota SK, Jammula S, Kota SK, Meher LK, Modi KD. Necrobiosis lipoidica diabeticorum: a case-based review of literature. *Indian J Endocrinol Metab.* 2012;16(4):614-620. PMID: 22837927

Female Reproduction Board Review

Kathryn A. Martin, MD

1 ANSWER: C) Type 2 diabetes

Menopausal hormone therapy reduces the risk of developing type 2 diabetes (Answer C). The best evidence for this comes from the Women's Health Initiative. Menopausal hormone therapy improves β-cell insulin secretion, glucose effectiveness, and insulin sensitivity, as measured in clinical settings. This reduction was seen in a follow-up analysis from the Women's Health Initiative.

When younger postmenopausal women (ages 50-59 or <10 years since menopause) take menopausal hormone therapy, its benefits outweigh its risks. However, menopausal hormone therapy does not reduce the risks of stroke (Answer A) or pulmonary embolism (Answer D) at any age. In older women, it may have a harmful effect on cognitive function and dementia (Answer B), but its impact in younger menopausal women remains unclear.

Educational Objective

Explain the risk-benefit profile of estrogen and estrogen-progestin therapy in younger postmenopausal women (ages 50 to 59 years or <10 years since menopause).

Reference(s)

Margolis KL, Bonds DE, Rodabough RJ, et al; Women's Health Initiative Investigators. Effect of oestrogen plus progestin on the incidence of diabetes in postmenopausal women: results from the Women's Health Initiative Hormone Trial. *Diabetologia.* 2004;47(7):1175-1187. PMID: 15252707

Mauvais-Jarvis F, Manson JE, Stevenson J, Fonseca VA. Menopausal hormone therapy and type 2 diabetes prevention: evidence, mechanisms, and clinical implications. *Endocr Rev.* 2017;38(3): 173-188. PMID: 28323934

Stuenkel CA, Davis SR, Gompel A, et al. Treatment of symptoms of the menopause: an Endocrine Society clinical practice guideline. *J Clin Endocrinol Metab.* 2015;100(11):3975-4011. PMID: 26444994

2 ANSWER: B) 21-Hydroxylase antibodies

This patient has spontaneous primary ovarian insufficiency (POI). Additional evaluation is needed once this condition is diagnosed. Although the etiology of POI remains unknown in most cases, a number of tests should be done once a diagnosis of POI is established. These investigations include karyotype analysis (primarily to diagnose Turner syndrome), genetic testing for the fragile X premutation (approximately 6% of cases of POI are associated with premutations in the *FMR1* gene, the gene responsible for the fragile X syndrome and fragile X–associated tremor/ataxia syndrome). Women with the premutation often have POI, but the main concern is expansion to a full mutation in male offspring, causing intellectual disability and a number of other features.

Approximately 3% of women with spontaneous POI have asymptomatic autoimmune adrenal insufficiency—the diagnosis of POI typically precedes that of adrenal insufficiency by several years. As a screen for the presence of asymptomatic autoimmune adrenal insufficiency, serum 21-hydroxylase antibodies (Answer B) and usually adrenal cortical antibodies should be measured in all women with a 46,XX karyotype at the time spontaneous POI is diagnosed. Women with adrenal autoimmunity detected by the presence of autoantibodies have a 50% risk of developing adrenal insufficiency. These women should then be evaluated for the presence of adrenal insufficiency by measuring 8-AM serum cortisol and plasma ACTH. Testing for 21-hydroxylase antibodies may serve the dual purpose of screening for autoimmune adrenal insufficiency and making the diagnosis of autoimmune oophoritis. Autoimmune oophoritis is characterized by theca-cell destruction; granulosa cells are preserved.

Inhibin B levels (Answer A) are normal in women with autoimmune POI, but are low in women with other types of POI. Therefore, affected women present with serum LH concentrations that are higher than FSH concentrations. Measurement of serum ovarian antibodies (Answer D) (using an indirect immuno-fluorescence assay using cynomolgus monkey ovary) has poor predictive value for autoimmune POI. The prevalence of ovarian antibodies is similar (30%-50%) in normal cycling women and women with sponta-neous POI. IGF-1 measurement (Answer C) would not provide useful clinical information about POI.

Educational Objective
Diagnose the etiology of primary ovarian insufficiency.

Reference(s)
Bakalov VK, Anasti JN, Calis KA, et al. Autoim-mune oophoritis as a mechanism of follicular dysfunction in women with 46,XX spontaneous premature ovarian failure. *Fertil Steril.* 2005; 84(4):958-965. PMID: 16213850

Welt CK, Hally JE, Adams JM, Taylor AE. Re-lationship of estradiol and inhibin to the follicle-stimulating hormone variability in hypergonadotropic hypogonadism or premature ovarian failure. *J Clin Endocrinol Metab.* 2005; 90(2):826-830. PMID: 15562017

Novosad JA, Kalantaridou SN, Tong ZB, Nelson LM. Ovarian antibodies as detected by indirect immunofluorescence are unreliable in the di-agnosis of autoimmune premature ovarian fail-ure: a controlled evaluation. *BMC Womens Health.* 2003;3(1):2. PMID: 12694633

ANSWER: A) Menopausal transition (perimenopause)
This woman is experiencing typical symptoms of the menopausal transition or perimenopause. Many cycles are anovulatory and serum estradiol levels are ex-tremely high at times, followed by a rapid drop. FSH concentrations vary depending on estradiol levels and whether there has been a recent ovulation. Obesity alone (Answer C) can be associated with a change in menstrual cycles, but it would not explain her high serum estradiol or vasomotor symptoms. Symptoms during the menopausal transition may include breast

soreness when estradiol levels are extremely high, and hot flashes/night sweats when estradiol levels fall. Se-rum progesterone concentrations would be much higher with pregnancy (Answer B). The high estradiol value is not enough to raise suspicion for a granulosa-cell tumor (Answer D). Women with such tumors often have abdominal pain (the tumors are large), bleeding, and endometrial hyperplasia.

Educational Objective
Identify the characteristic clinical and biochemical findings of the menopausal transition.

Reference(s)
Harlow SD, Gass M, Hall JE, et al; STRAW + 10: addressing the unfinished agenda of staging re-productive aging. Executive summary of the Stages of Reproductive Aging Workshop + 10: addressing the unfinished agenda of staging re-productive aging. *J Clin Endocrinol Metab.* 2012; 97(4):1159-1168. PMID: 22344196

Burger HG, Hale GE, Robertson DM, Dennerstein L. A review of hormonal changes during the menopausal transition: focus on findings from the Melbourne Women's Midlife Health Project. *Hum Reprod Update.* 2007;13(6):559-565. PMID: 17630397

ANSWER: B) Midcycle LH surge
At the time of the midcycle surge (Answer B), both LH and estradiol levels are high. FSH increases as well, but the magnitude of rise is small compared with that of LH. This patient has lost slightly more than 10% of her body weight, which often results in restoration of ovulatory cycles in women with polycystic ovary syndrome. Thus, it appears that she may be ovulatory again and may not require ovulation induction. How-ever, it would be best for her to lose more weight to further improve pregnancy outcomes.

When a woman with polycystic ovary syndrome (Answer C) is anovulatory, basal LH, FSH, and es-tradiol levels are lower than those described here. Se-rum LH is typically higher than FSH, and may be as high as 20 mIU/mL (20 IU/L). In contrast, serum LH is much higher at the midcycle surge (serum concen-trations can be greater than 100 mIU/mL (>100 IU/L). In women with primary ovarian insufficiency (Answer A), FSH is higher than LH (with the exception of autoimmune oophoritis) and estradiol is very low. The progesterone level would be very high in pregnancy (Answer D).

Educational Objective

Identify the characteristic biochemical findings of the preovulatory midcycle LH surge.

Reference(s)

Adams JM, Taylor AE, Schoenfeld DA, Crowley WF Jr, Hall JE. The midcycle gonadotropin surge in normal women occurs in the face of an unchanging gonadotropin-releasing hormone pulse frequency. *J Clin Endocrinol Metab*. 1994;79(3): 858-864. PMID: 7521353

ANSWER: C) Transdermal 17β-estradiol, 50 to 200 mcg once or twice weekly

Transdermal estradiol (Answer C) is the optimal estrogen preparation for transgender women, as it has the lowest rate of vascular risks. This is most important for patients with risk factors for venous thromboembolism. Either an antiandrogen or a GnRH agonist should be added to the estrogen regimen to lower serum androgens—this allows lowering of the estrogen dosage. Oral estradiol is only appropriate for patients at low risk for venous thromboembolism. Ethinyl estradiol, 50 to 100 mcg daily, (Answer A) is too potent an estrogen, too high of a dosage, is associated with cardiovascular complications (particularly venous thromboembolism), and is not recommended for use in this population. Conjugated estrogens, 1.25 mg daily (Answer D), is too low a dosage, and is less appealing than 17β-estradiol to most patients. Although transdermal 17β-estradiol is the optimal regimen, oral 17β-estradiol, 2 to 6 mg daily (Answer B) is a commonly used regimen because of its lower expense.

Educational Objective

Differentiate among the estrogen regimens for transgender women who choose hormonal therapy.

Reference(s)

Hembree WC, Cohen-Kettenis PT, Gooren L, et al. Endocrine treatment of gender dysphoric/gender-incongruent persons: an Endocrine Society clinical practice guideline. *J Clin Endocrinol Metab*. 2017;102(11):3869-3903. PMID: 28945902

Deutsch MB, Feldman JL. Updated recommendations from the world professional association for transgender health standards of care. *Am Fam Physician*. 2013;87(2):89-93. PMID: 23317072

ANSWER: C) Sleep apnea

Polycystic ovary syndrome is a common disorder that occurs in 6% to 8% of women. Affected patients usually present with hirsutism, acne, and irregular menses. Sixty percent of affected women become obese. In addition to being at increased risk for impaired glucose tolerance and type 2 diabetes mellitus with a risk 5 to 10 times that of age-matched control women, women with polycystic ovary syndrome are also at high risk for sleep apnea. Given this patient's history of daytime sleepiness, the most likely diagnosis is sleep apnea (Answer C).

Although she has gained weight and reports fatigue, she has no other features that strongly suggest hypercortisolism (Answer D). Type 2 diabetes mellitus (Answer A) is also a possibility, but sleepiness would not be the main feature. Depression (Answer B) affects many women with polycystic ovary syndrome, and insomnia can be a symptom, but daytime sleepiness strongly suggests sleep apnea.

Educational Objective

Counsel patients about the increased risk of sleep apnea associated with polycystic ovary syndrome.

Reference(s)

McCartney CR, Marshall JC. Clinical practice. Polycystic ovary syndrome. *N Engl J Med*. 2016; 375(1):54-64. PMID: 27406348

Legro RS, Arslanian SA, Ehrmann DA, et al; Endocrine Society. Diagnosis and treatment of polycystic ovary syndrome: an Endocrine Society clinical practice guideline. *J Clin Endocrinol Metab*. 2013;98(12):4565-4592. PMID: 24151290

Ehrmann DA. Metabolic dysfunction in PCOS: relationship to obstructive sleep apnea. *Steroids*. 2012;77(4):290-294. PMID: 22178788

Tasali E, Chapotot F, Leproult R, Whitmore H, Ehrmann DA. Treatment of obstructive sleep apnea improves cardiometabolic function in young obese women with polycystic ovary syndrome. *J Clin Endocrinol Metab*. 2011;96(2):365-374. PMID: 211234494

7 ANSWER: A) Dementia

This patient is an excellent candidate for estrogen. The results of the Women's Health Initiative are not relevant to her, as the mean age of the patients in that study was 63 years and she is only 41. She should be approached like any woman with primary ovarian insufficiency and be treated with estrogen until the average age of menopause (50 or 51 years). She has severe symptoms that are interfering with her quality of life and her ability to function, so estrogen is indicated.

Menopausal hormone therapy (until the average age of menopause) is suggested for women who undergo early bilateral oophorectomy or who have primary ovarian insufficiency. The goal is to reduce the risk of health disorders associated with early estrogen deficiency (coronary disease, dementia [Answer A], osteoporosis). The risks of migraine headaches (Answer B), autoimmune disorders (Answer C), and osteoarthritis (Answer D) have not been associated with early menopause.

Observational data suggest that some of the long-term health consequences of bilateral oophorectomy can be reduced by taking estrogen therapy. After age 50 years, the use of menopausal hormone therapy prevents bone loss and osteoporosis, but there is not strong evidence that it is reliably effective for the prevention of other long-term diseases (coronary heart disease, dementia).

Educational Objective

Describe the potential health consequences of early oophorectomy and estrogen deficiency on women and the role of estrogen therapy to minimize those risks.

Reference(s)

Stuenkel CA, Davis SR, Gompel A, et al. Treatment of symptoms of the menopause: an Endocrine Society clinical practice guideline. *J Clin Endocrinol Metab*. 2015;100(11):3975-4011. PMID: 26444994

Rocca WA, Grossardt BR, de Andrade M, Malkasian GD, Melton LJ 3rd. Survival patterns after oophorectomy in premenopausal women: a population-based cohort study. *Lancet Oncol*. 2006;7(10):821-828. PMID: 17012044

8 ANSWER: C) Prednisone

Nonclassic congenital adrenal hyperplasia (CAH) is a cause of hyperandrogenic anovulation with a clinical presentation that is similar or identical to that of polycystic ovary syndrome (hirsutism with irregular menses). In women with nonclassic CAH, basal morning serum 17-hydroxyprogesterone concentrations (during the follicular phase of the menstrual cycle) are usually greater than 200 ng/dL (>6.1 nmol/L) (high-normal or high).

For anovulatory women with nonclassic CAH who are pursuing fertility, most experts suggest glucocorticoid therapy as the initial treatment (rather than clomiphene citrate or letrozole [Answer D]—the drugs used in polycystic ovary syndrome). However, clomiphene citrate and other assisted reproduction techniques may be added if glucocorticoid therapy alone is ineffective. Dexamethasone (Answer A) is not inactivated by placental 11β-hydroxysteroid dehydrogenase type 2 (fetal exposure occurs). Therefore, hydrocortisone or prednisone (Answer C) is a better option. A common regimen is prednisone, 5 mg daily; clomiphene citrate can be added if ovulation has not occurred with prednisone alone. Alternatively, the prednisone dosage can be increased to 7.5 mg daily before adding clomiphene.

Metformin (Answer B) had been used in women with polycystic ovary syndrome as a strategy to restore ovulatory cycles. However, metformin is no longer recommended because ovulatory and live birth rates are considerably lower than those observed with clomiphene citrate and letrozole.

Educational Objective

Recommend the best treatment of nonclassic congenital adrenal hyperplasia.

Reference(s)

Moran C, Azziz R, Weintrob N, et al. Reproductive outcome of women with 21-hydroxylase-deficient nonclassic adrenal hyperplasia: a multicenter study. *J Clin Endocrinol Metab*. 2006; 91(9):3451-3456. PMID: 16822826

Bidet M, Bellanné-Chantelot C, Galand-Portier MB, et al. Fertility in women with nonclassical congenital adrenal hyperplasia due to 21-hydroxylase deficiency. *J Clin Endocrinol Metab*. 2010;95(3):1182-1190. PMID: 20080854

Finkielstain GP, Kim MS, Sinaii N, et al. Clinical characteristics of a cohort of 244 patients with congenital adrenal hyperplasia. *J Clin Endocrinol Metab.* 2012;97(12):4429-4438. PMID: 22990093

Speiser PW, Arlt W, Auchus RJ, et al. Congenital adrenal hyperplasia due to steroid 21-hydroxylase deficiency: an Endocrine Society clinical practice guideline. *J Clin Endocrinol Metab.* 2018;103(11): 4043-4088. PMID: 30272171

9 ANSWER: A) Transdermal estradiol, 0.05 mg patch twice weekly

Of the options listed, transdermal estradiol, 0.05 mg twice weekly (Answer A), would be the optimal choice; lower starting dosages are often used (eg, 0.025 mg), but the dosage of 0.05 mg twice weekly will relieve her symptoms more quickly. A low-dosage oral contraceptive (Answer B) would be a good option for a perimenopausal woman with symptoms who also desired contraception. However, oral contraceptives are not ideal for obese perimenopausal women, as both age and obesity increase the risk of venous thromboembolism. In addition, she already has an intrauterine device in place, so contraception is not required. Gabapentin (Answer C) is a nonhormonal alternative therapy that is less effective than estrogen. Conjugated estrogens (Answer D) are a possibility, but the dose of 0.3 mg daily would be unlikely to relieve her symptoms.

Educational Objective
Recommend the best treatment option in a perimenopausal woman with severe hot flashes (in the late transition).

Reference(s)
Stuenkel CA, Davis SA, Gompel A, et al. Treatment of symptoms of the menpause: an Endocrine Society clinical practice guideline. *J Clin Endocrinol Metab.* 2015;100(11):3975-4011. PMID: 26444994

The NAMS 2017 Hormone Therapy Position Statement Advisory Panel. The 2017 hormone therapy position statement of The North American Menopause Society. *Menopause.* 2017; 24(7):728-753. PMID: 28650869

10 ANSWER: B) Thyroid function tests, hemoglobin A$_{1c}$ measurement, liver enzymes

Turner syndrome occurs in 1 in 2500 live births and is associated with growth failure, pubertal delay, and cardiac abnormalities. In addition, affected patients are at risk for a number of comorbidities, including type 2 diabetes, elevated liver enzymes, autoimmune thyroid disease, celiac disease, hearing loss, orthodontic problems, and psychosocial disorders. Cardiac MRI is the most important test because congenital cardiac abnormalities are present in up to 50% of patients and include coarctation of the aorta, bicuspid aortic valve, and partial anomalous pulmonary venous return. Echocardiography is also sometimes used as part of the routine follow-up of women with Turner syndrome (but it is not performed annually).

Current practice guidelines recommend annual visits for women with Turner syndrome. In addition to measuring blood pressure, calculating BMI, and performing a full skin examination, the following assessments are recommended: thyroid function tests, hemoglobin A$_{1c}$ measurement, and liver enzymes (AST, ALT, gamma-glutamyl transferase, alkaline phosphatase) (Answer B). Screening for other comorbidities (eg, celiac disease [Answer C] or renal disorders [Answer A]) is performed at less frequent intervals. Complete blood cell count (Answer D) is not recommended routinely.

Educational Objective
Recommend appropriate evaluation for girls with gonadal dysgenesis.

Reference(s)
Gravholt CH, Andersen NH, Conway GS, et al; International Turner Syndrome Consensus Group. Clinical practice guidelines for the care of girls and women with Turner syndrome: proceedings from the 2016 Cincinnati International Turner Syndrome Meeting. *Eur J Endocrinol.* 2017;177(3):G1-G70. PMID: 28705803

Davenport ML. Approach to the patient with Turner syndrome. *J Clin Endocrinol Metab.* 2010; 95(4):1487-1495. PMID: 20375216

Pinsker JE. Clinical review: Turner syndrome: updating the paradigm of clinical care. *J Clin Endocrinol Metab.* 2012;97(6):994-1003. PMID: 22472565

11 ANSWER: B) Increased oiliness of the skin and acne

Testosterone therapy has many masculinizing effects in transgender men. Some of the effects are noticeable in the first 6 months of treatment (eg, increased oiliness of the skin [Answer B], clitoral enlargement, cessation of menses, vaginal atrophy), while others are not observed until 6 to 12 months of therapy (eg, deepening of the voice [Answer A], scalp hair loss [Answer D], increased body hair [Answer C], and increased muscle mass and strength). The maximum effect can take up to 5 years for outcomes such as facial and body hair growth, muscle mass and strength, and fat redistribution.

Educational Objective

Counsel transgender men regarding the time course of the masculinizing effects of testosterone therapy.

Reference(s)

Hembree WC, Cohen-Kettenis PT, Gooren L, et al. Endocrine treatment of gender-dysphoric/ gender-incongruent persons: an Endocrine Society clinical practice guideline. *J Clin Endocrinol Metab.* 2017;102(11):3869-3903. PMID: 28945902

Spack NP. Management of transgenderism. *JAMA.* 2013;309(5):478-484. PMID: 23385274

12 ANSWER: C) 46,XY

This patient is phenotypically female, with excellent breast development but an absent uterus and high LH and FSH levels. This is the presentation of a patient with complete androgen insensitivity syndrome, and her karyotype is most likely 46,XY.

In androgen insensitivity syndrome, an individual with this karyotype presents with a female phenotype because testosterone is unable to activate its receptor. This is confirmed by the absence of a cervix, as the mullerian ducts are needed for development of the upper one-third of the vagina, cervix, uterus, and fallopian tubes. Serum testosterone levels in these women are high and distinguish androgen insensitivity syndrome from the even more rare congenital absence of the uterus and vagina (mullerian agenesis), which would present with absent menarche but normal pubertal development because of normal ovarian function. Such patients have a 46,XX karyotype (Answer B). In androgen insensitivity syndrome, pubic and axillary hair is sparse because of lack of androgen in combination with estrogen action. Aromatization of testosterone in peripheral tissues results in high estrogen as well. Individuals with complete androgen insensitivity syndrome function as phenotypic females, although they are unable to bear children. The testes are often located in the groin and should be removed because of the potential for tumor formation (2%-5%).

The other karyotypes are not consistent with this patient's presentation. Women with Turner syndrome (gonadal dysgenesis) have a 45,X karyotype. They have ovarian failure, short stature, and many comorbidities, including cardiovascular anomalies. Lastly, a 46,XXY karyotype is the underlying cause of Klinefelter syndrome (men with hypergonadotropic hypogonadism).

Educational Objective

Diagnose complete androgen insensitivity syndrome.

Reference(s)

Hughes IA, Davies JD, Bunch TI, Pasterski V, Mastroyannopoulou K, MacDougall J. Androgen insensitivity syndrome. *Lancet.* 2012;380(9851): 1419-1428. PMID: 22698698

Tadokoro-Cuccaro R, Hughes IA. Androgen insensitivity syndrome. *Curr Opin Endocrinol Diabetes Obes.* 2014;21(6):499-503. PMID: 25354046

13 ANSWER: C) Start a low-dosage continuous estrogen-progestin oral contraceptive (20 mcg ethinyl estradiol; 1 mg norethindrone acetate)

Approximately 40% to 50% of perimenopausal women experience depression and/or anxiety symptoms during the menopausal transition. The symptoms are responsive to estrogen, but many women need both estrogen and an antidepressant (a selective serotonin reuptake inhibitor). This patient has hot flashes and perimenopausal depression, which often coexist in this population. Her psychopharmacologist has started her on a selective serotonin reuptake inhibitor, citalopram, and her dosage has been titrated up to 30 mg daily. However, she still does not feel like herself. She has vasomotor symptoms, but she may have persistent depression symptoms as well. Although not FDA-approved for the treatment of perimenopausal depression, estrogen therapy has been shown to be effective in this population. Of note, estrogen is not effective for postmenopausal women with depression. Given her vasomotor symptoms, some form of estrogen would be the best option.

Increasing the citalopram dosage further (Answer B) is not the best next step, and neither is referring her to cognitive behavioral therapy (Answer D). Oral estradiol with cyclic micronized progesterone (Answer A) would relieve her hot flashes, but the cyclic progesterone could exacerbate her mood symptoms. Therefore, the best option is a low-dosage oral contraceptive (Answer C). This provides the estrogen, which will treat her vasomotor symptoms. It must be given continuously, however, or her vasomotor symptoms will recur during the pill-free interval. In addition, she may have premenstrual mood symptoms on a cyclic pill regimen; a continuous regimen would preclude this.

Educational Objective
Identify and treat depression during the menopausal transition.

Reference(s)
Maki PM, Kornstein SG, Joffe H, et al; Board of Trustees for The North American Menopause Society (NAMS) and the Women and Mood Disorders Task Force of the National Network of Depression Centers. Guidelines for the evaluation and treatment of perimenopausal depression: summary and recommendations. *Menopause.* 2018;25(10):1069-1085. PMID: 30179986

Stuenkel CA, Davis SA, Gompel A, et al. Treatment of symptoms of the menopause: an Endocrine Society clinical practice guideline. *J Clin Endocrinol Metab.* 2015;100(11):3975-4011. PMID: 26444994

Gordon JL, Girdler SS. Hormone replacement therapy in the treatment of perimenopausal depression. *Curr Psychiatry Rep.* 2014;16(12): 517. PMID: 25308388

14 ANSWER: A) Combined estrogen-progestin oral contraceptive: ethinyl estradiol, 20 mcg, and norethindrone, 1 mg

Hirsutism in women is defined as excessive terminal hair growth in a male pattern. With the Ferriman-Gallwey scoring method, a score of 8 or higher is indicative of hirsutism in white women. The Endocrine Society clinical practice guidelines on the Evaluation and Treatment of Hirsutism in Premenopausal Women, published in 2018, recommend screening androgen levels in women with any degree of hirsutism. Testosterone levels do not always correlate with the severity of the hirsutism. When associated with other symptoms and signs, evaluation for polycystic ovary syndrome, Cushing syndrome, congenital adrenal hyperplasia, hyperprolactinemia, and, rarely, ovarian or adrenal tumors is appropriate.

Most women with hirsutism eventually receive a multipronged treatment approach: ovarian androgen suppression (oral contraceptive), androgen blockade with an androgen-receptor antagonist (spironolactone), and direct hair removal (laser or electrolysis). For most women, the Endocrine Society guidelines suggest an oral contraceptive (Answer A) as initial therapy. A low-dosage formulation (20 mcg ethinyl estradiol) can be used and can be increased to 30/35 mcg if there is not significant improvement after 6 months. All oral contraceptives appear to be equally effective for treating hirsutism, but some progestins have been associated with higher risk of venous thromboembolism (drospirenone, desogestrel, gestodene). Oral contraceptives reduce hirsutism via several mechanisms, including suppression of gonadotropins (the stimulus to ovarian androgen production); increase in SHBG, which decreases free testosterone levels; and some suppression of adrenal androgens. In addition, they optimize menstrual cycle regularity and flow and provide contraception. After 6 months of oral contraceptive therapy, spironolactone is often added if the patient wants a better cosmetic result. The eventual dosage is 50 to 100 mg twice daily.

Spironolactone alone (Answer C) is not recommended in premenopausal women because it can cause irregular menses and has the theoretical risk of inducing ambiguous genitalia in a male fetus if taken during early pregnancy. Flutamide (Answer B) is a pure antiandrogen with effectiveness similar to that of spironolactone, but it is more costly than spironolactone and has a risk of hepatic toxicity. Photoepilation

(Answer D) is an effective therapy, but it should be used in conjunction with pharmacologic therapy to minimize growth of new terminal hairs.

Educational Objective

Recommend therapy for hirsutism.

Reference(s)

Van Zuuren EJ, Fedorowicz Z. Interventions for hirsutism excluding laser and photoepilation therapy alone: abridged Cochrane systematic review including GRADE assessments. *Br J Dermatol.* 2016;175(1):45-61. PMID: 26892495

Martin KA, Anderson RR, Chang RJ, et al. Evaluation and treatment of hirsutism in premenopausal women: an Endocrine Society clinical practice guideline. *J Clin Endocrinol Metab.* 2018;103(4):1-25. PMID: 29522147

Hagag P, Steinschneider M, Weiss M. Role of the combination spironolactone-norgestimate-estrogen in hirsute women with polycystic ovary syndrome. *J Reprod Med.* 2014;59(9-10):455-463. PMID: 25330687

15 ANSWER: D) Letrozole

Women with polycystic ovary syndrome can have intermittent ovulation or anovulation, hyperandrogenism, and insulin resistance. Before planning for fertility, lifestyle should be optimized with diet and exercise. A relatively small amount of weight loss sometimes restores ovulatory cycles. Addition of metformin as an insulin sensitizer can help regulate cycles and suppress androgens, and it may make lifestyle intervention more effective.

Historically, if fertility was desired, clomiphene citrate (Answer A) (50 mg on cycle days 5 through 9) was prescribed to induce ovulation. Clomiphene citrate is more effective than metformin therapy (Answer C) to achieve live births. In addition, results from recent meta-analyses suggest that combination therapy with clomiphene and metformin may be more useful to increase live births. Although clomiphene citrate is a potential approach to induce ovulation, the recent Reproductive Network Trial comparing the second-generation aromatase inhibitor letrozole (Answer D) with clomiphene citrate demonstrated a convincingly higher rate of ovulation induction and live births with letrozole, especially in obese women with polycystic ovary syndrome.

Progesterone suppositories (Answer B) are sometimes prescribed for women with hypothalamic amenorrhea and inadequate luteal phase—not for women with polycystic ovary syndrome. They improve menstrual cyclicity, but they have not been shown to increase rates of ovulation induction.

Educational Objective

Compare treatment effectiveness of clomiphene citrate with that of aromatase inhibitors for ovulation induction in women with polycystic ovary syndrome who would like to become pregnant.

Reference(s)

Palomba S. Aromatase inhibitors for ovulation induction. *J Clin Endocrinol Metab.* 2015;100(5): 1742-1747. PMID: 25710566

Legro RS, Brzyski RG, Diamond MP, et al; NICHD Reproductive Medicine Network. Letrozole versus clomiphene for infertility in the polycystic ovary syndrome [published correction appears in *N Engl J Med.* 2014;317(15):1465]. *N Engl J Med.* 2014;371(2):119-129. PMID: 25006718

Franik S, Kremer JA, Nelen WL, Farquhar C, Marjoribanks J. Aromatase inhibitors for subfertile women with polycystic ovary syndrome: summary of a Cochrane review. *Fertil Steril.* 2015;103(2):353-355. PMID: 2545536

Fauser BC, Tarlatzis BC, Rebar RW, et al. Consensus on women's health aspects of polycystic ovary syndrome (PCOS): the Amsterdam ESHRE/ASRM-Sponsored 3rd PCOS Consensus Workshop Group. *Fertil Steril.* 2012;97(1):28-38. PMID: 22153789

Azziz R, Carmina E, Dewailly D, et al; Androgen Excess Society. Positions statement: criteria for defining polycystic ovary syndrome as a predominantly hyperandrogenic syndrome: an Androgen Excess Society guideline. *J Clin Endocrinol Metab.* 2006;91(11):4237-4245. PMID: 16940456

Legro RS, Arslanian SA, Ehrmann DA, et al; Endocrine Society. Diagnosis and treatment of polycystic ovary syndrome: An Endocrine Society clinical practice guideline. *J Clin Endocriol Metab.* 2013;98(12):4565-4592. PMID: 24151290

16 ANSWER: D) Depression and anxiety

Polycystic ovary syndrome is a common disorder that occurs in 6% to 8% of women. Affected patients usually present with hirsutism, acne, and irregular menses. They are also at increased risk for type 2 diabetes mellitus, dyslipidemia, and hypertension. Despite an increase in metabolic syndrome and cardiac risk factors, studies have not yet shown an increased risk of coronary heart disease (Answer B) in women with polycystic ovary syndrome. Therefore, routine screening for coronary heart disease is not recommended.

Women with polycystic ovary syndrome are more likely to have mood disorders (eg, depression and anxiety [Answer D]) than weight-matched women without polycystic ovary syndrome. They are also at risk for eating disorders (binge eating). A number of expert societies, including the Endocrine Society, suggest screening all women with polycystic ovary syndrome for depression and anxiety. One approach is to use validated screening tools such as the Patient Health Questionnaire (PHQ-9) for depression and the Generalized Anxiety Disorder 7 (GAD-7) scale for anxiety disorders.

Neither celiac disease (Answer A) nor autoimmune thyroid disease (Answer C) has been associated with polycystic ovary syndrome, so screening for these comorbidities is not indicated.

Educational Objective

Recommend screening for depression and anxiety in women with polycystic ovary syndrome.

Reference(s)

McCartney CR, Marshall JC. Clinical Practice. Polycystic ovary syndrome. *N Engl J Med.* 2016; 375(1):54-64. PMID: 27406348

Legro RS, Arslanian SA, Ehrmann DA, et al; Endocrine Society. Diagnosis and treatment of polycystic ovary syndrome: an Endocrine Society Clinical Practice Guideline. *J Clin Endocrinol Metab.* 2013;98(12):4565-4592. PMID: 24151290

Teede HJ, Misso ML, Costello MH, et al; International PCOS Network. Recommendations from the international evidence-based guideline for the assessment and management of polycystic ovary syndrome. *Fertil Steril.* 2018; 110(3):364-379. PMID: 30033227

17 ANSWER: B) Start a serotonin reuptake inhibitor

Women with premenstrual syndrome experience a wide variety of cyclic and recurrent physical, emotional, behavioral, and cognitive symptoms that start in the luteal phase and diminish and stop after the onset of menses. Major symptoms include affective symptoms such as depression, angry outbursts, irritability, and anxiety and somatic symptoms such as breast pain, bloating, swelling, and headache. Referral to a therapist (Answer A) may be helpful, but this has not been shown to be beneficial for this symptom complex. Antidepressants such as amitriptyline (Answer C) have been supplanted by newer targeted drugs and thus a tricyclic antidepressant is not the best option. Initiation of a selective serotonin reuptake inhibitor (Answer B) that targets mood directly is currently the treatment of choice. Controlled studies confirm that abrogation of ovulation with oral contraceptives administered continuously or with a 4-day pill-free interval are also effective. A cyclic estrogen-progestin oral contraceptive (Answer D) refers to those with a 7-day pill-free interval. Although they may be effective for premenstrual dysphoric disorder, they have not yet been well studied in this setting.

Educational Objective

Recommend treatment options for women with premenstrual dysphoria.

Reference(s)

Schmidt PJ, Martinez PE, Nieman LK, et al. Premenstrual dysphoric disorder symptoms following ovarian suppression: triggered by change in ovarian steroid levels but not continuous stable levels. *Am J Psychiatry.* 2017;174(10):980-989. PMID: 28427285

Shobeiri F, Araste FE, Ebrahimi R, Jenabi E, Nazari M. Effect of calcium on premenstrual syndrome: a double-blind randomized clinical trial. *Obstet Gynecol Sci.* 2017;60(1):100-105. PMID: 28217679

Management of premenstrual syndrome: green-top guideline No. 48. *BJOG.* 2017;124(3):e73-e105. PMID: 27900828

Brown J, O'Brien PM, Marjoribanks J, Wyatt K. Selective serotonin reuptake inhibitors for premenstrual syndrome. *Cochrane Database Syst Rev.* 2009:CD001396. PMID: 19370564

Jarvis CI, Lynch AM, Morin AK. Management strategies for premenstrual syndrome/premenstrual dysphoric disorder. *Ann Pharmacother*. 2008;42(7):967-978. PMID: 18559957

18 ANSWER: D) Serum triglycerides = 499 mg/dL (SI: 5.64 mmol/L)

This patient is a good candidate for menopausal hormone therapy. She is only 51 years old, is newly menopausal, and is in reasonably good health. Most expert societies recommend 17β-estradiol as the estrogen for perimenopausal and postmenopausal women; the route of administration depends on the individual patient. The transdermal route has a number of advantages. Unlike oral estrogens, it is not associated with an increased risk of venous thromboembolism or stroke, nor does it increase serum triglycerides. In this patient's case, her elevated triglyceride value of 499 mg/dL (5.64 mmol/L) (Answer D) is a factor in choosing her menopausal hormone regimen.

Both oral and transdermal estrogen tend to lower LDL-cholesterol levels, so a LDL-cholesterol value of 110 mg/dL (2.85 mmol/L) (Answer B) would not be the most important factor for choosing therapy. Menopausal hormone therapy can be given to postmenopausal women with glucose intolerance or type 2 diabetes, so a hemoglobin A_{1c} measurement (Answer C) is not essential for deciding on a hormone regimen for this patient. In the Women's Health Initiative, the number of new cases of type 2 diabetes was lower in women who took hormone therapy. A serum estradiol value of 26 pg/mL (95.4 pmol/L) (Answer A) is typical for a postmenopausal woman before starting therapy. Once treatment is started, routine monitoring of serum estradiol levels is not recommended; estrogen dosages are adjusted based on the patient's symptoms. Therefore, this is not an important test result to have at baseline when choosing therapy.

Educational Objective
Choose the appropriate menopausal hormone regimen based on the individual patient.

Reference(s)
Stuenkel CA, Davis SR, Gompel A, et al. Treatment of symptoms of the menopause: an Endocrine Society clinical practice guideline. *J Clin Endocrinol Metab*. 2015;100(11):3975-4011. PMID: 26444994

Whayne TF. Hypertriglyceridemia: an infrequent, difficult-to-predict, severe metabolic and vascular problem associated with estrogen administration. *Curr Vasc Pharmacol*. 2019 [Epub ahead of print] PMID: 30843488

Fonseca VA. Menopausal hormone therapy and type 2 diabetes prevention: evidence, mechanisms and clinical implications. *Endocr Rev*. 2017;38(3):173-188. PMID: 28323934

19 ANSWER: D) Preeclampsia

Recent guidelines have reviewed the treatment options for and complications of pregnancy in women with Turner syndrome. The most catastrophic risks are aortic dissection or rupture. Pregnancy should be avoided in women with an ascending aortic size index greater than 2.5 cm/m^2 or an ascending aortic size index of 2 to 2.5 cm/m^2 with associated risk factors for aortic dilatation.

More common risks are related to body size, metabolic issues, and hypertension, which is associated with an increased risk of preeclampsia (Answer D). Other rare but possible risks include stroke and, very rarely, a ruptured aorta. The prevalence of adrenal insufficiency (Answer B), ruptured spleen (Answer C), or placenta accreta (Answer A) is not reported to be increased during pregnancy in women with gonadal dysgenesis.

Educational Objective
List potential complications of pregnancy in women with gonadal dysgenesis.

Reference(s)
Gravholt CH, Andersen NH, Conway GS, et al; International Turner Syndrome Consensus Group. Clinical practice guidelines for the care of girls and women with Turner syndrome: proceedings from the 2016 Cincinnati International Turner Syndrome Meeting. *Eur J Endocrinol*. 2017;177(3):G1-G70. PMID: 28705803

Davenport ML. Approach to the patient with Turner syndrome. *J Clin Endocrinol Metab.* 2010; 95(4):1487-1495. PMID: 20375216

Ross JL, Quigley CA, Cao D, Feuillan P, Kowal K, Chipman JJ, et al. Growth hormone plus childhood low-dose estrogen in Turner's syndrome. *N Engl J Med.* 2011;364(13):1230-1242. PMID: 21449786

Pinsker JE. Clinical review: Turner syndrome: updating the paradigm of clinical care. *J Clin Endocrinol Metab.* 2012;97(6):E994-E1003. PMID: 22472565

20 ANSWER: B) FSH, estradiol, and prolactin

Functional hypothalamic amenorrhea is a diagnosis of exclusion. Excessive stress, exercise, low weight, and eating disorders may alter the GnRH pulse generator, thereby altering the necessary switch of pulse frequency and amplitude across the menstrual cycle to induce ovulation and ensure regular periods. Hyperprolactinemia due to mild thyroid dysfunction, medications, or prolactin-secreting pituitary tumors can turn off the GnRH pulse generator and present as hypothalamic amenorrhea. Estrogen is low in the settings of hypothalamic amenorrhea and hyperprolactinemia, but it would be high if the patient were pregnant. The best laboratory tests to order next are measurements of FSH, estradiol, and prolactin (Answer B).

Androgens (Answer A) should be measured in a patient who has acne and hirsutism. A stimulated 17-hydroxyprogesterone measurement (Answer C) is the best test to assess for congenital adrenal hyperplasia, but there is no reason to suspect that diagnosis in this vignette because the patient did not describe hyperandrogenic symptoms or early pubic hair. Progesterone (Answer D) is measured to assess ovulation and luteal-phase function in women attempting fertility. Cushing syndrome may result in amenorrhea due to inhibition of gonadotropin secretion by excess cortisol, and its measurement (Answer E) is not indicated in this case.

Educational Objective
Recommend appropriate hormone testing on the basis of the history, examination findings, and presentation in amenorrheic women.

Reference(s)

Gordon CM, Ackerman KE, Berga SL, et al. Functional hypothalamic amenorrhea: an Endocrine Society clinical practice guideline. *J Clin Endocrinol Metab.* 2017;102(5):1413-1439. PMID: 28368518

Gordon CM. Clinical practice. Functional hypothalamic amenorrhea. *N Engl J Med.* 2010;363(4):365-371. PMID: 20660404

Caronia LM, Martin C, Welt CK, et al. A genetic basis for functional hypothalamic amenorrhea. *N Engl J Med.* 2011;364(3):215-225. PMID: 21247312

Melmed S, Casanueva FF, Hoffman AR, et al; Endocrine Society. Diagnosis and treatment of hyperprolactinemia: an Endocrine Society clinical practice guideline. *J Clin Endocrinol Metab.* 2011;96(2):273-288. PMID: 21296991

Male Reproduction Board Review
Frances J. Hayes, MB BCh, BAO

1 ANSWER: D) Serum prolactin measurement

This patient has secondary hypogonadism (low serum testosterone and inappropriately normal gonadotropin levels). Given that his testes are adult sized and he is normally virilized, he has acquired secondary hypogonadism after the onset of puberty. The differential diagnosis of postpubertal secondary hypogonadism includes pituitary macroadenoma, Cushing syndrome, hyperprolactinemia, opioid use, and iron-overload syndromes (including hemochromatosis). Given the frequency with which hyperprolactinemia can cause hypogonadotropic hypogonadism, prolactin should be measured (Answer D) in all men with secondary hypogonadism.

In this patient, measurement of late-night salivary cortisol (Answer A) is not indicated because of the absence of any features suggestive of glucocorticoid excess (he has normal weight and blood pressure and no striae or evidence of proximal myopathy).

The major indication for karyotype analysis (Answer B) in men with hypogonadism is to confirm a diagnosis of Klinefelter syndrome, the most common genetic cause of primary hypogonadism. Given that this patient does not have primary hypogonadism, screening for Klinefelter syndrome by karyotyping is not indicated.

Testicular ultrasonography (Answer C) can be helpful in identifying a testicular tumor in a patient with gynecomastia. However, in the case described where there is no gynecomastia and the testes are normal on clinical examination, ultrasonography would not add any useful information.

Educational Objective

Measure prolactin in the evaluation of men with secondary hypogonadism.

Reference(s)

Schlechte JA. Clinical impact of hyper-prolactinaemia. *Baillieres Clin Endocrinol Metab.* 1995;9(2):359-366. PMID: 7625989

Bhasin S, Brito JP, Cunningham GR, et al. Testosterone therapy in men with hypogonadism: an Endocrine Society clinical practice guideline. *J Clin Endocrinol Metab.* 2018;103(5):1715-1744. PMID: 29562364

2 ANSWER: A) Hereditary hemochromatosis

This patient has secondary hypogonadism (symptoms and/or signs of hypogonadism, low serum testosterone, and low or inappropriately normal gonadotropin levels). Considering that his testes are adult size and he is normally virilized, one can conclude he has acquired secondary hypogonadism after the onset of puberty. The differential diagnosis of postpubertal, acquired secondary hypogonadism includes pituitary macroadenoma, Cushing syndrome, hyperprolactinemia, opioid use, and iron overload syndromes such as hemochromatosis. Hand arthralgias, chondrocalcinosis, hyperpigmentation, and secondary hypogonadism are the earliest manifestations of iron overload syndromes. In men, hereditary hemochromatosis (Answer A) often causes these sequelae in the third and fourth decades. Later in the disease course, patients may experience heart failure, cirrhosis, and diabetes mellitus. Acquired forms of iron overload syndromes (eg, due to multiple transfusions) may also cause disease earlier. Hemochromatosis is inherited in an autosomal recessive manner and has a prevalence of about 0.4% in populations of northern European descent, but it has much lower clinical penetrance, and disease severity is highly variable. Pathogenic variants in the *HFE* gene are responsible, and the most common genotype is homozygosity for the Cys282Tyr (C282Y) mutation. Assessment of transferrin saturation is the most useful initial test for hemochromatosis; a transferrin saturation less than 45% is enough to exclude the diagnosis. In the appropriate clinical setting, C282Y homozygosity suffices to diagnose hemochromatosis, but liver biopsy with iron staining remains the criterion standard for diagnosis.

Opioid abuse (Answer B) can cause hypogonadotropic hypogonadism, but it would not cause arthralgias. While the patient has a 5-mm pituitary lesion, incidentally discovered microadenomas are seen in 10% to 38% of patients on MRI. Given that this patient has no clinical features of glucocorticoid excess on history and physical examination, screening for Cushing disease (Answer C) is not indicated. In patients with marked hyperprolactinemia due to a large macroadenoma (Answer D), serum prolactin levels can be read as normal unless serial dilution of serum is done to assess for the "hook effect." However, this phenomenon would not be seen with a 5-mm pituitary adenoma.

Educational Objective
Diagnose hemochromatosis as a cause of secondary hypogonadism.

Reference(s)
Bhasin S, Brito JP, Cunningham GR, et al. Testosterone therapy in men with hypogonadism: an Endocrine Society clinical practice guideline. *J Clin Endocrinol Metab.* 2018;103(5):1715-1744. PMID: 29562364

McDermott JH, Walsh CH. Hypogonadism in hereditary hemochromatosis. *J Clin Endocrinol Metab.* 2005;90(4):2451-2455. PMID: 15657376

Moyer TP, Highsmith WE, Smyrk TC, Gross JB Jr. Hereditary hemochromatosis: laboratory evaluation. *Clin Chim Acta.* 2011;412(17-18):1485-1492. PMID: 21510925

van Bokhoven MA, van Deursen CT, Swinkels DW. Diagnosis and management of hereditary haemochromatosis. *BMJ.* 2011;342:c7251. PMID: 21248018

3 ANSWER: B) Congenital hypogonadotropic hypogonadism

This patient has prepubertal hypogonadism as evidenced by his failure to develop secondary sexual characteristics or an increase in testicular size. Laboratory tests show profound secondary hypogonadism with otherwise normal pituitary function and prolactin levels. His presentation is thus consistent with idiopathic hypogonadotropic hypogonadism (Answer B). Distinguishing between constitutional delay of growth and puberty (Answer A) and congenital hypogonadotropic hypogonadism can be challenging in younger adolescent boys. However, the absence of any signs of puberty by age 18 years, by definition, rules out congenital hypogonadotropic hypogonadism. Pathogenic variants in the *PROP1* gene (Answer C) are one of the most common causes of both familial and sporadic congenital combined pituitary hormone deficiency (GH, TSH, LH, FSH). Thus, the fact that the patient's pituitary hormone profile is normal apart from gonadotropin deficiency rules out an abnormality in *PROP1*. While complete failure of pubertal development has been reported in patients with pathogenic variants in the leptin receptor gene (Answer D), the most striking phenotypic feature of these patients is morbid obesity, which this patient does not have.

Educational Objective
Construct the differential diagnosis of a patient with congenital hypogonadotropic hypogonadism.

Reference(s)
Palmert MR, Dunkel L. Clinical practice. Delayed puberty. *N Engl J Med.* 2012;366(5):443-453. PMID: 22296078

Hayes FJ, Seminara SB, Crowley WF Jr. Hypogonadotropic hypogonadism. *Endocrinol Metab Clin North Am.* 1998;27(4):739-763. PMID: 9922906

Young J. Approach to the male patient with hypogonadotropic hypogonadism. *J Clin Endocrinol Metab.* 2012;97(3):707-718. PMID: 22392951

Costa-Barbosa FA, Balasubramanian R, Keefe KW, et al. Prioritizing genetic testing in patients with Kallmann syndrome using clinical phenotypes. *J Clin Endocrinol Metab.* 2013;98(5):E943-E953. PMID: 23533228

ANSWER: B) Klinefelter syndrome

On a statistical basis, the most common cause of congenital primary gonadal failure is Klinefelter syndrome (Answer B), which has an incidence of approximately 1 in 600. There is wide variability in the phenotypic spectrum depending largely on the degree of mosaicism. However, gynecomastia and small, firm testes, as described in this vignette, are common presenting features. Gonadotropin concentrations are invariably elevated (FSH > LH) in men with Klinefelter syndrome (and other causes of primary hypogonadism) because of impaired negative feedback by both sex steroids and inhibin B. Most patients have testosterone values in the low-normal range or just below the lower end of normal. SHBG concentrations tend to be elevated in affected men because of increased estrogen production rates. Given that 98% or more of circulating testosterone is protein bound, the free testosterone fraction tends to be disproportionately lower than the total testosterone concentration in men with Klinefelter syndrome. The diagnosis is confirmed by karyotype analysis, which shows a 47,XXY pattern in more than 80% of cases. This patient's karyotype showed 47,XXY/46,XY mosaicism, which explains why his testes are larger than those in many patients with Klinefelter syndrome and also why his testosterone level is still in the normal range.

Inactivating pathogenic variants in the gene encoding the FSH receptor (Answer A) are a rare cause of primary gonadal failure. Men harboring such mutations present with small testes and elevated FSH levels such as in the case described. However, unlike this patient, their LH levels are not elevated and they do not develop gynecomastia.

High biotin dosages (Answer C) can falsely lower FSH levels if measured using a sandwich biotin-streptavidin capture assay. However, in this case, FSH levels were high rather than low and assay interference would not explain the clinical picture of small testes and gynecomastia.

The incidence of mumps orchitis (Answer D) has declined dramatically since the introduction of the childhood vaccination program. However, in situations where parents decide not to have their children vaccinated, outbreaks of mumps can still occur. Orchitis is the most common complication of mumps in postpubertal men, affecting about 20% to 30% of patients. Thirty to fifty percent of affected testicles show some degree of atrophy. Mumps orchitis results in severe pain, swelling, and tenderness at the affected site and is often associated with high fever, nausea, vomiting, and abdominal pain.

Educational Objective

Construct the differential diagnosis of primary hypogonadism and gynecomastia.

Reference(s)

Groth KA, Skakkebæk A, Høst C, Gravholt CH, Bojesen A. Clinical review: Klinefelter syndrome--a clinical update. *J Clin Endocrinol Metab.* 2013;98(1):20-30. PMID: 23118429

Braunstein GD. Clinical practice: Gynecomastia. *N Engl J Med.* 2007;357(12):1229-1237. PMID: 17881754

Samarasinghe S, Meah F, Singh V, et al. Biotin interference with routine clinical immunoassay: understand the causes and mitigage the risk. *Endocr Pract.* 2017;23(8):989-998. PMID: 28534685

ANSWER: A) Measure free testosterone by equilibrium dialysis

This patient's clinical presentation with decreased libido, erectile dysfunction, and fatigue is highly suggestive of hypogonadism. His physical examination also reveals gynecomastia. Despite this, 2 total testosterone values, both measured by liquid chromatography/tandem mass spectrometry, are in the high-normal range. In such clinical scenarios, where the clinical phenotype is incongruent with biochemical results, clinicians should consider alterations in serum SHBG levels as a potential explanation. Certain clinical conditions are associated with elevated serum SHBG levels. These include aging, liver disease, hyperthyroidism, medications (anticonvulsant drugs, estrogen), and HIV infection. Although the exact mechanism behind SHBG elevation in HIV remains unclear, increased inflammatory milieu in these patients has been posited as one of the mechanisms (SHBG is an acute-phase reactant). As longevity is increasing in persons with HIV, quality-of-life issues in this patient population are gaining considerable attention. Furthermore, the prevalence of hypogonadism in men with HIV is higher than in the general population; therefore, an accurate diagnosis is important.

Thus, in cases such as this where the history is suggestive of hypogonadism and a disorder known to impact SHBG levels is present, measurement of free testosterone (Answer A) is required to diagnose androgen deficiency. Reliable methods of free testosterone measurement include (1) measurement by equilibrium dialysis (considered the gold standard, but not routinely available in commercial laboratories); and (2) calculated free testosterone (derived from total testosterone and SHBG measurements using law of mass action equations). This patient's free testosterone level (measured by equilibrium dialysis) was low at 4.8 ng/dL (1.7 nmol/L) because of a markedly elevated SHBG level of 20.0 µg/mL (178 nmol/L), allowing a diagnosis of hypogonadism to be confirmed.

Epitestosterone is a biologically inactive 17-epimer of testosterone that is cosecreted by the Leydig cells of the testes. The urinary testosterone-to-epitestosterone ratio (Answer B) is measured in the evaluation of men suspected of androgen abuse. However, exogenous use of testosterone by this patient would be associated with suppressed gonadotropin levels.

Men with partial androgen insensitivity syndrome resulting from pathogenic variants in the gene encoding the androgen receptor (Answer C) may also present with symptoms and signs of hypogonadism in association with an elevated serum testosterone level. However, patients with partial androgen insensitivity syndrome tend to have additional clinical manifestations, including perineoscrotal hypospadias and infertility. Importantly, gonadotropin levels in such patients are elevated due to impaired testosterone negative feedback, unlike the gonadotropin profile of patients with HIV infection who typically have secondary hypogonadism.

Measuring estradiol (Answer D) would not be very helpful in this patient, as his high SHBG levels would also tend to cause a high estradiol level. If he were taking estrogen or had an estrogen-secreting tumor as the cause of his gynecomastia, testosterone levels would be low rather than high.

Educational Objective

Diagnose androgen deficiency in men with HIV who experience alterations in the concentration of serum SHBG.

Reference(s)

Antonio L, Wu FC, O'Neill TW, et al; European Male Ageing Study Group. Low free testosterone is associated with hypogonadal symptoms and signs in men with normal testosterone levels. *J Clin Endocrinol Metab.* 2016;101(7):2647-2657. PMID: 26909800

Shea JL, Wong PY, Chen Y. Free testosterone: clinical utility and important analytical aspects of measurement. *Adv Clin Chem.* 2014;63:59-84. PMID: 24783351

Moreno-Pérez O, Escoín C, Serna-Candel C, et al. The determination of total testosterone and free testosterone (RIA) are not applicable to the evaluation of gonadal function in HIV-infected males. *J Sex Med.* 2010;7(8):2873-2883. PMID: 20626606

6 ANSWER: C) *NR0B1* (formerly *DAX1*) (nuclear receptor subfamily 0 group B member 1)

The development of hypogonadotropic hypogonadism in a patient with primary adrenal insufficiency should raise suspicion for adrenal hypoplasia congenita, an X-linked recessive disease due to pathogenic variants in the *NR0B1* gene (also known as *DAX1*) (Answer C). The age at presentation and the severity of adrenal insufficiency are variable. Although adrenal insufficiency is most often diagnosed in childhood as in this vignette (some cases even presenting in the neonatal period), the onset may be delayed until adulthood. Pathogenic variants in the *NR0B1* gene affect function of all levels of the hypothalamic-pituitary-gonadal axis, as well as the adrenal glands. There is a broad phenotypic spectrum for males with adrenal hypoplasia congenita. Unlike most patients with idiopathic hypogonadotropic hypogonadism, those with adrenal hypoplasia congenita fail to initiate spermatogenesis when treated with gonadotropin therapy due to the concomitant testicular defect.

Patients with partial hypopituitarism due to a pathogenic variant in the *PROP1* gene (Answer A) could present with hypogonadotropic hypogonadism and adrenal insufficiency, but the latter would be secondary as opposed to primary. A pathogenic variant in the *AIRE* gene (Answer B) causing autoimmune polyglandular endocrine deficiency syndrome could cause primary adrenal insufficiency, but associated hypogonadism would be primary rather than secondary.

A pathogenic variant in the *ANOS1* gene (formerly *KAL1*) (Answer D) results in Kallmann syndrome, which is the association of hypogonadotropic hypogonadism with anosmia. It is not the correct diagnosis for this patient, as he has a normal sense of smell and Kallmann syndrome does not cause primary adrenal insufficiency.

Educational Objective
Describe the clinical and biochemical presentation of adrenal hypoplasia congenita.

Reference(s)
Jadhav U, Harris RM, Jameson JL. Hypogonadotropic hypogonadism in subjects with DAX1 mutations. *Mol Cell Endocrinol.* 2011;346(1-2):65-73. PMID: 21672607

Lin L, Achermann JC. Inherited adrenal hypoplasia: not just for kids! *Clin Endocrinol (Oxf).* 2004;60(5):529-537. PMID: 15104553

Reutens AT, Achermann JC, Ito M, et al. Clinical and functional effects of mutations in the DAX-1 gene in patients with adrenal hypoplasia congenita. *J Clin Endocrinol Metab.* 1999;84(2):504-511. PMID: 10022408

7 ANSWER: A) Start testosterone replacement therapy

The diagnosis of hypogonadism made by the patient's primary care physician is correct based on the presence of symptoms of hypogonadism in association with 2 low morning testosterone measurements. While the patient is eager to initiate testosterone therapy in the hope of improving his symptoms, it is the physician's responsibility to ensure that he is an appropriate candidate and that the risk-to-benefit ratio favors treatment.

Starting a phosphodiesterase inhibitor (Answer B) would help his erectile dysfunction, but it would not address his fatigue or decreased libido and would not correct his hypogonadism. This patient is young and is otherwise healthy apart from hypogonadism, and he has no contraindication to testosterone therapy. Therefore, starting testosterone replacement (Answer A) is reasonable.

An important objective of the baseline evaluation in men being considered for testosterone replacement therapy is to identify and exclude those who have a history of prostate cancer or are at high risk for developing prostate cancer. Given this patient's young age, normal prostate examination, and absence of risk factors for prostate cancer such as African American heritage or having a first-degree relative with prostate cancer, his risk of prostate cancer is low and screening by measuring PSA (Answer C) is not recommended.

Most organizations that provide prostate cancer screening guidelines strongly encourage informing the patient of the potential benefits and risks and engaging him in shared decision-making regarding screening with PSA measurement and digital rectal examination. The Endocrine Society clinical practice guidelines recommend that clinicians consider screening and monitoring for all men with hypogonadism who are 55 to 69 years of age for whom testosterone replacement therapy is being considered if they are in excellent health and have a life expectancy of more than 10 years. Screening should start at age 40 years in men who are at increased risk for high-grade cancers, such as those of African American ethnicity and men with a first-degree male relative with diagnosed prostate cancer. Men younger than 40 years do not need prostate monitoring because the risk of prostate cancer is very low in this population. The risk of death due to prostate cancer in men diagnosed when they are older than 70 years is not considered high enough to warrant monitoring. The baseline assessment of prostate cancer risk should consider risk factors such as age, family history (increased risk in men who have a first-degree relative with prostate cancer), ethnicity (increased risk in men of African American ancestry), biopsy history, elevated PSA levels, and abnormal prostate examination results.

As a general rule, patients who have a palpable prostate nodule or induration or a PSA level greater than 4.0 ng/mL (>4.0 µg/L) need further urologic evaluation before testosterone therapy is initiated. However, in subgroups of men considered to be at increased risk for prostate cancer, such as African American patients or men with a first-degree relative with prostate cancer, the baseline PSA level at which referral to a urologist is recommended is greater than 3.0 ng/mL (>3.0 µg/L).

While Klinefelter syndrome is a common cause of hypogonadism in young men (incidence of approximately 1 in 600), it causes primary gonadal failure. Therefore, performing karyotype analysis (Answer D) to screen for Klinefelter syndrome in a patient with normal gonadotropin levels is not indicated.

Educational Objective

Determine whether a patient is an appropriate candidate for testosterone replacement therapy.

Reference(s)

Bhasin S, Brito JP, Cunningham GR, et al. Testosterone therapy in men with hypogonadism: an Endocrine Society clinical practice guideline. *J Clin Endocrinol Metab.* 2018;103(5):1715-1744. PMID: 29562364

8 ANSWER: C) Recheck his PSA level

Although this patient's PSA level remains within the reference range and he has no lower urinary tract symptoms, the magnitude of its change is higher than one would expect. However, PSA levels are known to fluctuate in an individual and also have considerable test-retest variability. Therefore, the most appropriate next step is to confirm that there has been a significant increase by rechecking his PSA level (Answer C). If the repeated PSA value is normal, testosterone therapy can be continued and a urology referral is not necessary. However, a confirmed increase in PSA of greater than 1.4 ng/mL (>1.4 µg/L) over the course of a year in a man on testosterone therapy cannot be attributed to random variation alone and should therefore prompt referral to a urologist for consideration of prostate biopsy (Answer B). A systematic review of prostate risk during testosterone therapy found that the average PSA increase after initiation of testosterone therapy is 0.3 ng/mL and 0.44 ng/mL in young and old men, respectively. A cutoff of 1.4 ng/mL has been adopted on the basis of the findings of a clinical trial that evaluated the effectiveness of finasteride vs placebo on lower urinary tract symptoms and prostate volume in men with benign prostatic hyperplasia. In that study, the upper limit of the 90% confidence interval for the change in PSA level in the placebo arm was 1.4 ng/mL (1.4 µg/L). Hence, on the basis of the findings of the finasteride study and the fact that the average increase in PSA levels on testosterone therapy is less than 0.5 ng/mL (<0.5 µg/L) (regardless of patient age), the Endocrine Society's clinical practice guidelines recommend that patients with a PSA increase of greater than 1.4 ng/mL (>1.4 µg/L) during testosterone therapy should be referred for urologic consultation. It is important to understand that this increase of 1.4 ng/mL (1.4 µg/L) in PSA concentration does not indicate prostate cancer, but only serves as a trigger for further evaluation.

This patient has experienced symptomatic improvement on his current testosterone dosage, and his on-treatment testosterone concentration is normal. Therefore, discontinuing treatment (Answer A) is not indicated now. Although this patient's PSA level has increased, he does not have lower urinary tract symptoms. Therefore, treatment with a 5α-reductase inhibitor (Answer D) is not warranted.

Educational Objective

Outline the appropriate prostate monitoring for middle-aged and older patients receiving testosterone replacement.

Reference(s)

Bhasin S, Brito JP, Cunningham GR, et al. Testosterone therapy in men with hypogonadism: an Endocrine Society clinical practice guideline. *J Clin Endocrinol Metab.* 2018;103(5):1715-1744. PMID: 29562364

9 ANSWER: A) Increased risk of detecting subclinical prostate cancer

There have been no randomized clinical trials large enough to have adequate statistical power to determine whether testosterone administration increases risk of prostate cancer. However, testosterone therapy does increase the risk of detecting subclinical prostate cancer (Answer A) because of increased surveillance and testosterone-induced increase in PSA levels, which may lead to an increased likelihood of prostate biopsy. Because of the high prevalence of subclinical prostate cancer in older men, more biopsies in men receiving testosterone therapy leads to the detection of a greater number of subclinical prostate cancers.

Clinical trials have shown that testosterone therapy does not worsen lower urinary tract symptoms (Answer B) in men with hypogonadism who do not have severe symptoms before treatment.

A systematic review of prostate risk during testosterone therapy found that the increase in PSA after initiation of testosterone therapy is modest (Answer C), averaging 0.3 ng/mL (0.3 µg/L) and 0.44 ng/mL (0.44 µg/L) in young and old men, respectively.

There is no relationship between testosterone therapy and risk of prostatitis (Answer D).

Most organizations that provide guidelines for prostate cancer screening strongly encourage informing the patient of the potential benefits and risks and engaging him in shared decision-making regarding screening with PSA levels and digital rectal examination. The Endocrine Society clinical practice guidelines do not advocate screening all hypogonadal men for prostate cancer, but do recommend that clinicians consider screening and monitoring for all men with hypogonadism who are 55 to 69 years of age for whom testosterone replacement therapy is being considered if they are in excellent health and have a life expectancy of more than 10 years. This screening and monitoring should start at age 40 years in men who are at increased risk for high-grade cancers, such as those of African American ethnicity and men with a first-degree male relative with diagnosed prostate cancer. Men younger than 40 years do not need prostate monitoring because the risk of prostate cancer is very low in this population. The risk of death due to prostate cancer in men diagnosed when they are older than 70 years is not considered high enough to warrant monitoring. The baseline assessment of prostate cancer risk should consider risk factors such as age, family history (increased risk in men who have a first-degree relative with prostate cancer), ethnicity (increased risk in men with African American ancestry), history of biopsy, elevated PSA levels, and abnormal prostate examination results.

Educational Objective

Outline the impact of testosterone therapy on prostate health in middle-aged and older men.

Reference(s)

Bhasin S, Singh AB, Mac RP, Carter B, Lee MI, Cunningham GR. Managing the risks of prostate disease during testosterone replacement therapy in older men: recommendations for a standardized monitoring plan. *J Androl.* 2003;24(3): 299-311. PMID: 12721204

Kathrins M, Doersch K, Nimeh T, Canto A, Niederberger C, Seftel A. The relationship between testosterone-replacement therapy and lower urinary tract symptoms: a systematic review. *Urology.* 2016;88:22-32. PMID: 26616095

Bhasin S, Brito JP, Cunningham GR, et al. Testosterone therapy in men with hypogonadism: an Endocrine Society clinical practice guideline. *J Clin Endocrinol Metab.* 2018;103(5):1715-1744. PMID: 29562364

10 ANSWER: C) Measure testosterone 2 to 8 hours after the gel has been applied

Gel delivery systems are the preferred form of testosterone replacement therapy for many hypogonadal patients because they provide an easy and convenient way to restore and maintain testosterone levels in the physiologic range, have minimal adverse effects, and have favorable pharmacokinetics. Endocrine Society guidelines recommend that when monitoring patients being treated with a testosterone gel, the testosterone concentration should be assessed 2 to 8 hours after gel application (Answer C). Many patients apply the gel at home and then arrive in the lab early in the day to have their blood drawn before to going to work, which has the potential to give an erroneously high testosterone reading. Therefore, reducing the dosage (Answer B) in this patient who was previously stable on this dosage is not appropriate without first rechecking the testosterone level and ensuring that the sample was drawn under the right conditions. Stopping testosterone therapy (Answer A) is not appropriate, as this patient has derived benefit from testosterone therapy and would become hypogonadal again if it were discontinued due to the ongoing need for opioid therapy. While he has a history of opioid use, if he were truly abusing androgens and using a higher than prescribed dosage for a period, one would expect to see increased hematocrit, which, in his case, has been stable over the past year.

This patient expressed a clear preference for a transdermal route of testosterone administration when treatment options were initially discussed. Switching him to an intramuscular preparation (Answer D) at this point would offer no advantage and would most likely have a negative effect on adherence.

Educational Objective

Appropriately monitor hypogonadal patients receiving replacement with a testosterone gel.

Reference(s)

Bhasin S, Brito JP, Cunningham GR, et al. Testosterone therapy in men with hypogonadism: an Endocrine Society clinical practice guideline. *J Clin Endocrinol Metab.* 2018;103(5):1715-1744. PMID: 29562364

11 ANSWER: C) Cough and shortness of breath following the injection

A long-acting intramuscular formulation comprising testosterone undecanoate was approved for the treatment of male hypogonadism in the United States in 2014. This preparation has the advantage of having a superior pharmacokinetic profile compared with other injectable formulations such as enanthate and cypionate, and it has the ability to maintain testosterone levels more consistently in the normal range over a 10-week period. The absence of marked swings in serum testosterone levels means that fluctuations in mood and energy (Answer A) are not typical adverse effects.

The US FDA has stipulated that all injections of testosterone undecanoate must be administered in an office or hospital setting by a trained health care provider and that the patient be monitored for adverse effects for 30 minutes after the injection. The restrictions associated with use of this drug result from reported cases of pulmonary oil microembolism (1.5 cases/10,000 injections) and anaphylaxis (0.4 cases/10,000 injections). Symptoms of pulmonary oil microembolism include the urge to cough, dyspnea (Answer C), throat tightening, chest pain, dizziness, and syncope. These symptoms have been reported with all testosterone injections, but are reported to be more common with testosterone undecanoate because of the larger injection volume (3 mL compared with 1 mL or less for the shorter-acting formulations).

Skin irritation (Answer D) can occur in as many as 50% of patients whose hypogonadism is treated with a testosterone patch, but this adverse effect is not seen with intramuscular testosterone undecanoate.

When ingested orally, testosterone is broken down by the liver and has the potential to cause liver damage, including cholestatic jaundice, peliosis hepatis, and hepatomas. However, testosterone formulations administered intramuscularly are not hepatotoxic, so abnormal liver function (Answer B) is incorrect.

Educational Objective
Counsel patients about potential adverse effects of the long-acting intramuscular formulation of testosterone undecanoate.

Reference(s)
Wang C, Harnett M, Dobs AS, Swerdloff RS. Pharmacokinetics and safety of long-acting testosterone undecanoate injections in hypogonadal men: an 84-week phase III clinical trial. *J Androl.* 2010;31(5):457-465. PMID: 20133964

Bhasin S, Brito JP, Cunningham GR, et al. Testosterone therapy in men with hypogonadism: an Endocrine Society clinical practice guideline. *J Clin Endocrinol Metab.* 2018;103(5):1715-1744. PMID: 29562364

12 ANSWER: D) Measure a trough testosterone level

Testosterone esters, including enanthate and cypionate, have been used for the treatment of male hypogonadism for more than 7 decades. They have the advantage of being the least expensive of the testosterone replacement modalities and they predictably restore testosterone levels to the normal range. However, they have unfavorable pharmacokinetics characterized by significant fluctuation in serum testosterone between peak and trough values. When administered by a deep intramuscular injection, testosterone is slowly released from this oily suspension into the circulation over a period of weeks. The esters are typically injected at 2-week intervals with levels reaching peak concentrations 24 to 48 hours after the injection followed by a gradual decline to the low-normal range before the next injection is due. When the interval between injections is extended to every 3 weeks, peak concentrations tend to be supraphysiologic and testosterone levels may fall to the hypogonadal range by the time the next injection is administered. Such wide excursions in serum testosterone concentrations can, in turn, cause undesirable swings in mood, libido, and energy levels.

Checking a trough testosterone level (Answer D) is correct, as it will ascertain whether his current regimen is insufficient to maintain a testosterone level within the therapeutic range for the entire 2 weeks. If a low trough testosterone level is confirmed, his regimen can be altered by either increasing the dose or shortening the interval between injections.

Recommending an antidepressant (Answer A) is not appropriate given that the patient is feeling better overall and that his symptoms are limited to the few days before each injection.

The pharmacokinetics of testosterone cypionate are similar to those of testosterone enanthate. Hence, switching esters (Answer B) will not address his problem.

Given that the patient fulfilled criteria for hypogonadism and feels better overall since he started injections, discontinuing testosterone therapy at this point (Answer C) is not appropriate and efforts should be focused instead on optimizing his treatment regimen.

Educational Objective
Describe the pharmacokinetics of injectable testosterone esters and manage potential adverse effects.

Reference(s)
Bhasin S, Brito JP, Cunningham GR, et al. Testosterone therapy in men with hypogonadism: an Endocrine Society clinical practice guideline. *J Clin Endocrinol Metab.* 2018;103(5):1715-1744. PMID: 29562364

Snyder PJ, Lawrence DA. Treatment of male hypogonadism with testosterone enanthate. *J Clin Endocrinol Metab.* 1980;51(6):1335-1339. PMID: 6777395

13 ANSWER: B) Normal testosterone, normal LH, high FSH

One of the most common long-term adverse effects of chemotherapy in men is gonadal dysfunction. After 1 year of follow-up, azoospermia is seen in 90% of men with Hodgkin lymphoma who have received more than 3 courses of an alkylating agent such as cyclophosphamide. Therefore, all men about to undergo gonadotoxic chemotherapy should be offered the option of sperm cryopreservation.

In the testis, the cells within the seminiferous tubules of the germinal epithelium have the highest mitotic and meiotic indices, and are thus most susceptible to the toxic effects of chemotherapy. Damage to the seminiferous tubules decreases secretion of inhibin B from Sertoli cells. This drop in inhibin B, which is the major nonsteroidal regulator of FSH, leads to a 5- to 10-fold increase in FSH levels. By contrast, Leydig cells are less sensitive to the gonadal toxicity of chemotherapeutic agents than the germinal epithelium, which is why LH and testosterone levels are typically maintained within the normal range. In some situations, there may be evidence of subclinical Leydig-cell dysfunction, characterized by testosterone levels that are at the lower end of the normal range in association with elevated LH levels.

Based on this differential sensitivity of the cells of the testes to chemotherapy, the typical hormone profile of a patient with azoospermia following cyclophosphamide is that of normal testosterone, normal LH, and high FSH, which makes Answer B correct. Answer A is incorrect because in the setting of azoospermia, testosterone and LH levels are typically normal, but the FSH level would be elevated. Answer C depicts the hormone milieu of hypogonadotropic hypogonadism, which is what one would see following toxicity to the hypothalamus or pituitary rather than the testis. Answer C reflects a combination of both central (low LH, low testosterone) and peripheral defects in the hypothalamic-pituitary-gonadal axis and is incorrect, as the reproductive effects of cyclophosphamide are confined to the testis.

Educational Objective
Explain the impact of cytotoxic chemotherapy on gonadal function and fertility in men.

Reference(s)
Howell SJ, Shalet SM. Spermatogenesis after cancer treatment: damage and recovery. *J Natl Cancer Inst Monogr.* 2005;34:12-17. PMID: 15784814

Jahnukainen K, Ehmcke J, Hou M, Schlatt S. Testicular function and fertility preservation in male cancer patients. *Best Pract Res Clin Endocrinol Metab.* 2011;25(2):287-302. PMID: 21397199

Hayes FJ, Pitteloud N, DeCruz S, Crowley WF Jr, Boepple PA. Importance of inhibin B in the regulation of FSH secretion in the human male. *J Clin Endocrinol Metab.* 2001;86(11):5541-5546. PMID: 11701733

14 ANSWER: A) Y-Chromosome microdeletion

This patient has nonobstructive azoospermia based on a normal semen volume and pH. He has normal LH and testosterone levels indicating normal Leydig-cell function, but he has an elevated FSH level due to lack of negative feedback from undetectable inhibin B, which suggests a selective defect in the seminiferous tubule compartment of the testis. This presentation is most likely due to a microdeletion in the Y-chromosome (Answer A), the second most common genetic cause of male infertility after Klinefelter syndrome. The male-specific region on the long arm of the Y chromosome has a locus known as the azoospermia factor (AZF) that contains genes needed for spermatogenesis. This AZF locus contains 3 regions: AZFa, AZFb, and AZFc. Deletions of the entire AZFa region result in complete atrophy of the tubular compartment, with only Sertoli cells seen on testicular biopsy, making sperm retrieval for intracytoplasmic sperm injection virtually impossible. Large deletions in the AZFb region also result in Sertoli-cell–only syndrome. Pathogenic variants in the AZFc region are the most common and account for 80% of Y-chromosome microdeletions. AZFc deletions are compatible with residual spermatogenesis, with oligospermia being a common presentation. These men may be candidates for intracytoplasmic sperm injection. Infertile men who do not have obstructive azoospermia, hypogonadotropic hypogonadism, or a karyotype abnormality should be tested for Y-chromosome microdeletions.

Kallmann syndrome (Answer B) is a condition characterized by congenital hypogonadotropic hypogonadism in association with anosmia or hyposmia. This patient's history of normal puberty, normal testes size, and elevated FSH levels are not consistent with this condition. This patient does not have mosaic Klinefelter syndrome (Answer C) given his normal testicular size and karyotype. Congenital bilateral absence of the vas deferens due to a mutation in the cystic fibrosis transmembrane conductance regulator gene (CFTR) is a relatively frequent cause of infertility in men with obstructive azoospermia. However, given that this patient has a normal semen volume and pH, congenital absence of the vas deferens (Answer D) would not explain his presentation.

Educational Objective

Describe the presentation of Y-chromosome microdeletions and outline the differential diagnosis of nonobstructive azoospermia.

Reference(s)

Vogt PH, Edelmann A, Kirsch S, et al. Human Y chromosome azoospermia factors (AZF) mapped to different subregions in Yq11. *Hum Mol Genet*. 1996;5(7):933-943. PMID: 8817327

Pryor JL, Kent-First M, Muallem A, et al. Microdeletions in the Y chromosome of infertile men. *N Engl J Med*. 1997;336(8):534-539. PMID: 9023089

Stahl PJ, Schlegel PN. Genetic evaluation of the azoospermic or severely oligozoospermic male. *Curr Opin Obstet Gynecol*. 2012;24(4):221-228. PMID: 22729088

15 ANSWER: B) Arrange for transrectal ultrasonography

The vas deferens is normally palpable as a thin, ropelike structure within the spermatic cord. In this case, imaging using transrectal ultrasonography (Answer B) confirmed the clinical suspicion of bilateral absence of the vas deferens. This patient turned out to have pathogenic variants in the *CFTR* gene, which is associated with cystic fibrosis. Congenital absence of the vas deferens, without the typical pulmonary and pancreatic manifestations of cystic fibrosis, is associated with compound heterozygosity for a classic (severe) *CFTR* variant and a mild *CFTR* variant. Given the autosomal recessive mode of inheritance of cystic fibrosis, screening of the female partner and genetic counseling are key components of this patient's management to determine the risk of transmitting this condition to offspring or of having a child with cystic fibrosis. When the records of his semen analyses were retrieved, they were consistent with an obstructive cause of azoospermia as evidenced by an ejaculate volume of 1 mL, absent fructose, and low pH (normal >7.2). The patient's initial low testosterone level could be explained by his obesity and was not low enough to cause azoospermia.

Adding FSH injections (Answer A) would not be appropriate given his normal testicular size and endogenous FSH levels. Increasing his hCG dosage (Answer C) would not be appropriate because his testosterone level is already near the upper end of the normal range. Use of donor sperm (Answer D) is not indicated in this patient, as the problem is not in sperm production and the patient's own sperm could be readily retrieved by testicular sperm extraction.

Educational Objective

Explain the association between congenital bilateral absence of the vas deferens and infertility.

Reference(s)

Anawalt BD. Approach to male infertility and induction of spermatogenesis. *J Clin Endocrinol Metab.* 2013;98(9):3532-3542. PMID: 24014811

Kolettis PN. The evaluation and management of the azoospermic patient. *J Androl.* 2002;23(3):293-305. PMID: 12002427

16 ANSWER: D) hCG injections

The 3 key elements of this case are: (1) the patient has secondary, rather than primary, hypogonadism; (2) the cause of his central defect is a pituitary, rather than hypothalamic, lesion; and (3) his hypogonadism is acquired rather than congenital. In men with primary hypogonadism, fertility options are typically limited to assisted reproductive techniques such as intracytoplasmic sperm injection, use of donor sperm, or adoption. In contrast, men whose infertility is due to secondary hypogonadism can have spermatogenesis induced with hormonal therapy in the form of either exogenous gonadotropins (hCG ± FSH) or GnRH. Therefore, this patient who has hypogonadotropic hypogonadism is an appropriate candidate for medical therapy.

The site of the defect in the hypothalamic-pituitary-gonadal axis dictates which form of medical therapy is most appropriate to stimulate spermatogenesis in a given patient. GnRH (Answer C) is administered subcutaneously through a portable infusion pump every 120 minutes, and it stimulates the gonadotrope cells in the anterior pituitary to stimulate LH and FSH, which in turn stimulate the testes to make testosterone and sperm. Thus, an intact pituitary gland is a prerequisite for GnRH to effectively induce spermatogenesis, so this treatment is not appropriate for a patient who has had a hypophysectomy. In contrast, gonadotropin therapy is effective in patients with both pituitary and hypothalamic disease, as gonadotropins act directly on the testes.

Gonadotropin therapy to induce spermatogenesis consists of subcutaneous administration of hCG alone or in combination with FSH. hCG bears strong structural homology to LH, and acting through the LH receptor on Leydig cells it increases both intratesticular and systemic testosterone production. In men who become hypogonadal after normal puberty has been completed and thus have normal testicular size, treatment with hCG alone is adequate to stimulate spermatogenesis. In contrast, patients who have congenital hypogonadotropic hypogonadism and prepubertal testes (<4 mL) need combination therapy with both hCG and FSH to stimulate growth of the seminiferous tubules. Thus, in this patient with acquired hypogonadism and testes of 20 mL, monotherapy with hCG (Answer D) is the correct answer and combination therapy with both hCG and FSH (Answer B) is incorrect.

Clomiphene citrate (Answer A) is a selective estrogen-receptor modulator, which can increase testosterone secretion by blocking estrogen-mediated negative feedback in the hypothalamus, thus increasing endogenous gonadotropins. However, it would not be effective in someone whose pituitary gland has been removed. In addition, clomiphene is not FDA-approved for the treatment of male hypogonadotropic hypogonadism and there are concerns that long-term use of estrogen blockade may negatively impact libido, bone health, and insulin sensitivity.

Educational Objective

Recommend appropriate treatment to restore fertility in a man with acquired hypogonadotropic hypogonadism.

Reference(s)

Burris AS, Rodbard HW, Winters SJ, Sherins RJ. Gonadotropin therapy in men with isolated hypogonadotropic hypogonadism: the response to human chorionic gonadotropin is predicted by initial testicular size. *J Clin Endocrinal Metab.* 1988;66(6):1144-1151. PMID: 3372679

King TF, Hayes FJ. Long-term outcome of idiopathic hypogonadotropic hypogonadism. *Curr Opin Endocrinol Diabetes Obes.* 2012;19(3):204-210. PMID: 22499222

17 ANSWER: C) Estrogen-secreting testicular tumor

This patient has tender gynecomastia. Breast tenderness suggests benign breast growth of recent onset (<6 months). He has a low testosterone concentration and low gonadotropin concentrations but the most striking abnormality is a 3-fold increase in estradiol levels. Increased estradiol levels may reflect increased testicular secretion of estradiol, increased extraglandular aromatization of estrogen precursors secreted by the adrenal glands, increased extraglandular aromatase activity, or exposure to exogenous estrogens. Testicular tumors can cause gynecomastia by a number of mechanisms. The production of hCG by germ-cell tumors can stimulate the production of testosterone and estradiol by normal testicular tissue. In this case, the patient's negative β-hCG level rules out a germ-cell tumor. Unlike germ-cell tumors, Leydig-cell tumors can secrete estradiol directly and in as many as 50% of cases, gynecomastia precedes the development of a palpable testicular mass, but the tumor is usually detectable by ultrasonography. In this patient, the elevated estradiol level, suppressed gonadotropins due to estrogen-mediated negative feedback, and low testosterone levels are best explained by an estrogen-secreting testicular tumor (Answer C).

Anabolic steroid use (Answer A) would cause gonadotropin suppression, but it would not explain the hormone profile as most are nonaromatizable and do therefore do not increase estradiol levels. If the patient were also taking testosterone, it would increase his estradiol levels, but in that case his testosterone level would be high rather than low.

Finasteride (Answer B) modestly raises serum testosterone concentrations by blocking the conversion of testosterone to dihydrotestosterone, so it would not explain this patient's gynecomastia or hormone profile.

The patient's TSH level is not provided. However, his presentation is not consistent with hyperthyroidism (Answer D) given his normal thyroid examination, absence of clinical features of hyperthyroidism, and the fact that his testosterone level is low rather than high-normal, as would be expected in the hyperthyroid state due to high SHBG levels.

Educational Objective

Identify the clinical and biochemical features of an estrogen-secreting Leydig-cell tumor.

Reference(s)

Case Records of the Massachusetts General Hospital. Weekly clinicopathological conferences. Case 12-2000. A 60-year-old man with persistent gynecomastia after excision of a pituitary adenoma [published correction appears in *N Engl J Med.* 2000;343(1):76]. *N Engl J Med.* 2000;342(16);1196-1204. PMID: 10770986

Amory JK, Wang C, Swerdloff RS, et al. The effect of 5alpha-reductase inhibition with dutasteride and finasteride on semen parameters and serum hormones in healthy men [published correction appears in *J Clin Endocrinol Metab.* 2007;92(11): 4379]. *J Clin Endocrinol Metab.* 2007;92(5):1659-1665. PMID: 17299062

Braunstein GD. Clinical practice. Gynecomastia. *N Engl J Med.* 2007;357(12):1229-1237. PMID: 17881754

18 ANSWER: B) Persistent postpubertal gynecomastia

The pathophysiology of gynecomastia involves an imbalance between free estrogen and free androgen actions in the breast tissue. During mid-to-late puberty, relatively more estrogen may be produced by the testes and peripheral tissues before testosterone secretion reaches adult levels, resulting in the gynecomastia that commonly occurs during this period. Most adolescents presenting with isolated gynecomastia have physiologic pubertal gynecomastia, which generally appears at 13 or 14 years of age, lasts for 6 months or less, and then regresses. Although the diagnosis is evident in most cases, a thorough history that includes review of medications, environmental exposures, and illicit drug use and physical examination are necessary. The case described fits the diagnosis of pubertal gynecomastia (Answer B), but unlike most cases, it has failed to regress and is causing significant psychological distress. Surgical resection should be considered for adolescents with physiologic gynecomastia that is greater than 4 cm in diameter, has not responded to medical therapy, persists for more than 1 year or after the patient is age 17 years, or is associated with embarrassment that interferes with normal daily activities.

FSH levels are invariably elevated in men with Klinefelter syndrome, even mosaic forms (Answer A), so this patient's FSH level of 3.0 mIU/mL (3.0 IU/L) effectively rules out this diagnosis. Leydig-cell tumors (Answer C) are a rare but important cause of gynecomastia. They are frequently too small to be found on clinical examination but are usually identified on ultrasonography. They cause gynecomastia by increasing estradiol levels, so they would not explain the breast enlargement in this patient with normal estradiol levels. There are a number of case reports of gynecomastia arising from inadvertent exposure to estrogens (Answer D). If this were the case in this patient, his LH level would be suppressed, as would his endogenous estradiol.

Educational Objective
Diagnose persistent postpubertal gynecomastia.

Reference(s)
Braunstein GD. Clinical practice. Gynecomastia. *N Engl J Med.* 2007;357(12):1229-1237. PMID: 17881754

Guss CE, Divasta AD. Adolescent gynecomastia. *Pediatr Endocrinol Rev.* 2017;14(4):371-377. PMID: 28613047

19 ANSWER: B) Switch her regimen to a GnRH agonist with a 0.05-mg estradiol patch

In male-to-female transgender patients, estrogen therapy is needed to develop female sexual characteristics. In patients with an intact hypothalamic-pituitary-gonadal axis, the estrogen dosage needed is supraphysiologic given the need to suppress testosterone secretion. However, combined use of a GnRH agonist with estrogen allows physiologic doses of estrogen to be used, as testosterone secretion is already suppressed. Estrogen therapy can result in marked hypertriglyceridemia. However, the lipid effects of estrogen depend on the route of administration, with the transdermal route having less effect on HDL cholesterol and triglycerides than the oral route. Given this patient's history of hypertriglyceridemia, she is not a suitable candidate for oral estrogen and the most appropriate hormone regimen would be a GnRH agonist and a low-dosage estrogen patch (Answer B), which can be titrated based on clinical response and triglyceride levels. Ethinyl estradiol (Answer D) would not be a good choice because of its negative effects on triglycerides, as well as the fact that it increases the risk of venous thromboembolism significantly more so than 17β-estradiol.

Using spironolactone alone without an estrogen (Answer A) would not provide adequate suppression and blockade of androgen action for the desired physical effects.

Given that the patient has been living as a woman for more than 2 decades, and considering the increased risk of depression and suicide in the transgender population, withholding further hormone therapy (Answer C) would most likely negatively affect her mental health. In addition, estrogen therapy was not her only risk factor for hypertriglyceridemia.

Educational Objective
Guide the hormonal care of a transgender patient with hypertriglyceridemia.

Reference(s)
Hembree WC, Cohen-Kettenis PT, Gooren L, et al. Endocrine treatment of gender-dysphoric/gender-incongruent persons: an Endocrine Society clinical practice guideline. *J Clin Endocrinol Metab.* 2017;102(11):3869-3903. PMID: 28945902

Aljenedil S, Hegele RA, Genest J, Awan Z. Estrogen-associated severe hypertriglyceridemia with pancreatitis. *J Clin Lipidol.* 2017;11(1):297-300. PMID: 28391900

Lufkin EG, Ory SJ. Relative value of transdermal and oral estrogen therapy in various clinical situations. *Mayo Clin Proc.* 1994;69(2):131-135. PMID: 8309263

Rosenthal SM. Approach to the patient: transgender youth: endocrine considerations. *J Clin Endocrinol Metab.* 2014;99(12):4379-4389. PMID: 25140398

20 ANSWER: D) Partial androgen insensitivity syndrome

This patient's presentation with hypospadias, cryptorchidism, small testes, gynecomastia, high-normal testosterone level, and elevated gonadotropin concentrations is consistent with partial androgen insensitivity (PAIS) (Answer D). The phenotypic spectrum of PAIS ranges from that of a phenotypic female at the most severe end of the spectrum (complete androgen resistance) to that of a virilized male with oligospermia at the mildest end of the spectrum. PAIS is due to a pathogenic variant in the androgen receptor gene located on the X chromosome. In some cases, there may be a history of a family member presenting with primary amenorrhea or an inguinal hernia as a neonate. In the patient described, the testosterone level is not as high as one typically sees in a patient with PAIS. This is most likely due to suppression of his hypothalamic-pituitary-gonadal axis by pneumonia.

One of the key clinical features that helps to refine the differential diagnosis in this case is the presence of hypospadias. In patients with hypospadias, the urethral opening occurs on the underside of the penis rather than the tip due to insufficient testosterone production in the first trimester of pregnancy when sexual differentiation is occurring. Thus, while a patient with Klinefelter syndrome could present with cryptorchidism, gynecomastia, small testes, and a high-normal testosterone level if he is being treated with testosterone (Answer A), it would not explain his decreased body hair or hypospadias, as testosterone production is normal in utero in a patient with Klinefelter syndrome.

5α-Reductase deficiency (Answer B) is a rare autosomal recessive disorder in which patients with a 46,XY karyotype have impaired virilization during embryogenesis due to defective conversion of testosterone to dihydrotestosterone. These patients often present with ambiguous genitalia and may be reared as girls in childhood. However, patients with a milder phenotype may present with hypospadias. Two of the features that help to distinguish this condition from PAIS are the absence of gynecomastia and gonadotropins in the low-normal range. Thus, 5α-reductase deficiency (Answer B) would not explain this patient's presentation.

Polyglandular autoimmune syndrome type 2 (Answer C) is an autoimmune disorder that impacts multiple endocrine organs and most commonly results in type 1 diabetes, Addison disease, and hypothyroidism. While primary hypogonadism can be part of the presentation of polyglandular autoimmune syndrome type 2 and this patient indeed has a diagnosis of hypothyroidism, he does not have any of the other manifestations and it would not explain his cryptorchidism or hypospadias.

Educational Objective
Diagnose partial androgen insensitivity and construct a differential diagnosis for hypospadias.

Reference(s)
Mongan NP, Tadokoro-Cuccaro R, Bunch T, Hughes IA. Androgen insensitivity syndrome. *Best Pract Res Clin Endocrinol Metab.* 2015; 29(4):569-580. PMID: 26303084

Okeigwe I, Kuohung W. 5-Alpha reductase deficiency: a 40-year retrospective review. *Curr Opin Endocrinol Diabetes Obes.* 2014;21(6):483-487. PMID: 25321150

Obesity & Lipids Board Review

Andrea D. Coviello, MD

1 ANSWER: D) *FTO* (fat mass and obesity associated)

While lifestyle and environmental factors are extremely important in weight gain, genetic factors are also important. Genome-wide association studies have identified a number of gene loci that are important determinants of BMI. The single gene most commonly associated with typical human obesity is *FTO* (Answer D). This association has been documented in a number of different populations. Individuals with the at-risk allele weigh 4.4 to 6.6 lb (2-3 kg) more than those without the allele. A large number of studies have tried to determine the mechanisms by which the at-risk alleles in the *FTO* gene produce increased BMI. Most of the physiologic data suggest this occurs through a predisposition for increased food intake. However, a recent study using the most definitive methods applied to date provides strong evidence that DNA near the *FTO* gene interacts with other genes at a distance to foster the development of adipocyte precursors to either white or brown/beige adipocytes.

Pathogenic variants in the genes encoding the melanocortin 4 receptor (*MC4R*), leptin (*LEP*), and the leptin receptor (*LEPR*) (Answers A, B, and C) have been found in humans and are associated with obesity. However, these pathogenic variants are uncommon (*MC4R*) or rare (*LEP* and *LEPR*), typically involve consanguinity, and are associated with extreme obesity that develops in childhood. This is not the phenotype of the patient described in this vignette.

Educational Objective

Identify the common gene variants that predispose to obesity.

Reference(s)

Loos RJ, Yeo GS. The bigger picture of FTO: the first GWAS-identified obesity gene. *Nat Rev Endocrinol.* 2014;10(1):51-61. PMID: 24247219

Qi Q, Downer MK, Kilpelainen TO, et al. Dietary intake, FTO genetic variants, and adiposity: a combined analysis of over 16,000 children and adolescents. *Diabetes.* 2015;64(7):2467-2476. PMID: 25720386

Claussnitzer M, Dankel SN, Kim KH, et al. FTO obesity variant circuitry and adipocyte browning in humans. *N Engl J Med.* 2015;373(10):895-907. PMID: 26287746

2 ANSWER: C) Decreased energy expenditure

Weight regain after successful weight loss is very common. The body adapts to weight loss in several ways. There is a shift in the hormones that regulate appetite and satiety. The premeal hunger hormone ghrelin is higher and the satiety hormones such as GLP-1, cholecystokinin, and peptide YY are lower than before weight loss. This shift in appetite regulation favors weight regain. The shift in hormones stimulates the corresponding anorexigenic (satiety) and orexigenic (hunger) pathways differently, favoring increased appetite and weight regain. Although she is most likely experiencing increased appetite (Answer D) and decreased satiety (Answer B) after successful weight loss, her food diary shows she has been able to maintain her target caloric intake over time.

Total energy expenditure is linearly related to lean body mass. To maintain weight stability, total daily energy intake must be the same as total daily energy expenditure. The components of total energy expenditure include resting metabolic rate, the thermic effect of feeding, and energy expended in physical activity. In addition, total energy expenditure decreases (Answer C) with both a drop in resting energy expenditure and voluntary energy expenditure with physical activity, creating a state of improved "energy efficiency." Resting energy expenditure represents the majority of energy expenditure in a day at 50% to 70% of total energy expenditure. Thermic energy expenditure is about 10%, and voluntary physical activity energy expenditure can vary between 20% and 30% for most people. Although initially increases in physical activity result in increased energy expenditure (Answer A), over time the body becomes more energy efficient and uses less energy for the same amount of physical activity.

Resting energy expenditure and total energy expenditure will fall with weight loss because of a loss in lean body mass in addition to loss of fat mass. In part, a reduction in the energy expended in physical activity is the result of mechanically moving less weight. However, a number of studies have demonstrated that there is an even greater fall in total and resting energy expenditure than would be predicted from loss of lean body mass alone. Therefore, the decrease in resting energy expenditure has the greatest magnitude of effect in terms of tendency for weight regain if nutrient/energy intake has not increased.

Educational Objective

Explain the changes in energy expenditure that occur with weight loss.

Reference(s)

Sumithran P, Prendergast LA, Delbridge E, et al. Long-term persistence of hormonal adaptations to weight loss. *N Engl J Med.* 2011;365(17):1597-1604. PMID: 22029981

Leibel RL, Rosenbaum M, Hirsch J. Changes in energy expenditure resulting from altered body weight [published correction appears in *N Engl J Med.* 1995;333(6):399]. *N Engl J Med.* 1995; 332(10):621-628. PMID: 7632212

Goldsmith R, Joanisse DR, Gallagher D, et al. Effects of experimental weight perturbation on skeletal muscle work efficiency, fuel utilization, and biochemistry in human subjects. *Am J Physiol Regul Integr Comp Physiol.* 2010;298(1): R79-R88. PMID: 19889869

Lichtman SW, Pisarska K, Berman ER, et al. Discrepancy between self-reported and actual caloric intake and exercise in obese subjects. *N Engl J Med.* 1992;327(27):1893-1898. PMID: 1454084

3 ANSWER: C) Glipizide

Drug-induced weight gain is a common clinical problem. A number of drug classes can cause this problem, including antidiabetes medications, antipsychotic agents, antidepressant agents, mood stabilizers, glucocorticoids, and progestational agents. Several management options are available for patients who have drug-induced weight gain. One is to reduce the dosage of the offending medication or to reconsider the value of that medication and potentially to stop it. Alternatively, a behavioral weight-management program can be instituted. Finally, the problematic medication can be stopped and an alternative medication can be prescribed. For example, a GLP-1 agonist or an SGLT-2 inhibitor can be used in place of, or in addition to, a sulfonylurea.

Of the available antihypertensive medications, β-adrenergic blockers such as metoprolol are associated with weight gain, while ACE inhibitors (Answer A), angiotensin-receptor blockers, calcium-channel blockers, and diuretics are not.

Many diabetes medications are associated with weight gain—up to 10 to 20 lb (4.5-9.1 kg) in the first 6 to 12 months—including the anabolic hormone insulin, insulin secretagogues such as the sulfonylurea glipizide (Answer C), meglitinides, and thiazolidinediones such as pioglitazone. Metformin (Answer B) is weight neutral in general, although it is associated with mild weight loss in some patients. DPP-4 inhibitors and α-glucosidase inhibitors are weight neutral and GLP-1 receptor agonists promote weight loss in addition to blood glucose control. SGLT-2 inhibitors are associated with mild weight loss in the context of glucosuria and water loss.

More recently, antihistamines have been recognized as weight promoting. The more potent the antihistamine, the more likely the patient is to gain weight with long-term use. The H1-antihistamines such as cetirizine are the most likely to be associated with weight gain.

Statins (Answer D) are not associated with significant weight gain.

Other medication classes that can lead to weight gain include glucocorticoids, antidepressants, antipsychotic agents, and hormonal contraceptives. Of the antidepressants, the selective serotonin reuptake inhibitors sertraline, citalopram, and escitalopram (Answer E) are weight neutral. Fluoxetine and bupropion are associated with weight loss.

Educational Objective

Identify weight-promoting and weight-neutral medications among commonly prescribed medications for adults.

Reference(s)

Apovian CM, Aronne LJ, Bessesen DH, et al; Endocrine Society. Pharmacological management of obesity: an Endocrine Society clinical practice guideline. *J Clin Endocrinol Metab.* 2015;100(2): 342-362. PMID: 25590212

Answer: B) Liraglutide

Liraglutide, 3.0 mg daily, (Answer B) is approved for patients with a BMI of 27 kg/m^2 or greater with an obesity-related comorbidity (of which this patient has multiple). The most common adverse effects of liraglutide are gastrointestinal in nature and include nausea in about 30% to 40% of patients, vomiting, abdominal pain, and diarrhea or constipation. Gastrointestinal adverse effects are significant enough in approximately 6% of patients in clinical trials to prompt them to stop the medication. Gallbladder disease occurs in about 5% of patients on liraglutide compared with placebo and is to be used in caution in someone who has had known gallstones. However, this patient already had a cholecystectomy, so this is not a risk for her.

Lorcaserin (Answer A) is a selective serotonin reuptake inhibitor specific to 5-HT2C serotonin receptors. It should not be used in patients already on a selective serotonin reuptake inhibitor (this patient is taking escitalopram). Additionally, one of the most common adverse effects of lorcaserin is headache. This patient already suffers from migraines; lorcaserin would not be a good choice in this context.

Topiramate (Answer D) is a medication that is FDA approved for epilepsy and migraine headaches, which makes it a potentially attractive choice for this patient given her history of migraines. Although there are a number of studies in which it was used specifically for weight loss, it is not FDA approved for this purpose. However, there is strong evidence that it produces a 6% to 8% weight loss that is sustained at 1 year. However, topiramate is associated with the formation of kidney stones due its acid-base effects and urine metabolite excretion. Topiramate is contraindicated in patients with kidney stones. The combination of phentermine

and topiramate (Answer C) is also contraindicated for this patient due to her history of kidney stones.

Naltrexone/bupropion (Answer E) is contraindicated in patients with uncontrolled hypertension, which makes it a suboptimal choice for this patient.

Educational Objective

Appropriately select weight-loss medications on the basis of a patient's clinical circumstances and current medications.

Reference(s)

Rosenstock J, Hollander P, Gadde KM, Sun X, Strauss R, Leung A; OBD-202 Study Group. A randomized, double-blind, placebo-controlled, multicenter study to assess the efficacy and safety of topiramate controlled release in the treatment of obese type 2 diabetic patients. *Diabetes Care.* 2007;30(6):1480-1486. PMID: 17363756

Eliasson B, Gudbjörnsdottir S, Cederholm J, Liang Y, Vercruysse F, Smith U. Weight loss and metabolic effects of topiramate in overweight and obese type 2 diabetic patients: randomized double-blind placebo-controlled trial. *Int J Obes (London).* 2007;31(7):1140-1147. PMID: 17264849

Apovian CM, Aronne LJ, Bessesen DH, et al; Endocrine Society. Pharmacological management of obesity: an Endocrine Society clinical practice guideline. *J Clin Endocrinol Metab.* 2015;100(2):342-362. PMID: 25590212

ANSWER: C) Cholelithiasis

The most effective treatment currently available for weight loss is bariatric surgery. However, aggressive energy restriction with a very low-calorie diet is almost as effective as gastric banding. Very low-calorie diets are restricted to fewer than 800 kcal per day. Very low-calorie diets are high in protein to maximally preserve lean body mass, which may be a problem in this patient with chronic kidney disease. Very low-calorie diets produce, on average, 17% to 18% weight loss over 3 months. However, 25% of patients on such a diet for 2 months develop gallbladder disease, particularly acute cholecystitis due to cholelithiasis (Answer C), frequently requiring surgery (6% of patients on a very low-calorie diet for 2 months require surgery). The increase in gallbladder disease is believed to be due to decreased gallbladder contractility. The greater the rate and magnitude of weight loss, the greater the risk of gall-bladder disease. This patient already has known gall-stones, which would put her at even higher risk for cholecystitis and potentially gallstone pancreatitis.

Very low-calorie diets have also been shown to produce dramatic improvements in glucose levels in persons with type 2 diabetes (thus, Answer E is incorrect). Fatty liver disease is generally improved with weight loss, particularly with diets lower in fats (thus, Answer A is incorrect), which can also effectively lower triglycerides and improve dyslipidemia (thus, Answer B is incorrect). Hypertension generally improves with weight loss (thus, Answer D is incorrect). Concerns remain about the long-term maintenance of weight loss with this strategy. Long-term weight loss with very low-calorie diets tends to be the same as that for low-calorie diets.

Educational Objective
Counsel patients about the benefits and risks of very low-calorie diets.

Reference(s)
Tsai AG, Wadden TA. The evolution of very-low-calorie diets: an update and meta-analysis. *Obesity (Silver Spring)*. 2006;14(8):1283-1293. PMID: 16988070

ANSWER: D) Gastric band erosion
Patients who had gastric banding procedures many years ago often fail to follow-up with their surgeon. Endocrinologists who follow these patients for diabetes or other comorbid illnesses may be the only physicians who see them in long-term follow-up. For this reason, it is important for endocrinologists to recognize some of the long-term complications of gastric banding and gastric bypass operations. In particular, endocrinologists should be aware of the anatomy produced by the different bariatric surgical procedures and consider the possibility of a mechanical or anatomic problem when they see patients with new symptoms who have had bariatric surgical procedures.

The symptoms that this patient describes are typical for a gastric band erosion (Answer D). In this complication, the gastric band erodes through the stomach wall. Band erosion may present as unexplained weight regain with abdominal pain, or may present with signs of infection and inflammation as

the gastric wall is perforated at the site of the erosion, with gastric contents tracking along the filling catheter to the subcutaneous port site. Gastric band erosion typically occurs in the first year after surgery, but can present 2 to 5 years after implantation. Staple line dehiscence (Answer B) and anastomotic leaks (Answer C) are complications of gastric bypass operations, thus they could not occur in the described patient because a gastric banding procedure does not have any staple lines or intestinal anastomoses. Food impaction in a band (Answer E) typically occurs shortly after a band adjustment and subsequent solid food intake without adequate chewing. Affected patients present to the emergency department with abdominal pain and the inability to keep anything down, including saliva. The condition can be treated endoscopically. While a patient could conceivably manipulate the injection port (Answer A), there is no incentive to do this and he/she would not have the symptoms described.

Educational Objective
Describe the clinical features of common complications of bariatric surgical procedures.

Reference(s)
Levine MS, Carucci LR. Imaging of bariatric surgery: normal anatomy and postoperative complications. *Radiology*. 2014;270(2):327-341. PMID: 24471382

Aarts EO, van Wageningen B, Berends F, Janssen I, Wahab P, Groenen M. Intragastric band erosion: experiences with gastrointestinal endoscopic removal. *World J Gastroenterol*. 2015;21(5):1567-1572. PMID: 25663775

O'Brien PE, MacDonald L, Anderson M, Brennan L, Brown WA. Long-term outcomes after bariatric surgery: fifteen-year follow-up of adjustable gastric banding and a systematic review of the bariatric surgical literature. *Ann Surg*. 2013;257(1):87-94. PMID: 23235396

7. ANSWER: A) Deletion in the 15q11.2-q13 chromosomal region (Prader-Willi syndrome)

Although a number of conditions can cause serious childhood obesity, this patient's phenotype is typical for Prader-Willi syndrome (PWS). PWS is a multisystem disorder that is caused by the lack of expression of paternally inherited imprinted genes in the chromosomal region 15q11.2-q13 (Answer A). Typical features include hypotonia, poor feeding after birth, learning disabilities, growth retardation, behavioral problems, hypothalamic hypogonadism, and cryptorchidism. The initial genetic test, DNA methylation analysis, is important for making a definitive diagnosis.

The most common monogenic form of early-onset obesity involves pathogenic variants in the gene that encodes the melanocortin 4 receptor (*MC4R*) (Answer B). The melanocortin 4 receptor is involved in hypothalamic signaling along the neural pathway that responds to leptin. Individuals with *MC4R* pathogenic variants do not have the hypotonia, early poor feeding, or characteristic appearance as described in the patient in this vignette, but rather are hyperphagic from birth. They also have normal reproductive function in contrast to the patient in this vignette. Individuals who have pathogenic variants in the genes encoding leptin or the leptin receptor (Answer C) have hypothalamic hypogonadism and subtle impairments in GH and immune function. Bardet-Biedl syndrome (Answer E) and Alstrom syndrome (Answer D) are both ciliopathies. Bardet-Biedl syndrome is characterized by truncal obesity, polydactyly, rod-cone dystrophy, cognitive impairment, male hypogonadotrophic hypogonadism, female genitourinary malformations, and renal abnormalities. By contrast, Alstrom syndrome is characterized by insulin resistance and the development of type 2 diabetes in childhood. Vision and sensory neural hearing problems are common, as is polycystic ovary syndrome and hyperandrogenism in affected female patients. This suggests that cilia are somehow important in body weight regulation and insulin sensitivity. Polydactyly occurs in Bardet-Biedl syndrome, but not in Alstrom syndrome. Individuals with leptin receptor pathogenic variants, Alstrom syndrome, or Bardet-Biedl syndrome do not have the hypotonia, poor feeding, and phenotypic features described in this patient.

Educational Objective
Diagnose Prader-Willi syndrome and describe the clinical features of the genetic causes of severe childhood obesity.

Reference(s)
Goldstone AP, Holland AJ, Hauffa BP, Hokken-Koelega AC, Tauber M; speakers contributors at the Second Expert Meeting of the Comprehensive Care of Patients with PWS. Recommendations for the diagnosis and management of Prader-Willi syndrome [published correction appears in *J Clin Endocrinol Metab.* 2010;95(12): 5465]. *J Clin Endocrinol Metab.* 2008;93(11): 4183-4197. PMID: 18697869

Farooqi S, O'Rahilly S. Genetics of obesity in humans. *Endocr Rev.* 2006;27(7):710-718. PMID: 17122358

Ranadive SA, Vaisse C. Lessons from extreme human obesity: monogenic disorders. *Endocrinol Metab Clin North Am.* 2008;37(3):733-751. PMID: 18775361

Girard D, Petrovsky N. Alström syndrome: insights into the pathogenesis of metabolic disorders. *Nat Rev Endocrinol.* 2011;7(2):77-88. PMID: 21135875

8. ANSWER: D) Biliopancreatic diversion

Patients commonly ask their endocrinologists for advice on the risks and benefits of bariatric surgery. It is important, therefore, for clinical endocrinologists to have a sense of both the amount of weight loss that a patient might expect from the commonly performed bariatric surgical procedures, as well as the potential problems associated with each.

The laparoscopic banding procedure (Answer C) was popular for a number of years because it was relatively easy for the surgeon to perform and had low perioperative risk. Because it was potentially reversible, it satisfied many patients' desire to not have their "plumbing changed." However, it is now clear that the weight loss with laparoscopic banding is less (18%-22% of baseline weight) than that of other procedures and that mechanical problems are more common with this procedure over the long run.

Sleeve gastrectomy (Answer A) is gaining in popularity because it does not require ongoing adjustment (as does the band), results in more weight loss (22%-25%), and is relatively easy for the surgeon to perform.

Despite these advantages, recent studies have shown that the sleeve gastrectomy is not as effective as gastric bypass in either producing weight loss or improving glucose control in patients with type 2 diabetes.

Roux-en-Y gastric bypass (Answer B) provides the most weight loss (25%-28%) of the first 3 operations listed and often dramatically improves glucose levels in patients with type 2 diabetes. However, it results in a lifelong need for vitamin supplementation and most likely puts patients at risk for metabolic bone disease.

Biliopancreatic diversion (Answer D) is a more extensive operation that is not often performed. It is important for endocrinologists to be aware of this procedure, however, as they may see patients who are thinking of having it or who have had it. It is associated with the greatest degree of weight loss (32%-35%) and has the largest effect on glucose levels, but it is not widely used because of more frequent complications and adverse effects including severe and potentially difficult to treat vitamin deficiencies.

The endoscopically placed duodenal sleeve (Answer E) is an experimental device that mimics the duodenal bypass that is part of the gastric bypass procedure. In animal studies done in rodent models of diabetes, it appears to have beneficial effects on glucose control. The limited data available in humans suggest about a 13% weight loss 6 months after placement.

Educational Objective
Describe the expected weight loss associated with different bariatric surgical procedures.

Reference(s)
Dumon KR, Murayama KM. Bariatric surgery outcomes. *Surg Clin North Am.* 2011;91(6):1313-1338. PMID: 22054156

Chang SH, Stoll CR, Song J, Varela JE, Eagon CJ, Colditz GA. The effectiveness and risks of bariatric surgery: an updated systematic review and meta-analysis, 2003-2012. *JAMA Surg.* 2014; 149(3):275-287. PMID: 24352617

Padwal R, Klarenbach S, Wiebe N, et al. Bariatric surgery: a systematic review and network meta-analysis of randomized trials. *Obes Rev.* 2011; 12(8):602-621. PMID: 21438991

9 ANSWER: D) Acarbose

Gastric bypass surgery has a dramatic effect on carbohydrate metabolism. Forty to fifty percent of patients who have diabetes preoperatively do not require medication for diabetes after surgery. Diabetes resolves in many of these individuals within weeks of the operation. It appears that the exposure of the distal bowel to food results in exaggerated secretion of GLP-1, which may facilitate the improvement in glucose control seen after surgery. Postprandial hypoglycemia is an uncommon late complication of gastric bypass surgery that is increasingly recognized. It appears that in some individuals, perhaps in response to ongoing stimulation by GLP-1, β-cell proliferation occurs, resulting in islet hyperplasia associated with excessive insulin secretion and endogenous hyperinsulinemic hypoglycemia. Some patients may develop multiple small insulinomas.

The management of this condition is controversial. Dietary changes alleviate symptoms in 50% to 70% of affected individuals. Thus, dietary modification is the initial treatment choice. These patients can be managed by reducing the intake of carbohydrates, consuming low–glycemic index carbohydrates, and always eating carbohydrates in the context of a mixed meal. If symptoms persist, the best choice is to start oral acarbose (Answer D) with meals, which helps to delay carbohydrate release and metabolism resulting in less insulin secretion after meals.

While partial pancreatectomy (Answer B) was suggested in initial series, pancreatectomy has become a treatment of last resort. It appears that the condition recurs in many individuals who have a subtotal pancreatectomy, and those who have more aggressive pancreatic surgery can develop pancreatic diabetes. For this reason, pancreatectomy is currently used only if other treatments fail and the patient remains debilitated by frequent episodes of hypoglycemia that limit functional capacity.

Octreotide (Answer C) has been used effectively to reduce hypoglycemia, but it requires either intravenous administration acutely or subcutaneous injections at home, which makes it a second-line medication. GLP-1 receptor agonists (Answer A) are believed to help reduce insulin-mediated hypoglycemia by slowing gastric emptying, but they also stimulate insulin release from β cells. GLP-1 receptor agonists currently require subcutaneous injection at home. The successful use of

GLP-1 receptor agonists in this setting remains anecdotal and cannot be recommended as first-line therapy.

Educational Objective
Manage hyperinsulinemic hypoglycemia that develops after gastric bypass surgery.

Reference(s)
Service GJ, Thompson GB, Service FJ, Andrews JC, Collazo-Clavell ML, Lloyd RV. Hyperinsulinemic hypoglycemia with nesidioblastosis after gastric bypass surgery. *N Engl J Med.* 2005; 353(3):249-254. PMID: 16034010

Rariy CM, Rometo D, Korytkowski M. Post-gastric bypass hypoglycemia. *Curr Diab Rep.* 2016;16(2): 19. PMID: 26868861

10 ANSWER: A) Same amount of weight loss

Many approaches to diet regimens for weight loss exist, including versions of the low-carbohydrate diet, low glycemic–index diet, ketogenic diet, low-fat/high-fiber diet, and, more recently, intermittent fasting diets. Intermittent fasting refers to fasting for 12 hours or longer. Time-restricted feeding involves restricting food intake to certain timeframes—usually between 6 and 12 hours a day. Alternate day fasting refers to alternating one day of fasting with one day of unrestricted eating. Alternate day modified fasting denotes an eating pattern where one consumes 25% or less of caloric needs on the "fasting" day and unrestricted eating on nonfasting days. Lastly, periodic fasting refers to fasting for 1 to 2 days a week and eating unrestricted 5 to 6 days per week. The premise behind intermittent fasting is that caloric restriction on fasting days leads to a shift in fuel metabolism from carbohydrates and glucose after glycogen stores are depleted and moves to lipolysis and the generation of ketones bodies. Intermittent fasting has been shown to improve glucose and lipid metabolism, reduce inflammation, reduce liver fat, and reduce blood pressure, although heart rate variability has been shown to increase. Overall though, intermittent fasting results in similar weight loss to caloric restriction when total caloric intake is taken into account (thus, Answer A is correct and Answers B, C, and D are incorrect).

Educational Objective
Explain the rationale behind intermittent fasting diets and their efficacy for weight loss and improved health.

Reference(s)
Anton SD, Moehl K, Donahoo WT, et al. Flipping the metabolic switch: understanding and applying the health benefits of fasting. *Obesity (Silver Spring).* 2018;26(2):254-268. PMID: 29086496

Trepanowski JF, Kroeger CM, Barnosky A, et al. Effect of alternate day fasting on weight loss, weight maintenance, and cardioprotection among metabolically healthy, obese adults: a randomized clinical trial. *JAMA Internal Med.* 2017;177(7):E1-E19. PMID: 28459931

Catenacci VA, Pan Z, Ostendorf D, et al. A randomized pilot study comparing zero-calorie alternate-day fasting to daily caloric restriction in adults with obesity. *Obesity (Silver Spring).* 2016; 24(9):1874-1883. PMID: 27569118

11 ANSWER: A) Vitamin B_{12}

Roux-en-Y gastric bypass is associated with thiamin deficiency, B_{12} deficiency, and, less commonly, zinc deficiency that typically causes a rash and diarrhea. Note that laparoscopic banding procedures do not bypass any intestinal segment and therefore do not cause malabsorption. Lap banding is not associated with vitamin or mineral deficiencies. Biliopancreatic diversion (duodenal switch) can cause significant malabsorption and vitamin and mineral deficiencies as late complications due to depleted body stores.

Vitamin B_{12} deficiency (Answer A) can cause neurologic symptoms and signs as found in this patient, as well as megaloblastic anemia, but the body stores a sizeable amount of B_{12} in the liver. Vitamin B_{12} deficiency does not usually occur until 6 to 24 months after bariatric surgery. Sleeve gastrectomy can be associated with B_{12} deficiency, but it is not as common after this procedure as it is with gastric bypass. Vitamin B_{12} is an essential micronutrient that the body cannot produce; it must be ingested. Vitamin B_{12} is found in animal-based foods including dairy, eggs, fish, meat, poultry. Persons following a vegan diet may not get vitamin B_{12} unless they take a supplement or eat a fortified food such as cereal. Vitamin B_{12} deficiency can occur in other gastrointestinal disorders, including pernicious anemia, malabsorption from inflammatory bowel disease, gastrectomy, small-bowel bypass, or bowel resection. Vitamin B_{12} deficiency presents with glossitis, angular stomatitis, and neurologic changes with paresthesias in a stocking and glove distribution, loss of vibratory sense, progressive weakness, ataxia, and ultimately dementia if untreated.

Thiamine deficiency (Answer C) causes neuronal death due to metabolic dysfunction of astrocytes within the central nervous system. The classic triad of this condition is confusion, ataxia, and nystagmus. A wide range of other abnormalities can be seen, including cranial nerve dysfunction, peripheral neuropathies, seizures, and psychosis. Because thiamine is a water-soluble vitamin, body stores can be depleted within days to weeks of inadequate intake. The condition typically presents 4 to 12 weeks after bariatric surgery but can occur as early as 2 weeks. Although most commonly reported following Roux-en-Y gastric bypass, Wernicke encephalopathy can occur after any type of bariatric surgery. The most common antecedent is persistent vomiting, which then severely limits thiamine intake. Other less common precipitating factors are intravenous glucose or parenteral nutrition administration without thiamine supplementation. The condition is important to recognize, as treatment with parenteral thiamine (100 mg daily for 7 to 14 days, or 500 mg 3 times daily for 3 days) must be administered to prevent serious persistent morbidity.

Folate deficiency (Answer B) is uncommon and typically presents as anemia. Zinc deficiency (Answer D) is rare. It is associated with skin and hair findings and is primarily seen as a late complication after biliary pancreatic diversion.

Educational Objective
Differentiate among the vitamin deficiencies that can occur after gastric bypass surgery.

Reference(s)
Aasheim ET. Wernicke encephalopathy after bariatric surgery, a systematic review. *Ann Surg.* 2008;248(5):714-720. PMID: 18948797

Serra A, Sechi G, Singh S, Kumar A. Wernicke encephalopathy after obesity surgery: a systematic review. *Neurology.* 2007;69(6):615. PMID: 17679686

Mechanick JI, Kushner RF, Sugerman HJ, et al; American Association of Clinical Endocrinologists; Obesity Society; American Society for Metabolic & Bariatric Surgery. American Association of Clinical Endocrinologists, The Obesity Society, and American Society for Metabolic & Bariatric Surgery medical guidelines for clinical practice for the perioperative nutritional, metabolic, and nonsurgical support of the bariatric surgery patient [published correction appears in *Obesity (Silver Spring).* 2010;18(3):649]. *Obesity (Silver Spring).* 2009;17(Suppl 1):S1-S70. PMID: 19319140

12 ANSWER: D) DXA scan for bone mineral density

Bariatric surgery alters macronutrient and micronutrient metabolism in complex ways that vary by procedure. Both glucose and lipid metabolism improve with remission of diabetes in a significant number of patients. There is also a decrease in cholesterol levels and, over time, a reduction in cardiovascular disease and mortality that has been shown in long-term observational studies (eg, Swedish BOLD registry). However, patients are at risk for many vitamin deficiencies after bariatric surgery, including vitamin D deficiency (most common), but also deficiencies of vitamin B_{12}, thiamine, folate, and minerals such as zinc. Alterations in metabolism associated with the ensuing weight loss also put patients at risk for gallstones, kidney stones, and osteoporosis. However, routine screening with right upper-quadrant ultrasonography (Answer B), abdominal plain films (Answer C), or 24-hour urine collection for measurement of calcium and creatinine (Answer E) is not recommended for asymptomatic patients. Similarly, screening asymptomatic patients for ischemic heart disease via a cardiac stress test (Answer A) is not recommended.

However, routine assessment of bone mineral density (Answer D) at baseline before bariatric surgery and 2 years after bariatric surgery is recommended because of the high prevalence of vitamin D deficiency with altered calcium metabolism. There is a high risk of bone loss after bariatric surgery with the development of osteoporosis in some patients and a significantly increased risk of fracture after gastric bypass.

Educational Objective

Recommend necessary health care screening for patients who have undergone bariatric surgery.

Reference(s)

Mechanick JI, Kushner RF, Sugerman HJ, et al; American Association of Clinical Endocrinologists; Obesity Society; American Society for Metabolic & Bariatric Surgery. American Association of Clinical Endocrinologists, The Obesity Society, and American Society for Metabolic & Bariatric Surgery medical guidelines for clinical practice for the perioperative nutritional, metabolic, and nonsurgical support of the bariatric surgery patient [published correction appears in *Obesity (Silver Spring)*. 2010;18(3):649]. *Obesity (Silver Spring)*. 2009;17(Suppl 1): S1-S70. PMID: 19319140

13 ANSWER: D) Lorcaserin

Weight loss is associated with improvements in glucose metabolism. It is unclear whether weight-loss medications vary in their impact on glycemic control outside of weight loss.

Both liraglutide, 3 mg daily, (not a choice) and lorcaserin, 10 mg twice daily (Answer D), improve glycemic control and have been shown to reduce progression to type 2 diabetes in patients who are overweight or obese over 3 years of follow-up. In the CAMELLIA-TIMI 61 study (Cardiovascular and Metabolic Effects of Lorcaserin in Overweight and Obese Patients-Thrombolysis in Myocardial Infarction 61) of approximately 12,000 participants in 8 countries, overweight and obese patients with cardiovascular disease or those at very high risk for cardiovascular disease were treated with lorcaserin, 10 mg twice daily, vs placebo with follow-up for a median of 3.3 years. At baseline, 33% had prediabetes and 10% were normoglycemic. Over 3.3 years, progression to type 2 diabetes was reduced 19% in patients with prediabetes at baseline (hazard ratio, 0.81; 95% confidence interval, 0.66-0.96) and reduced 23% among those with normoglycemia at baseline (hazard ratio, 0.77; 95% confidence interval, 0.63-0.94). Furthermore, in patients with diabetes, there was a 0.33% reduction in hemoglobin A_{1c} from a baseline of 7.0% (53 mmol/mol) at 1 year, which persisted at 3 years.

Phentermine (Answer A), phentermine/topiramate (Answer B), and naltrexone-bupropion (Answer C) have not been shown in randomized controlled trials to reduce progression to type 2 diabetes, although weight loss with any of these medications would be associated with improved glucose metabolism.

GLP-1 receptor agonists are now widely used in the treatment of type 2 diabetes to improve glycemic control. While all formulations are delivered by subcutaneous injection, the duration of action varies with twice-daily, once-daily, and now weekly formulations. Only one GLP-1 receptor agonist is currently approved for the treatment of overweight and obesity—liraglutide at a dosage of 3.0 mg daily. It is important to note that liraglutide is also FDA-approved in a formulation with a maximum dosage of 1.8 mg daily for treatment of type 2 diabetes.

The SCALE trial (Efficacy of Liraglutide for Weight Loss Among Patients With Type 2 Diabetes) examined the safety and efficacy of liraglutide, 3 mg daily. There was a 9.2% weight loss in the liraglutide group compared with a 3.5% weight loss in the placebo group by the end of the first year (intention-to-treat analysis: weight loss of 7.4% vs 3.0% from baseline, P <.0001). Participants with prediabetes randomly assigned to liraglutide or placebo were followed for an additional 2 years. For patients with prediabetes who participated in the extension trial for a total of 160 weeks of drug therapy, the liraglutide group lost about 7.1% of their baseline weight compared with 2.7% in the placebo group (P <.0001). At the end of 3 years of treatment, 6% of the placebo group progressed from prediabetes to type 2 diabetes compared with 2% of the liraglutide group, with a hazard ratio of 0.21 (95% confidence interval, 0.13-0.34) for a 79% reduction in risk of developing type 2 diabetes. Additionally, two-thirds of patients who had prediabetes and were taking liraglutide reverted to normoglycemia at 160 weeks compared with about one-third of patients on placebo. Liraglutide, 3.0 mg daily, is delivered by subcutaneous injection and was not offered as an answer choice in this vignette given the patient's preferences.

Educational Objective

Recall secondary effect profiles of weight-loss medications and choose medications accordingly.

Reference(s)

Apovian CM, Aronne LJ, Bessesen DH, et al; Endocrine Society. Pharmacological management of obesity: an Endocrine Society clinical practice guideline. *J Clin Endocrinol Metab.* 2015;100(2): 342-362. PMID: 25590212

Yanovski SZ, Yanovski JA. Long-term drug treatment for obesity: a systematic and clinical review. *JAMA.* 2014;311(1):74-86. PMID: 24231879

Bohula EA, Scirica BM, Inzucchi SE, et al; CAMELLIA-TIMI 61 Steering Committee Investigators. Effect of lorcaserin on prevention and remission of type 2 diabetes in overweight and obese patients (CAMELLIA-TIMI 61): a randomised, placebo-controlled trial. *Lancet.* 2018;392(10161):2269-2279. PMID: 30293771

le Roux CW, Astrup A, Fujioka K, et al; SCALE Obesity Prediabetes NN8022-1839 Study Group. 3 years of liraglutide versus placebo for type 2 diabetes risk reduction and weight management in individuals with prediabetes: a randomized, double-blind trial. *Lancet.* 2017;389(10077): 1399-1409. PMID: 28237263

Pi-Sunyer X, Astrup A, Fujioka K, et al; SCALE Obesity and Prediabetes NN8022-1839 Study Group. A randomized, controlled trial of 3.0 mg of liraglutide in weight management. *N Engl J Med.* 2015;373(1):11-22. PMID: 26132939

14 ANSWER: A) Lifestyle modification to achieve 5% to 10% weight loss

The overall prevalence of nonalcoholic fatty liver disease (NAFLD) and nonalcoholic steatohepatitis (NASH) is estimated to be 24% in North America with a projected global cost of $50 trillion by 2025. NAFLD/NASH are examples of obesity-associated organ damage; detailed in the Edomonton Obesity Staging System (EOSS). Patients with NASH are at increased risk for progression of cirrhosis with increasing fibrosis determined by liver biopsy (fibrosis stage 1 to 4). In 2016, NASH replaced hepatitis C infection as the main cause of liver transplant. NASH, even with fibrosis, is a dynamic condition with opportunities for both progression and remission. However, the natural course of NASH with stage 3 fibrosis is to progress to cirrhosis rather than regress. Currently, there are no FDA-approved medications to treat NAFLD/NASH, although there are many compounds in development. Pioglitazone has been shown to improve liver fibrosis based on liver biopsy and is commonly used in the setting of diabetes and NAFLD/NASH, although it is weight-promoting, which dampens enthusiasm for its long-term use.

The mainstay of therapy is lifestyle modification (Answer A) with changes in diet and increases in physical activity. Exercise independent of weight loss has been shown to result in regression of NASH. Weight loss of 5% to 10% of body weight results in significant regression in NASH as demonstrated by liver biopsy. Weight loss of 5% to 7% of body weight has been associated with regression by at least one stage of fibrosis in 50% of patients depending on BMI. Weight loss of 10% or more results in NASH regression in 97% of patients. No medication has been associated with this degree of NAFLD/NASH regression without weight loss.

A small randomized, placebo-controlled trial of liraglutide, 1.8 mg daily (Answer B) (dosing targeted to improved glycemic control), has been shown to result in NASH regression. Liraglutide, 1.8 mg daily, vs placebo for 48 weeks in patients with biopsy-proven NASH resulted in resolution of steatohepatitis as determined by liver biopsy in 9 of 23 patients (39%) in the liraglutide group vs 2 of 23 patients (9%) in the placebo group (LEAN trial, 2016). Moderate weight loss and improved glycemic control with liraglutide, 1.8 mg daily, resulted in less regression than did weight loss of 5% to 10% through lifestyle modification.

Improved glycemic control is associated with lowered triglycerides and is beneficial for fatty liver, but the effects of NASH regression with fibrosis have not been demonstrated with other diabetes medications. Canagliflozin (Answer C), an SGLT-2 inhibitor that promotes glucosuria, is associated with mild weight loss, improved glycemic control, and improved circulating markers of liver function, including ALT, AST, and γ-glutamyl transferase, but it has not been shown to lead to regression of NASH as determined by liver biopsy. Current research is focusing on SGLT inhibition to treat NAFLD and NASH, and it may become an important treatment modality for NAFLD/NASH in the future.

Metformin (Answer D) improves glycemic control and was shown to decrease progression from prediabetes to type 2 diabetes in the Diabetes Prevention Trial in conjunction with weight loss, but metformin alone has not been associated with improvement of NASH.

Educational Objective

Recommend an approach to weight management for obesity complicated by nonalcoholic liver disease and nonalcoholic steatohepatitis.

Reference(s)

Younossi Z, Tacke F, Arrese M, et al. Global perspectives on non-alcoholic fatty liver disease and non-alcoholic steatohepatitis. *Hepatology.* 2019;69(6):2672-2682. PMID: 30179269

Wong VW, Chan RS, Wong GL, et al. Community-based lifestyle modification programme for non-alcoholic fatty liver disease: a randomized controlled trial. *J Hepatol.* 2013;59(3):536-542. PMID: 23623998

Cusi K. Pioglitazone for the treatment of NASH in patients with prediabetes or type 2 diabetes mellitus. *Gut.* 2018;67(7):1371. PMID: 28408383

Boettcher E, Csako G, Pucino F, Wesley R, Loomba R. Meta-analysis: pioglitazone improves liver histology and fibrosis in patients with non-alcoholic steatohepatitis. *Aliment Pharmacol Ther.* 2012;35(1):66-75. PMID: 22050199

Armstrong MJ, Gaunt P, Aithal GP, et al. Liraglutide safety and efficacy in patients with non-alcoholic steatohepatitis (LEAN): a multicentre, double-blind, randomized, placebo-controlled trial phase 2 study. *Lancet.* 2016;387(10019):679-690. PMID: 26608256

Inoue M, Hayashi A, Taguchi T, et al. Effects of canagliflozin on body composition and hepatic fat content in type 2 diabetes patients with non-alcoholic fatty liver disease. *J Diabetes Investig.* 2019;10(4):1004-1011. PMID: 30461221

Leiter LA, Forst T, Polidori D, Balis DA, Xie J, Sha S. Effect of canagliflozin on liver function tests in patients with type 2 diabetes. *Diabetes Metab.* 2016;42(1):25-32. PMID: 26575250

Li B, Wang Y, Ye Z, et al. Effects of canagliflozin on fatty liver indexes in patients with type 2 diabetes: a meta-analysis of randomized controlled trials. *J Pharm Pharm Sci.* 2018;21(1):222-235. PMID: 29935547

15 ANSWER: B) Travoprost ophthalmic solution

Topiramate is a medication that is FDA-approved for the reduction of migraine headaches and seizures. Although a number of studies have been conducted in which it was used specifically for weight loss, it is not FDA-approved for weight loss, but it is commonly used off-label for this purpose. There is strong evidence that it produces a 6% to 8% weight loss that is sustained at 1 year. Topiramate is FDA-approved for weight loss in combination with phentermine (Qysmia) (phentermine/topiramate, 15/92 mg extended release formulation), which was approved in 2015. Topiramate is contraindicated in pregnancy due to the risk of birth defects, including cleft lip and cleft palate. It is also contraindicated in patients with glaucoma (Answer B) or hyperthyroidism or in patients who have used monoamine oxidase inhibitors antidepressants within the last 2 weeks.

Common adverse effects include paresthesias in the fingers and toes, dysgeusia (altered taste including metallic taste, particularly when drinking carbonated drinks), difficulty concentrating ("brain fog"), mood disturbances (depressed mood in some, rarely suicidal thoughts), trouble sleeping, and constipation. Topiramate shifts the acid-base status to become more acidic, resulting in a metabolic acidosis in some. Due to the shift toward acidemia, topiramate increases the risk of kidney stones and possibly osteoporosis through increased bone turnover. For this reason, topiramate should not be used in patients with kidney stones. Topiramate is contraindicated in patients with glaucoma (Answer B) due to acid-base shifts as well. There is a small risk of lactic acidosis with topiramate, so it should be used with caution with metformin, which is also associated with a small risk of lactic acidosis. However, prediabetes and metformin use (Answer D) are not contraindications to combination therapy with topiramate.

Topiramate is used to treat migraines and could be a preferable choice in someone who also suffers for chronic headaches. Metoprolol (Answer A) is not a contraindication for topiramate use. Fatty liver disease (mild liver disease) and pioglitazone (Answer C) are not contraindications for use of topiramate.

Educational Objective

List potential adverse effects of weight-loss medications and select medications appropriately in the context of other medical conditions.

Reference(s)

Apovian CM, Aronne LJ, Bessesen DH, et al; Endocrine Society. Pharmacological management of obesity: an Endocrine Society clinical practice guideline. *J Clin Endocrinol Metab*. 2015;100(2): 342-362. PMID: 25590212

Yanovski SZ, Yanovski JA. Long-term drug treatment for obesity: a systematic and clinical review. *JAMA*. 2014;311(1):74-86. PMID: 24231879

Rosenstock J, Hollander P, Gadde KM, Sun X, Strauss R, Leung A; OBD-202 Study Group. A randomized, double-blind, placebo-controlled, multicenter study to assess the efficacy and safety of topiramate controlled release in the treatment of obese type 2 diabetic patients. *Diabetes Care*. 2007;30(6):1480-1486. PMID: 17363756

Eliasson B, Gudbjörnsdottir S, Cederholm J, Liang Y, Vercruysse F, Smith U. Weight loss and metabolic effects of topiramate in overweight and obese type 2 diabetic patients: randomized double-blind placebo-controlled trial. *Int J Obes (London)*. 2007;31(7):1140-1147. PMID: 17264849

16 ANSWER: B) Hypothyroidism

When caring for a patient with hyperlipidemia, the clinician must consider and rule out secondary causes. This patient had relatively normal lipid levels 1 year ago and now has elevations of total and LDL cholesterol without much change in triglycerides or HDL cholesterol. The change over the last year suggests that the lipid abnormalities are not entirely genetic but due to something that has changed during this period. The changes described are typical of those seen with hypothyroidism (Answer B). LDL-cholesterol and total cholesterol levels increase as hypothyroidism worsens and are increased by 30% in frank hypothyroidism. Both subclinical hypothyroidism and overt hypothyroidism are associated with increased risk for cardiovascular disease.

Sleep apnea (Answer A) per se does not alter lipid levels unless it is a manifestation of another condition such as insulin resistance and type 2 diabetes. Weight gain (Answer C) and undiagnosed diabetes (Answer D) would typically be expected to increase triglyceride levels significantly and reduce HDL-cholesterol levels without much change in LDL cholesterol. This is not the case in this vignette.

Educational Objective

Identify hypothyroidism as a secondary cause of lipid abnormalities.

Reference(s)

Pearce EN. Update in lipid alterations in subclinical hypothyroidism. *J Clin Endocrinol Metab*. 2012; 97(2):326-333. PMID: 22205712

Duntas LH, Wartofsky L. Cardiovascular risk and subclinical hypothyroidism: focus on lipids and new emerging risk factors. What is the evidence? *Thyroid*. 2007;17(11):1075-1084. PMID: 17900236

Pearce EN. Hypothyroidism and dyslipidemia: modern concepts and approaches. *Curr Cardiol Rep*. 2004;6(6):451-456. PMID: 15485607

17 ANSWER: E) Sitosterolemia

The classic cause of tendon xanthomas is familial hypercholesterolemia (Answer D). In this condition, the xanthomas are due to the accumulation of cholesterol resulting from the high circulating levels of LDL cholesterol. Although the molecular defect is different, the pathophysiology of familial defective apolipoprotein B (Answer C) is the same—LDL-cholesterol levels are very high due to a defect in removal as the LDL receptor recognizes the LDL particle via apolipoprotein B. Tendinous xanthomas are seen in this condition as well. Familial defective apolipoprotein B occurs in about 1 in 1000, while the heterozygous form of familial hypercholesterolemia occurs in about 2 in 1000. The frequency of the heterozygous form of familial hypercholesterolemia and familial defective apolipoprotein B varies with ethnicity and geography. LDL-cholesterol levels are high in both conditions, but the levels overlap, making it difficult to phenotypically distinguish the 2 conditions.

However, the surprising feature of the patient in this vignette is the presence of tendon xanthomas with normal LDL-cholesterol levels. The degree of LDL-cholesterol elevation distinguishes familial hypercholesterolemia and heterozygous forms of familial hypercholesterolemia (in which there are moderate to marked elevations) from cerebrotendinous xanthomatosis (Answer A) and sitosterolemia (Answer E) (in which LDL-cholesterol levels are normal to modestly increased). Tendon xanthomas occur in patients with cerebrotendinous xanthomatosis because of the deposition of a steroid metabolite, cholestanol not cholesterol. Clinical signs and symptoms of cerebrotendinous xanthomatosis include adult-onset progressive neurologic dysfunction (ie, ataxia, dystonia, dementia, epilepsy, psychiatric disorders, peripheral neuropathy, and myopathy) and premature nonneurologic manifestations, including tendon xanthomas, childhood-onset cataracts, diarrhea, premature atherosclerosis, osteoporosis, and respiratory insufficiency. The described patient has none of these findings. Tendon xanthomas are also found in patients with sitosterolemia. Sitosterolemia has been associated with mutations in *ABCG8* and *ABCG5* that regulate sterol transport at the apical surface of hepatocytes and enterocytes. These transporters are necessary for the movement of sterols across membranes in the intestine and liver. This condition is associated with an increased risk of cardiovascular disease, but it responds well to dietary restriction of cholesterol and phytosterols. The clinical manifestations include xanthomas, premature atherosclerosis, hemolytic anemia, and macrothrombocytopenia due to abnormal membrane lipids. Neurologic signs and symptoms are not part of this condition. Ezetimibe may be useful in lowering serum levels of plant sterols. Familial combined hyperlipidemia (Answer B) is not associated with tendon xanthomas. The described patient is most likely to have sitosterolemia (Answer E).

Educational Objective
Differentiate among the primary lipid disorders that are associated with tendinous xanthomas.

Reference(s)
Escolà-Gil JC, Quesada H, Julve J, Martín-Campos JM, Cedó L, Blanco-Vaca F. Sitosterolemia: diagnosis, investigation, and management. *Curr Atheroscler Rep.* 2014;16(7):424. PMID: 24821603

Nie S, Chen G, Cao X, Zhang Y. Cerebrotendinous xanthomatosis: a comprehensive review of pathogenesis, clinical manifestations, diagnosis, and management. *Orphanet J Rare Dis.* 2014; 9(1):179. PMID: 25424010

Tsouli SG, Kiortsis DN, Argyropoulou MI, Mikhailidis DP, Elisaf MS. Pathogenesis, detection and treatment of Achilles tendon xanthomas. *Eur J Clin Invest.* 2005;35(4): 236-244. PMID: 15816992

18 ANSWER: A) Start rosuvastatin, 10 mg daily
As many as 5% to 10% of patients who are prescribed statin therapy report experiencing myalgias. This is a much greater prevalence than statin-induced myopathy, which the FDA defines as a creatine phosphokinase level greater than 10 times the upper normal limit, or rhabdomyolysis, defined as a creatine phosphokinase level greater than 10,000 U/L (>167 µkat/L). Rhabdomyolysis is an emergent condition that warrants the immediate cessation of statin therapy to prevent renal failure. However, this condition occurs in only 3 per 100,000 person-years.

Deciding what to do when patients have muscle pain, weakness, or cramps when taking a statin is a difficult clinical problem. A number of options are available and no clear clinical trial data define the best approach. Statins are currently the single best class of medications for cardiovascular disease prevention. As a result, the first goal is to try to keep a patient such as this one on the highest tolerated statin dosage possible. The best first approach is to prescribe a lower dosage of a statin that the patient has not tried before. For the described patient, that would be rosuvastatin, 10 mg daily (Answer A).

While it might be reasonable to rechallenge him with the previous dosage of atorvastatin (Answer D), this carries more risk of problems than trying a lower dose of a new statin. Another option that can be tried is alternate day or weekly statin use. However, no clinical trials show cardiovascular event reduction using this approach. While fenofibrate (Answer B), niacin (not a choice), and ezetimibe (Answer C) all can produce favorable effects on serum lipid levels, none of these has been shown to produce reductions in cardiovascular endpoints when used as a single agent, so prescribing any one of them would not be the next step until various approaches to prescribing statins have failed.

Both current PCSK9 inhibitors, evolocumab and alirocumab (Answer E), are approved by the US FDA for use in patients with clinical atherosclerotic cardiovascular disease and heterozygous familial hyperlipidemia, which this patient does not have. PCSK9 inhibitors have been studied in statin-intolerant patients with LDL-cholesterol levels in this patient's range (GAUSS-1 and GAUSS-2 studies), but statin intolerance alone is not currently an approved indication in the United States in the absence of clinical atherosclerotic cardiovascular disease or familial hyperlipidemia. However, once his highest dose of a tolerated statin is established, a PCSK9 inhibitor (evolocumab or alirocumab) can be added for greater LDL-cholesterol reduction and cardiovascular disease risk reduction.

Educational Objective
Recommend options for managing statin-associated muscle pain.

Reference(s)
Joy TR, Hegele RA. Narrative review: statin-related myopathy. *Ann Intern Med.* 2009;150(12):858-868. PMID: 19528564

Cornier MA, Eckel RH. Non-traditional dosing of statins in statin-intolerant patients-is it worth a try? *Curr Atheroscler Rep.* 2015;17(2):475. PMID: 25432858

Ahmad Z. Statin intolerance. *Am J Cardiol.* 2014; 113(10):1765-1771. PMID: 24792743

Stroes E, Colquhoun D, Sullivan D, et al; GAUSS-2 Investigators. Anti-PCSK9 antibody effectively lowers cholesterol in patients with statin intolerance: the GAUSS-2 randomized, placebo-controlled phase 3 clinical trial of evolocumab. *J Am Coll Cardiol.* 2014;63(23):2541-2548. PMID: 24694531

Sullivan D, Olsson AG, Scott R, et al. Effect of a monoclonal antibody to PCSK9 on low-density lipoprotein cholesterol levels in statin-intolerant patients: the GAUSS randomized trial. *JAMA.* 2012;308(23):2497-2506. PMID: 23128163

19 ANSWER: C) Liraglutide
Cardiovascular disease remains the primary cause of death for persons with diabetes mellitus, and aggressive approaches to prevent disease are warranted. Statins have been unequivocally shown to reduce coronary heart disease risk in patients with diabetes in randomized controlled trials and in post hoc analyses of such trials. The most common lipid abnormalities seen in patients with diabetes are increased triglyceride and reduced HDL-cholesterol levels, even after optimizing LDL-cholesterol reduction. Historically, lowering serum triglycerides has not been a focus of lipid-lowering therapy to reduce cardiovascular events. However, there is emerging evidence that triglyceride-rich lipoproteins are also atherogenic and contribute significantly to the "residual cardiovascular disease risk" observed in patients with diabetes. A number of ongoing studies address this important question, and new insights may emerge over time, but the currently available data suggest that the single best approach to cardiovascular risk reduction in patients with diabetes is reduction of LDL-cholesterol levels with a statin, which was the position of the 2013 American Heart Association/American College of Cardiology cholesterol-lowering guidelines. However, the 2018 American Heart Association/American College of Cardiology cholesterol management guidelines and the American Diabetes Association 2019 diabetes standards of care statement have both recognized the issue of addressing elevated triglycerides that remain elevated above target (>175 mg/dL [>1.98 mmol/L]). The 2018 American Heart Association guidelines recommend intensified lifestyle modification if triglycerides are greater than 150 mg/dL (>1.70 mmol/L) and consideration of additional lipid-lowering therapy if triglycerides are persistently greater than 175 mg/dL (>1.98 mmol/L). The 2019 American Diabetes Association guidelines target triglycerides less than 175 mg/dL (<1.98 mmol/L) as well and also recommend additional therapy for patients with triglyceride concentrations between 175 and 499 mg/dL (1.98-5.64 mmol/L) with weight loss, glycemic control, evaluation of secondary causes of high triglycerides, including hypothyroidism, liver disease, nephrotic syndrome, and medications. The addition of liraglutide, 1.8 mg daily subcutaneous injection (Answer C), would most likely improve this patient's glycemic control, assist with weight-loss efforts, and lower his triglyceride levels and is the best next step.

To date, randomized controlled trials have not demonstrated any cardiovascular benefit of triglyceride-lowering with fibrates (Answers A and B) or over-the-counter omega-3 fatty acids (Answer E) in patients with diabetes. A new purified omega-3 fatty acid preparation—icosapent ethyl—was shown to reduce the risk of major cardiovascular events in patients with well-controlled LDL cholesterol but triglyceride concentrations of 135 mg/dL or greater (≥1.53 mmol/L) with either established cardiovascular disease or diabetes and other cardiovascular disease risk factors.

However, the benefit was independent of the triglyceride level achieved, thus raising questions about the underlying mechanism leading to cardiovascular disease risk reduction. Icosapent ethyl requires a prescription and was not offered as a choice in this vignette.

Treatment of individuals with diabetes with a fibrate failed to show a reduction in primary cardiovascular endpoints in the Bezafibrate Infarction Prevention (BIP) trial and more recently in the Action to Control Cardiovascular Risk in Diabetes (ACCORD) trial. The ACCORD trial specifically assessed whether adding a fibrate to a statin conferred any additional cardiovascular benefits. The results were negative. These studies have been criticized for not selecting individuals with elevated triglycerides at baseline, and post hoc analyses suggest a benefit among those with high baseline triglyceride levels. The Fenofibrate Intervention and Event Lowering in Diabetes (FIELD) study enrolled nearly 10,000 patients with type 2 diabetes, of which about 3650 were women. This study also failed to demonstrate that fenofibrate reduced cardiovascular events.

Gemfibrozil (Answer A) should not be added to a statin due to the increased risk of myalgias, myositis, and rhabdomyolysis due to decreased statin clearance by the liver. Fenofibrate lowers triglycerides effectively and is the preferred agent in combination with a statin if one is to be used.

The AIM-HIGH study included a large number of patients with diabetes and examined the effectiveness of adding niacin (Answer D) to aggressive statin therapy. Despite the fact that niacin reduced triglyceride levels and increased HDL-cholesterol levels, the trial was stopped early because of a failure of niacin treatment to reduce cardiovascular endpoints and an unexpected increase in stroke rates.

Educational Objective

Recommend a treatment approach for moderate hypertriglyceridemia in patients with type 2 diabetes mellitus.

Reference(s)

Grundy SM, Stone NJ, Bailey AL, et al. 2018 AHA/ACC/AACVPR/AAPA/ABC/ACPM/ADA/AGS/APhA/ASPC/NLA/PCNA guideline on the management of blood cholesterol. *Circulation.* 2019;139(25):e1082-e1143. PMID: 30586774

Grundy SM, Stone NJ, Bailey AL, et al. 2018 AHA/ACC/AACVPR/AAPA/ABC/ACPM/ADA/AGS/APhA/ASPC/NLA/PCNA guideline on the management of blood cholesterol: executive summary. *Circulation.* 2019;139(25):e1046-e1081. PMID: 30565953

Bhatt DL, Steg PG, Miller M, et al; REDUCE-IT Investigators. Cardiovascular risk reduction with icosapent ethyl for hypertriglyceridemia. *N Engl J Med.* 2019;380(1):1-22. PMID: 30415628

Stone NJ, Robinson JG, Lichtenstein AH, et al; American College of Cardiology/American Heart Association Task Force on Practice Guidelines. 2013 ACC/AHA guideline on the treatment of blood cholesterol to reduce atherosclerotic cardiovascular risk in adults: a report of the American College of Cardiology/American Heart Association Task Force on Practice Guidelines [published correction appears in *Circulation.* 2014;129(25 Suppl 2): S46-S48]. *Circulation.* 2014;129(25 Suppl 2): S1-S45. PMID: 24222016

Cholesterol Treatment Trialists' (CTT) Collaboration, Baigent C, Blackwell L, et al. Efficacy and safety of more intensive lowering of LDL cholesterol: a meta-analysis of data from 170,000 participants in 26 randomised trials. *Lancet.* 2010;376(9753):1670-1681. PMID: 21067804

ACCORD Study Group, Ginsberg HN, Elam MB, et al. Effects of combination lipid therapy in type 2 diabetes mellitus [published correction appears in *N Engl J Med.* 2010;362(18):1748]. *N Engl J Med.* 2010;362(17):1563-1574. PMID: 20228404

Jun M, Foote C, Lv J, et al. Effects of fibrates on cardiovascular outcomes: a systematic review and meta-analysis. *Lancet.* 2010;375(9729):1875-1884. PMID: 20462635

Nordestgaard BG, Varbo A. Triglycerides and cardiovascular disease. *Lancet.* 2014;384(9943): 626-635. PMID: 25131982

20 ANSWER: B) Achilles tendon xanthomas

Familial hypercholesterolemia is relatively common with a prevalence of 1 in 250-500 persons depending on geographic region and ethnicity. Patients with familial hypercholesterolemia commonly have a pathogenic variant in the gene encoding the LDL receptor. Defective apolipoprotein B, the ligand for the receptor, and a defect in an intracellular adaptor protein cause a similar phenotype. Persons who are heterozygous have total cholesterol levels of 300 to 600 mg/dL (7.77-15.54 mmol/L), LDL-cholesterol levels greater than 200 mg/dL (>5.18 mmol/L), and early coronary artery disease. The homozygous form of familial hypercholesterolemia is associated with even high levels, which leads to atherosclerosis before age 20 to 30 years (sometimes in childhood). Liver transplant is often the treatment. Genetic testing does not alter therapy and is not usually performed unless other first-degree relatives have been diagnosed. Patients are diagnosed based on their clinical phenotype with pathognomonic physical findings and a characteristic lipid profile. Patients with familial hypercholesterolemia develop cholesterol deposits in the soft tissues, specifically tendon sheaths leading to thickened tendons over the knuckles of the hands and particularly thickened Achilles tendons (Answer B). It is not clear why lipid accumulates in the tendons, but it is thought to be secondary to recurrent inflammation and macrophage recruitment to where the tendon interacts with its overlying sheath. Cholesterol also deposits in the cornea around the iris, giving a blue-grey ringlike appearance (arcus cornealis) at an early age. This appearance can also occur with aging, so it becomes less specific in older patients (arcus senilis). High-dosage statin treatment is first-line therapy. Documenting the physical manifestations of familial hyperlipidemia will become increasingly important when considering adding a PCSK9 inhibitor, as some insurance groups are following the Dutch Lipid Criteria. These criteria use family history, including high cholesterol (>95th percentile in the patient's children), physical signs such as tendinous xanthoma and early-onset arcus cornealis, and genetic analysis (pathogenic variants in the *LDLR*, *APOB*, or *PCSK9* genes) if available.

Lipemia retinalis (Answer A) is the milky appearance of the retina and retinal vessels that accompanies severe hypertriglyceridemia, which this patient does not have. Eruptive xanthomas (Answer C) are acnelike papules on extensor surfaces of the arms and on the back and buttocks that present in the setting of severe hypertriglyceridemia. Palmar xanthomas (Answer D) are lipid depositions in the creases of the palms that occur with dysbetalipoproteinemia (formerly called type 3 hyperlipoproteinemia). Orange tonsils (Answer E) are the hallmark of Tangier disease, which is characterized by extremely low HDL-cholesterol levels, not high LDL-cholesterol levels, as in this patient with familial hyperlipidemia.

Educational Objective

Identify typical physical findings of familial hyperlipidemia to aid in diagnosis.

Reference(s)

Semenkovich CF, Goldberg AC, Goldberg IJ. Disorders of lipid metabolism. In: Melmed S, Polonsky KS, Larsen PR, Kronenberg HM, eds. *Williams Textbook of Endocrinology*. 12th ed. Philadelphia, PA: Elsevier Saunders; 2011:1633-1674.

21 ANSWER: D) Recommend statin therapy because he has had type 2 diabetes for more than 10 years and he has nephropathy

The 2018 American Heart Association guidelines on the treatment of cholesterol to reduce cardiovascular risk in adults represent a major change from the previous National Cholesterol Education Program Adult Treatment Panel III guidelines. These guidelines focused on evidence-based recommendations regarding which patients would benefit from statin treatment. The guidelines identify specific "statin benefit groups" on the basis of data available from large clinical intervention trials. Diabetes has long been considered a cardiovascular disease equivalent; the number one cause of death in persons with diabetes is cardiovascular disease, so aggressive preventive efforts seem warranted. However, the authors of the guidelines did not find enough evidence in clinical trials to definitively show that statin therapy is helpful in patients with diabetes who are younger than 40 years. The updated 2018 guidelines address the use of statins in patients younger than 40 years with diabetes who have a high lifetime risk of cardiovascular disease (approximately 50% for this patient). The 2018 guidelines note that patients younger than 40 with diabetes and added risk factors such as long duration of type 2 diabetes (>10 years) and complications such as nephropathy with albuminuria or chronic kidney disease stage 3 or higher should be on a moderate- or high-intensity statin (thus, Answer D is correct and Answer A is incorrect).

The 2018 American Heart Association/American College of Cardiology cholesterol management guidelines further risk stratify patients by their 10-year risk of having a cardiovascular event when considering statin therapy for primary prevention of cardiovascular disease into 4 groups. Ten-year cardiovascular disease risk is:

- Low if <5%
- Borderline if 5% to <7.5%
- Intermediate if 7.5% to <20%
- High if ≥20%

The specific wording in the guideline is that moderate-intensity statins are recommended for primary prevention in persons with diabetes aged 40 to 75 years who have an LDL-cholesterol level of 70 to 189 mg/dL (1.81-4.90 mmol/L). This patient has long-term type 2 diabetes complicated by albuminuria (a cardiovascular disease "risk enhancer"), so his 10-year risk less than 7.5% does not mean that a statin is not recommended for him. If this patient also has a 10-year atherosclerotic cardiovascular disease risk of 20% or greater, then high-intensity statin therapy should be considered (thus, Answer B is incorrect). The guidelines do not use lifetime risk to inform statin prescribing (thus, Answer C is incorrect).

Educational Objective
Determine which patients with diabetes mellitus would benefit from statin therapy according to the current 2018 American Heart Association guidelines for cholesterol management.

Reference(s)

Stone NJ, Robinson JG, Lichtenstein AH, et al; American College of Cardiology/American Heart Association Task Force on Practice Guidelines. 2013 ACC/AHA guideline on the treatment of blood cholesterol to reduce atherosclerotic cardiovascular risk in adults: a report of the American College of Cardiology/American Heart Association Task Force on Practice Guidelines [published correction appears in *Circulation*. 2014;129(25 Suppl 2): S46-S48]. *Circulation*. 2014;129(25 Suppl 2): S1-S45. PMID: 24222016

Stone NJ, Robinson JG, Lichtenstein AH, et al; 2013 ACC/AHA Cholesterol Guideline Panel. Treatment of blood cholesterol to reduce atherosclerotic cardiovascular disease risk in adults: synopsis of the 2013 American College of Cardiology/American Heart Association cholesterol guideline. *Ann Intern Med*. 2014; 160(5):339-343. PMID: 24474185

Grundy SM, Stone NJ, Bailey AL, et al. 2018 AHA/ACC/AACVPR/AAPA/ABC/ACPM/ADA/AGS/APhA/ASPC/NLA/PCNA Guideline on the Management of Blood Cholesterol. *Circulation*. 2018:CIR0000000000000625. PMID: 30586774

Grundy SM, Stone NJ, Bailey AL, et al. 2018 AHA/ACC/AACVPR/AAPA/ABC/ACPM/ADA/AGS/APhA/ASPC/NLA/PCNA Guideline on the Management of Blood Cholesterol: Executive Summary. *Circulation*. 2018: CIR0000000000000624. PMID: 30565953

22 ANSWER: D) Lipoprotein lipase deficiency

This patient has homozygous lipoprotein lipase deficiency (Answer D) and has a classic presentation with feeding difficulty beginning in childhood. Patients with lipoprotein lipase deficiency cannot breakdown triglycerides and have levels generally greater than 1000 mg/dL (>11.30 mmol/L). Triglyceride levels in this range are associated with abnormal lipid deposits in the skin (eruptive xanthomas as seen in the picture), and high circulating levels give a white-yellow "milky" appearance to the blood vessels in the retina.

This episode of severe hypertriglyceridemia and pancreatitis was probably precipitated by alcohol ingestion. Alcohol can severely elevate triglyceride levels in persons who have an underlying disorder in lipid metabolism. Alcohol has several effects on liver triglyceride metabolism, including reducing fatty acid oxidation and increasing de novo triglyceride production. Other factors that can significantly elevate triglycerides in genetically predisposed individuals include type 2 diabetes, use of estrogen-containing medications, and pregnancy.

This genetic disorder is especially common in French Canada because of a founder effect; the defect is thought to occur in 1 in 40 persons of French Canadian descent (compared with 1 in 1 million in the general population). Heterozygous forms of this enzyme deficiency are sometimes associated with hyperchylomicronemia and pancreatitis when superimposed on a second triglyceride-elevating stress, such as diabetes, pregnancy, or alcohol ingestion. Several other very rare causes of lipoprotein lipase inactivity have been discovered recently, and they lead to a similar hyperchylomicronemia phenotype.

Adipose triglyceride lipase is an intracellular enzyme that does not modulate plasma triglyceride levels (thus, Answer B is incorrect). This enzyme is required to release stored triglyceride from adipose and muscles. Hepatic lipase mediates removal of triglyceride from remnant lipoproteins and modulates HDL-cholesterol levels. Patients with hepatic lipase deficiency (Answer C) present with increased triglyceride and cholesterol levels without HDL-cholesterol reductions, but are not at risk of pancreatitis. Apolipoprotein B is a protein associated with increased LDL cholesterol and increased cardiovascular risk but not elevated triglycerides and pancreatitis (thus, Answer A is incorrect).

Pancreatic lipase is an enzyme secreted by the pancreas into the pancreatic ducts draining into the small intestine where it breaks down lipids emulsified by bile salts into fatty acids and glycerol for absorption into the circulation through the gut. Lipase is also secreted by oral and gastric mucosa. Lack of pancreatic lipase, sometimes from pancreatic insufficiency in patients with damage from chronic pancreatitis or in those with cystic fibrosis, leads to excessive amounts of fat in the stool and steatorrhea. Pancreatic lipase deficiency (Answer E) does not lead to elevated triglycerides or cause pancreatitis.

Educational Objective
Recognize primary and secondary causes of severe hypertriglyceridemia.

Reference(s)
Berglund L, Brunzell JD, Goldberg AC, et al; Endocrine Society. Evaluation and treatment of hypertriglyceridemia: an Endocrine Society clinical practice guideline. *J Clin Endocrinol Metab*. 2012;97(9):2969-2989. PMID: 22962670

Johansen CT, Kathiresan S, Hegele RA. Genetic determinants of plasma triglycerides. *J Lipid Res*. 2011;52(2):189-206. PMID: 21041806

Johansen CT, Wang J, McIntyre AD, et al. Excess of rare variants in non-genome-wide association study candidate genes in patients with hypertriglyceridemia. *Circ Cardiovasc Genet*. 2012;5(1):66-72. PMID: 22135386

23 ANSWER: A) Ezetimibe

This patient's clinical picture is consistent with familial hypercholesterolemia, which is associated with very high risk of cardiovascular disease. Fenofibrate (Answer B) and niacin (Answer D) have not been shown to reduce cardiovascular event rates when added to statin therapy. However, data from the IMPROVE-IT trial recently demonstrated that ezetimibe (Answer A) added to a regimen of simvastatin, 40 mg daily, resulted in a modest but significant 6.4% reduction in a composite cardiovascular endpoint.

Evolocumab (Answer C) is a monoclonal antibody that targets and degrades the protein PCSK9 that was approved by the US FDA in 2015. PCSK9 circulates in the blood and alters the liver's handling of LDL cholesterol by stimulating degradation of LDL receptors, which allows less LDL to be cleared from the circulation. Inhibition of PCSK9 with evolocumab lowers circulating LDL by 50% to 60% and significantly lowers the risk of cardiovascular disease. It is specifically approved for use in addition to diet and maximally tolerated statin therapy in adult patients with heterozygous or homozygous familial hypercholesterolemia. The other US FDA–approved medication in this class is alirocumab. Although a PCSK9 inhibitor will lower LDL cholesterol more than ezetimibe, the recently updated 2018 American Heart Association/American College of Cardiology cholesterol management guidelines state that ezetimibe should be added before a PCSK9 inhibitor. This recommendation is due in part to a cost-effectiveness analysis that showed that PSCK9 inhibitors cost approximately $150,000 per QUALY (quality-adjusted life year—the general threshold for value is ≤~$50,000 per QUALY). The best next step would be to add ezetimibe, although this patient will most likely benefit from the subsequent addition of a PCSK9 inhibitor. An additional treatment option for patients with familial hypercholesterolemia is lipopheresis, although this is not widely available.

Educational Objective
Explain current recommendations for the addition of lipid-lowering pharmacologic agents to statin therapy

for LDL-cholesterol lowering and cardiovascular risk reduction.

Reference(s)

Cannon CP, Blazing MA, Giugliano RP, et al; IMPROVE-IT Investigators. Ezetimibe added to statin therapy after acute coronary syndromes. *N Engl J Med.* 2015;372(25):2387-2397. PMID: 26039521

Sabatine MS, Giugliano RP, Wiviott SD, et al; Open-Label Study of Long-Term Evaluation against LDL Cholesterol (OSLER) Investigators. Efficacy and safety of evolocumab in reducing lipids and cardiovascular events. *N Engl J Med.* 2015;372(16):1500-1509. PMID: 25773607

Ajufo E, Rader DJ. Recent advances in the pharmacological management of hypercholesterolemia. *Lancet Diabetes Endocrinol.* 2016;4(5):436-446. PMID: 27012540

Grundy SM, Stone NJ, Bailey AL, et al. 2018 AHA/ ACC/AACVPR/AAPA/ABC/ACPM/ADA/ AGS/APhA/ASPC/NLA/PCNA guideline on the management of blood cholesterol. *Circulation.* 2019;139(25):e1082-e1143. PMID: 30586774

Grundy SM, Stone NJ, Bailey AL, et al. 2018 AHA/ ACC/AACVPR/AAPA/ABC/ACPM/ADA/ AGS/APhA/ASPC/NLA/PCNA guideline on the management of blood cholesterol: executive summary. *Circulation.* 2019;139(25):e1046-e1081. PMID: 30565953

24 ANSWER: B) Cholesteryl ester transfer protein deficiency

The patient's presentation is classic for cholesterol ester transfer protein (CETP) deficiency (Answer B). CETP catalyzes the exchange of triglyceride and cholesterol ester between triglyceride-rich lipoprotein particles and HDL particles. In normal individuals, the result is a net transfer of triglyceride to HDL, which leads to increased catabolism and reduced HDL-cholesterol levels. Persons with CETP deficiency have very high levels of HDL cholesterol. This condition is more common in individuals of Asian ancestry. Given this underlying physiology, pharmaceutical companies have developed CETP inhibitors. However, these medications to date have not been shown to reduce cardiovascular disease risk despite raising HDL-cholesterol levels significantly.

Alcohol use (Answer A) can raise HDL-cholesterol levels mildly, but typically not to this degree, and alcohol use is often associated with increases in triglycerides. Several medical conditions, including multiple myeloma and other paraproteinemias, can result in problems with the laboratory measurement of HDL cholesterol (Answer C), but in these cases, HDL cholesterol is low, not high. Apolipoprotein A1 is a major protein component and its deficiency (Answer D) can lead to low HDL cholesterol. Lipoprotein lipase deficiency (Answer E) is associated with low, not high, HDL-cholesterol levels and very high triglycerides.

Educational Objective

Differentiate among the causes of high HDL cholesterol and describe the clinical features of cholesterol ester transfer protein deficiency.

Reference(s)

de Grooth GJ, Klerkx AH, Stroes ES, Stalenhoef AF, Kastelein JJ, Kuivenhoven JA. A review of CETP and its relation to atherosclerosis. *J Lipid Res.* 2004;45(11):1967-1974. PMID: 15342674

Niesor EJ. Different effects of compounds decreasing cholesteryl ester transfer protein activity on lipoprotein metabolism. *Curr Opin Lipidol.* 2011;22(4):288-295. PMID: 21587074

Pownall HJ. Alcohol: lipid metabolism and cardioprotection. *Curr Atheroscler Rep.* 2002; 4(2):107-112. PMID: 11822973

Rader DJ, Hovingh GK. HDL and cardiovascular disease. *Lancet.* 2014;384(9943):618-625. PMID: 25131981

25 ANSWER: C) Stop gemfibrozil

Serum total cholesterol, HDL-cholesterol, LDL-cholesterol, and triglyceride levels increase during pregnancy (in normal women, the increases are by 75%, 40%, 70%, and 300%, respectively). The mean values for total cholesterol and triglycerides during pregnancy are 317 mg/dL (8.21 mmol/L) and 300 mg/dL (3.39 mmol/L), respectively. After delivery, lipids slowly return to prepregnancy levels. In women with underlying disorders of triglyceride metabolism, levels may rise during pregnancy to a degree that puts the mother at risk for pancreatitis, which could have serious implications for both the mother and the fetus. In addition, the development of gestational diabetes could increase the risk of marked hypertriglyceridemia.

Drugs used for the treatment of lipid disorders should generally be stopped before conception, including gemfibrozil (thus, Answer C is correct and Answer A is incorrect) and fenofibrate (thus, Answer B is incorrect). Statins are teratogenic and contra-indicated in pregnancy (thus, Answer D is incorrect). Ideally, all medications should be avoided during pregnancy, particularly during the first trimester when embryogenesis and tissue differentiation occur. Omega-3 fatty acids have been used to treat hypertriglyceridemia during pregnancy, but the available data suggest that they are not very effective. However, omega-3 fatty acids may be the treatment of choice in the first trimester.

Observational studies and case reports suggest that fibrates may be used safely and effectively during pregnancy after the first trimester. Fenofibrate is more potent than omega-3 fatty acids, so it is most likely the best choice in the second and third trimesters.

When pancreatitis due to hypertriglyceridemia develops during pregnancy, a number of treatment approaches have been used. The standard approach of fasting, fluid administration, and pain control is the best first step. If hyperglycemia is present, then intravenous insulin can be administered. Other treatments that have been tried include intravenous heparin, plasma exchange, lipoprotein apheresis, and cesarean delivery if the pregnancy is far enough along.

Educational Objective

Develop an approach to treating severe hypertriglyceridemia during pregnancy.

Reference(s)

Amin T, Poon LC, Teoh TG, et al. Management of hypertriglyceridaemia-induced acute pancreatitis in pregnancy. *J Matern Fetal Neonatal Med.* 2015;28(8):954-958. PMID: 25072837

Crisan LS, Steidl ET, Rivera-Alsina ME. Acute hyperlipidemic pancreatitis in pregnancy. *Am J Obstet Gynecol.* 2008;198(5):e57-e59. PMID: 18359475

Whitten AE, Lorenz RP, Smith JM. Hyperlipidemia-associated pancreatitis in pregnancy managed with fenofibrate. *Obstet Gynecol.* 2011;117(2 Pt 2):517-519. PMID: 21252809

Nakao J, Ohba T, Takaishi K, Katabuchi H. Omega-3 fatty acids for the treatment of hypertriglyceridemia during the second trimester. *Nutrition.* 2015;31(2):409-412. PMID: 25592021

26 ANSWER: C) Apolipoprotein E genotyping

Increased triglycerides commensurate with increased cholesterol occur in 2 situations: familial combined hyperlipidemia and dysbetalipoproteinemia. The former is due to an increase in both VLDL and LDL and is a relatively common dyslipidemia, especially in patients with diabetes. However, the cholesterol concentration in this patient and her lack of obesity or thyroid disorder suggest that she has a primary genetic abnormality. She has palmar xanthomas and cholesterol and triglyceride levels greater than 600 mg/dL (>15.54 mmol/L and >6.78 mmol/L, respectively) that are approximately equal. This finding occurs in dysbetalipoproteinemia, a disorder that is usually associated with an APOE*E2/APOE*E2 genotype (Answer C). This molecular defect is autosomal recessive, but it occurs in 1% of the population. However, only 1 in 10,000 patients present with the phenotype of this disease. Therefore, it is assumed that there must be an additional underlying factor that leads to its manifestation. Apolipoprotein E is needed to clear many lipoprotein particles by the liver, and presumably a high-fat diet leads to large numbers of circulating remnant lipoproteins that are not efficiently cleared. Unlike LDL, the shortened apolipoprotein B48 in chylomicrons is unable to serve as a ligand for liver lipoprotein receptors, and remnant lipoproteins produced in the intestine use apolipoprotein E as the primary ligand for receptor-mediated uptake by the liver. As an alternative to genotyping, centrifugation analysis of VLDL particles should show that they are cholesterol enriched. Patients with dysbetalipoproteinemia respond well to fibric acids. Untreated, the disorder is associated with a marked increase in both cardiovascular and peripheral vascular disease. Of note, this is the same genetic locus that is associated with risk for Alzheimer disease (the APOE*E4/APOE*E4 genotype).

Apolipoprotein A1 (Answer A) is an important structural protein in HDL cholesterol particles. Apolipoprotein A1 deficiency leads to very low HDL-cholesterol levels (<20 mg/dL [<0.52 mmol/L]), but not the cholesterol profile in dysbetalipoproteinemia noted above. Measuring apolipoprotein A1 levels has been done for research purposes and low levels are associated with cardiovascular disease. However, measuring levels would not be helpful in this setting.

Assessment of LDL particle size (Answer B) would not add any information for her diagnosis.

Lipoprotein (a) (Answer D) is highly atherogenic and is associated with increased risk of cardiovascular disease, particularly premature cardiovascular disease. Lipoprotein (a) is an LDL particle with a large protein, apo (a), attached covalently to apolipoprotein B that can incorporate into the arterial wall and contribute to atherosclerosis. Lipoprotein (a) may be modestly elevated in familial hyperlipidemia, but very high levels are associated with a significant increase in atherosclerotic disease. Persons with a lipoprotein (a) level in the upper tertile have an increased risk of cardiovascular disease (odds ratio, 1.7; 95% confidence interval, 1.4-1.9) compared with persons whose level is in the lowest tertile. However, elevated lipoprotein (a) is not associated with any specific skin findings. Lipoprotein (a) gene analysis would not help to discern the cause of her elevated total cholesterol and triglycerides.

Educational Objective

Evaluate mixed hyperlipidemia and diagnose dysbetalipoproteinemia.

Reference(s)

Chahil TJ, Ginsberg HN. Diabetic dyslipidemia. *Endocrinol Metab Clin North Am.* 2006;35(3): 491-510. PMID: 16959582

Mahley RW, Huang Y, Rall SC Jr. Pathogenesis of type III hyperlipoproteinemia (dysbetalipoproteinemia). Questions, quandaries, and paradoxes. *J Lipid Res.* 1999;40(11):1933-1949. PMID: 10552997

Berglund L, Brunzell JD, Goldberg AC, et al; Endocrine Society. Evaluation and treatment of hypertriglyceridemia: an Endocrine Society clinical practice guideline. *J Clin Endocrinol Metab.* 2012;97(9):2969-2989. PMID: 22962670

27 ANSWER: A) Atorvastatin

An estimated 25% of people globally have nonalcoholic fatty liver disease (NAFLD) with the highest rates in the Middle East (32%) and the lowest rates in Africa (13%). Both obesity and type 2 diabetes are strong predictors for NAFLD. A subset of patients with NAFLD progress to nonalcoholic steatohepatitis (NASH) and ultimately cirrhosis. By 2020, NASH is expected to be the leading cause of liver transplant. Patients with NAFLD are also at increased risk for cardiovascular disease. Cardiovascular disease is the leading cause of death in persons with NAFLD, not death from liver-related causes. The American Association for the Study of Liver Disease recommends aggressive risk factor modification in patients with NAFLD to lower their cardiovascular disease risk, including treatment of dyslipidemia. Patients with NAFLD typically have dyslipidemia with high triglycerides, low HDL cholesterol, and increased small, dense LDL cholesterol.

The American Heart Association/American College of Cardiology 2013 guidelines state that this patient's clinical profile and 10-year cardiovascular disease risk score (diabetes, aged 40-75 years, LDL cholesterol 70-189 mg/dL, >7.5% risk of cardiovascular disease event in the next 10 years) suggests that he would benefit from a high-intensity statin. Furthermore, the presence of NAFLD puts him at even greater risk of a cardiovascular event than someone with a similar profile without NAFLD. The American Association for the Study of Liver Disease recommends the use of statins in the presence of fatty liver disease for the reduction of cardiovascular risk, as patients with NAFLD are not at increased risk of liver toxicity from statin use. Furthermore, secondary analysis from the IMPROVE-IT trial shows that patients with NAFLD may have greater cardiovascular disease risk reduction with dual therapy given that the study showed greater benefit in the subset with NAFLD with the addition of ezetimibe to simvastatin than with simvastatin alone. Data from at least one clinical trial (secondary endpoint) showed that ALT decreased in patients with NAFLD who were placed on a statin vs placebo.

While there has been concern for some time about the potential risk of treating individuals who have abnormal liver function tests with lipid-lowering drugs, there is no evidence that these drugs cause severe or progressive hepatic damage or that they cannot be safely used in patients with chronic liver disease. The GREACE study (Greek Atorvastatin and Coronary Heart Disease Evaluation) demonstrated that in individuals with liver function tests less than 3 times the upper normal limit, there are no adverse effects of lipid-lowering drugs on liver function tests over time and there are significant benefits to lipid-lowering therapy in cardiovascular disease risk reduction.

In the absence of serious or progressive liver disease, this patient first requires therapy with a statin (Answer A). Omega-3 fatty acids (Answer B), fenofibrate (Answer C), ezetimibe (Answer D), and niacin (Answer E) would not provide the cardiovascular disease risk reduction comparable to that of a statin. Since a statin is safe to use in this patient and it has the greatest benefits, it is the treatment of choice. He may gain additional benefit from the addition of ezetimibe to a statin, but a statin is the first best choice.

Educational Objective

Assess the benefits and risks of statin use in patients with fatty liver disease.

Reference(s)

Younossi ZM, Koenig AB, Abdelatif D, Fazel Y, Henry L, Wymer M. Global epidemiology of nonalcoholic fatty liver disease-meta-analytic assessment of prevalence, incidence, and outcomes. *Hepatology.* 2016;64:73-84. PMID: 26707365

Chalasani N, Younossi Z, Lavine JE, et al. The diagnosis and management of nonalcoholic fatty liver disease: practice guidance from the American Association for the Study of Liver Diseases. *Hepatology.* 2018;67(1):328-357. PMID: 28714183

Motamed N, Rabiee B, Poustchi H, et al. Non-alcoholic fatty liver disease (NAFLD) and 10-year risk of cardiovascular diseases. *Clin Res Hepatol Gastroenterol.* 2017;41(1):31-38. PMID: 27597641

Bril F, PoNrtillo Sanchez P, Lomonaco R, et al. Liver safety of statins in prediabetes or T2DM and nonalcoholic steatohepatitis: post hoc analysis of a randomized trial. *J Clin Endocrinol Metab.* 2017;102(8):2950-2961. PMID: 28575232

Athyros VG, Tziomalos K, Gossios TD, et al; GREACE Study Collaborative Group. Safety and efficacy of long-term statin treatment for cardiovascular events in patients with coronary heart disease and abnormal liver tests in the Greek Atorvastatin and Coronary Heart Disease Evaluation (GREACE) Study: a post-hoc analysis. *Lancet.* 2010;376(9756):1916-1922. PMID: 21109302

Demyen M, Alkhalloufi K, Pyrsopoulos NT. Lipid-lowering agents and hepatotoxicity. *Clin Liver Dis.* 2013;17(4):699-714. PMID: 24099026

28   ANSWER: C) Icosapent ethyl, 2 g twice daily

Many patients who are high risk for cardiovascular disease, including those with diabetes, have residual cardiovascular disease risk even after receiving appropriate therapy with statins and ezetimibe. Elevated triglycerides are atherogenic and represent residual cardiovascular disease risk beyond LDL cholesterol. Thus, making no changes in this patient's current therapy (Answer A) is not the best option. While fenofibrate (Answer D) and niacin ER (Answer E) lower triglycerides, they have not been shown to lower cardiovascular disease risk when added to appropriate medical therapy, including statins. Similarly, in aggregate, n-3 fatty acids have not been shown to lower cardiovascular disease risk. Gemfibrozil (Answer B) should not be used in combination with a statin.

Icosapent ethyl (Answer C) is a purified eicosapentaenoic acid ethyl ester (an omega-3 fatty acid). Although omega-3 fatty acids have been shown to lower triglycerides, in aggregate they have not been shown to lower the risk of cardiovascular disease. Over-the-counter omega-3 fatty acid preparations are not regulated and may contain a variety of fatty acids and other components. In January 2019, the REDUCE-IT trial published in the *New England Journal of Medicine* showed that adding icosapent ethyl, 2 g twice daily vs placebo to a statin in patients with persistent mildly elevated fasting triglycerides (135 to 500 mg/dL [1.52-5.65 mmol/L]) and an LDL-cholesterol concentration between 41 and 100 mg/dL (1.06-2.59 mmol/L) for a median of 4.9 years (n = 8179) lowered the risk of major cardiovascular events (cardiovascular death, or nonfatal myocardial infarction, stroke, coronary revascularization, or unstable angina) by 25% (17.2% vs 22%; hazard ratio, 0.75; 95% confidence interval, 0.68-0.83). Cardiovascular death was 4.3% in the icosapent ethyl group and 5.2% in the placebo group (hazard ratio, 0.80; 95% confidence interval, 0.66-0.98). There have been concerns about omega-3 fatty acids promoting arrhythmia and possibly increasing bleeding risk. Hospitalization for atrial fibrillation was higher in the icosapent ethyl treatment group than in the placebo group (3.1% vs 2.1%; P = .004), and there was a trend toward more serious bleeding in the icosapent ethyl treatment group compared with placebo (2.7% vs 2.1%; P = .06). More work is needed to fully characterize the risk of these potential adverse events in the context of potential benefits for cardiovascular disease risk reduction.

Treatment of individuals with diabetes with a fibrate failed to show a reduction in primary cardiovascular endpoints in the Bezafibrate Infarction Prevention trial (BIP) and more recently in the Action to Control Cardiovascular Risk in Diabetes trial (ACCORD). The ACCORD trial specifically assessed whether adding a fibrate to a statin conferred any additional cardiovascular benefits. The results were negative. These studies have been criticized for not selecting individuals with elevated triglycerides at baseline, and post hoc analyses suggest a benefit among those with high baseline triglyceride levels. The Fenofibrate Intervention and Event Lowering in Diabetes study (FIELD) enrolled nearly 10,000 patients with type 2 diabetes, of which about 3650 were women. This study also failed to demonstrate that fenofibrate reduced cardiovascular events. The AIM-HIGH study included a large number of patients with diabetes and examined the effectiveness of adding niacin to aggressive statin therapy. Despite the fact that niacin reduced triglyceride levels and increased HDL-cholesterol levels, the trial was stopped early because of a failure of niacin treatment to reduce cardiovascular endpoints, as well as an unexpected increase in stroke rates.

Educational Objective
Describe the benefits of the new n-3 fatty acid, purified eicosapentaenoic acid (EPA), for both triglyceride lowering and cardiovascular risk reduction for patients with triglyceride levels above target and residual risk of cardiovascular disease despite good response to statin treatment.

Reference(s)
Bhatt DL, Steg PG, Miller M, et al; REDUCE-IT Investigators. Cardiovascular risk reduction with icosapent ethyl for hypertriglyceridemia. *N Engl J Med*. 2019;380(1):1-22. PMID: 30415628

29 ANSWER: B) Elevated lipoprotein (a)
Additional biomarkers of increased cardiovascular risk beyond LDL cholesterol have been used to further quantify cardiovascular risk in patients who have persistent disease despite good response to lipid-lowering therapy, including non-HDL cholesterol, apolipoprotein B (Answer D), and lipoprotein (a) (Answer B).

Lipoprotein (a) (Answer B) is highly atherogenic and is associated with increased risk of cardiovascular disease, particularly premature cardiovascular disease. Lipoprotein (a) is an LDL particle with a large protein, apo (a), attached covalently to apolipoprotein B that can incorporate into the arterial wall and contribute to atherosclerosis. Lipoprotein (a) may be modestly elevated in familial hyperlipidemia, but very high levels are associated with a significant increase in atherosclerotic disease. Persons with a lipoprotein (a) level in the upper tertile have an increased risk of cardiovascular disease (odds ratio, 1.7; 95% confidence interval, 1.4-1.9) compared with persons whose level is in the lowest tertile.

Apolipoprotein B (Answer D) is a lipoprotein found on all atherogenic lipid particles, including LDL and triglyceride-rich particles. Non-HDL cholesterol has been suggested as a marker of cardiovascular risk because it also includes non-LDL (triglyceride risk) atherogenic particles. Apolipoprotein B and non-HDL cholesterol predict risk along with LDL cholesterol in patients with primarily elevated LDL cholesterol and elevated triglycerides as found in patients with type 2 diabetes. This patient does not have diabetes or elevated triglycerides, which suggest apolipoprotein B and non-HDL cholesterol are not likely to be additionally informative beyond his LDL-cholesterol level. Apolipoprotein B elevation can support a diagnosis of familial hyperlipidemia and is associated with high risk of cardiovascular disease, but his baseline LDL-cholesterol level was not typical of a patient with familial hyperlipidemia.

The 2013 American College of Cardiology/American Heart Association cholesterol lowering guidelines do not currently recommend measurement of biomarkers such as apolipoprotein B, lipoprotein (a), and high-sensitivity C-reactive protein for the purpose of primary risk stratification in addition to the lipid profile, but these measures may be used in select cases. Newer guidelines suggest additional markers may be used in select cases to further risk stratify patients, although clear pharmacologic strategies to lower cardiovascular disease risk by targeting lipoprotein (a) reduction are still lacking. However, the particle is effectively removed by apheresis.

Apolipoprotein A1 (Answer B) is an important structural lipoprotein in HDL particles. Genetic variants leading to the deficiency of apolipoprotein A1 result in very low HDL-cholesterol levels, generally less than 20 mg/dL (<0.52 mmol/L), and high risk of heart disease. This man's HDL-cholesterol level is greater than 40 mg/dL (>1.04 mmol/L), which is not consistent with apolipoprotein A1 deficiency.

ATP-binding cassette A1 (ABCA1) deficiency (Answer C), or Tangier disease, is a cause of very low HDL cholesterol and is associated with very early-onset cardiovascular disease, frequently when individuals are in their 20s and 30s. Tangier disease is associated with accumulation of cholesterol in lymphoid tissue giving a classic physical finding: orange tonsils. However, patients with ABCA1 deficiency typically have HDL-cholesterol levels less than 20 mg/dL (<0.52 mmol/L).

Educational Objective
Explain the cardiovascular risk associated with elevated lipoprotein (a).

Reference(s)
Stone NJ, Robinson JG, Lichtenstein AH, et al; American College of Cardiology/American Heart Association Task Force on Practice Guidelines. 2013 ACC/AHA guideline on the treatment of blood cholesterol to reduce atherosclerotic cardiovascular risk in adults: a report of the American College of Cardiology/ American Heart Association Task Force on Practice Guidelines [published correction appears in *Circulation*. 2014;129(25 Suppl 2): S46-S48]. *Circulation*. 2014;129(25 Suppl 2):S1-S45. PMID: 24222016

Danesh J, Collins R, Peto R. Lipoprotein(a) and coronary heart disease. Meta-analysis of prospective studies. *Circulation*. 2000;102(10): 1082-1085. PMID: 10973834

Kamstrup PR, Benn M, Tybjaerg-Hansen A, Nordestgaard BG. Extreme lipoprotein(a) levels and risk of myocardial infarction in the general population: The Copenhagen City Heart Study. *Circulation*. 2008;117(2):176-184. PMID: 18086931

Nordestagarrd BG, Chapman MJ, Ray K, et al; European Atherosclerosis Society Consensus Panel. Lipoprotein(a) as a cardiovascular risk factor: current status. *Eur Heart J*. 2010;31(23): 2844-2853. PMID: 20965889

Chalasani N, Younossi Z, Lavine JE, et al. The diagnosis and management of nonalcoholic fatty liver disease: practice guidance from the American Association for the Study of Liver Diseases. *Hepatology*. 2018;67(1):328-357. PMID: 2871418

30 ANSWER: B) Assessment of the coronary artery calcium score

Of these options, the test with the best predictive value for cardiovascular disease events in middle-aged men is the coronary artery calcium score (Answer B) obtained using CT imaging. Coronary calcium is thought to indicate response to inflammation in the artery. Although no screening test is perfect, this test is meant to detect early disease and the 5-year risk of coronary events. Moreover, a positive score is associated with better adherence to lifestyle modification. If this patient's calcium score is zero, he could reasonably decline statin therapy at this time. However, in younger patients (eg, those with familial hypercholesterolemia), this imaging fails to detect disease because atherosclerotic plaques in these patients are often not calcified. Furthermore, the updated 2018 American Heart Association/American College of Cardiology guidelines suggest using the coronary artery calcium score to further discriminate cardiovascular disease risk in patients with unclear risk or in whom the decision to start a statin is complex.

Although LDL-particle size (Answer A) has been promoted as an independent risk factor, small, dense LDL is highly correlated with hypertriglyceridemia, low HDL cholesterol, and metabolic syndrome (which this patient does not have). LDL-particle size will not likely add additional information to guide therapy decisions. Moreover, there are no guidelines for use of LDL-particle size distribution to alter therapy. Measurement of apolipoprotein B (Answer C) provides similar data to that from assessment of non-HDL cholesterol, which is already available at no extra cost. Antioxidants (Answer D) such as vitamin E are not risk factor indicators.

Other blood tests that might be performed with some justification include measurement of lipoprotein

(a) and high-sensitivity C-reactive protein. Although white blood cell counts are a well-established indicator of cardiac risk, but variability precludes their use as a screening test.

Educational Objective

Recommend determining a coronary artery calcium score as a possible tool to assess cardiovascular disease risk in patients with intermediate or unclear cardiovascular disease risk when addressing decisions about medical therapy.

Reference(s)

Stone NJ, Robinson JG, Lichtenstein AH, et al; American College of Cardiology/American Heart Association Task Force on Practice Guidelines. 2013 ACC/AHA guideline on the treatment of blood cholesterol to reduce atherosclerotic cardiovascular risk in adults: a report of the American College of Cardiology/ American Heart Association Task Force on Practice Guidelines [published correction appears in *Circulation*. 2014;129(25 Suppl 2): S46-S48]. *Circulation*. 2014;129(25 Suppl 2): S1-S45. PMID: 24222016

Grundy SM, Stone NJ, Bailey AL, et al. 2018 AHA/ ACC/AACVPR/AAPA/ABC/ACPM/ADA/ AGS/APhA/ASPC/NLA/PCNA guideline on the management of blood cholesterol. *Circulation*. 2019;139(25):e1082-e1143. PMID: 30586774

Grundy SM, Stone NJ, Bailey AL, et al. 2018 AHA/ ACC/AACVPR/AAPA/ABC/ACPM/ADA/ AGS/APhA/ASPC/NLA/PCNA guideline on the management of blood cholesterol: executive summary. *Circulation*. 2019;139(25):e1046- e1081. PMID: 30565953

Yusuf S, Bosch J, Dagenais G, et al; HOPE-3 Investigators. Cholesterol lowering in intermediate-risk persons without cardiovascular disease. *N Engl J Med*. 2016; 374(21):2021-2031. PMID: 27040132

Guerci AD, Arad Y, Agatston A. Predictive value of EBCT scanning. *Circulation*. 1998;97(25):2583- 2584. PMID: 9657482

Orakzai RH, Nasir K, Orakzai SH, et al. Effect of patient visualization of coronary calcium by electron beam computed tomography on changes in beneficial lifestyle behaviors. *Am J Cardiol*. 2008;101(7):999-1002. PMID: 18359321

Pituitary Board Review

Laurence Katznelson, MD

1 ANSWER: B) Lanreotide depot monthly

Somatostatin analogues are effective in managing acromegaly and are often used as first-line medical therapy. Somatostatin analogues are also very useful in patients with headache. Therefore, lanreotide depot, a somatostatin analogue, given monthly (Answer B) would be the initial treatment choice in this patient. Octreotide LAR (long-acting release) is another somatostatin analogue with similar efficacy and adverse effect profile to that of lanreotide depot.

Of medical therapies, pegvisomant has the highest likelihood of normalizing this patient's IGF-1 levels. However, in the most recent Endocrine Society guidelines, pegvisomant was recommended to be considered as first-line medical therapy when administered as daily, not weekly, dosing (Answer D). Also, somatostatin analogues may be superior to pegvisomant in the setting of significant headache. Repeated surgery (Answer C) is probably not indicated if the residual tumor is within the cavernous sinus, as additional surgery is unlikely to be curative. Although cabergoline (Answer A) may be useful in selected patients, it is mostly useful for patients with mildly elevated IGF-1 levels. This patient has a more significantly elevated IGF-1 level.

Educational Objective

Manage persistent acromegaly after transsphenoidal surgery.

Reference(s)

Katznelson L, Laws ER Jr, Melmed S, et al. Acromegaly: an endocrine society clinical practice guideline. *J Clin Endocrinol Metab*. 2014;99(11): 3933-3951. PMID: 25356808

Giustina A, Chanson P, Kleinberg D, et al; Acromegaly Consensus Group. Expert consensus document: a consensus on the medical treatment of acromegaly. *Nat Rev Endocrinol*. 2014;10(4): 243-248. PMID: 24566817

2 ANSWER: A) Pathogenic variant in the *PROP1* gene

This patient had childhood-onset GH deficiency, as well as hypothyroidism. He also has empty sella on MRI. Pathogenic variants in the genes encoding a number of transcription factors, including *POU1F1* (formerly *PIT1*) and *PROP1*, can cause disruption in the development of many pituitary cell types during embryogenesis, resulting in multiple pituitary hormone deficiencies. Pathogenic variants in *PROP1* (Answer A) result in a decrease in PROP 1, a transcription factor important for the development of the somatotroph, lactotroph, and thyrotroph lineages with deficiencies of their respective hormones. Some affected individuals also have delayed puberty. Combined pituitary hormone deficiency (GH, prolactin, TSH) has an incidence of about 1 in 8000 births, and 10% of patients have an affected family member. Between 25% and 50% of these cases are due to pathogenic variants in *POU1F1* or *PROP1*. In this patient, the history of previous GH and thyroid hormone treatment starting in childhood suggests a congenital combined pituitary hormone deficiency. In some children with PROP1 deficiency, there is early pituitary enlargement of uncertain cause, which results in sellar enlargement and subsequent loss of pituitary volume, leading to an empty sella. In most series, when patients with empty sellas have evaluations of pituitary function, between one-quarter and one-third have varying degrees of hypopituitarism.

Acute trauma causing pituitary infarction (Answer B) may reveal subsequent empty sella, but this patient does not have a history of trauma and his hypopituitarism predated his concussion. Sarcoidosis (Answer C) and Langerhans cell histiocytosis (Answer D) are infiltrative diseases of the hypothalamus and pituitary stalk and might present with stalk thickening rather than an empty sella. Both usually present with diabetes insipidus.

Hemochromatosis (Answer E) can cause iron deposition in the pituitary and usually affects the gonadotroph cells; it is not associated with an empty sella.

Educational Objective

Determine the cause of childhood-onset combined hypopituitarism.

Reference(s)

Prince KL, Walvoord EC, Rhodes SJ. The role of homeodomain transcription factors in heritable pituitary disease. *Nat Rev Endocrinol.* 2011;7(12): 727-737. PMID: 21788968

Mendonca BB, Osorio MG, Latronico AC, Estefan V, Lo LS, Arnhold IJ. Longitudinal hormonal and pituitary imaging changes in two females with combined pituitary hormone deficiency due to deletion of A301,G302 in the PROP1 gene. *J Clin Endocrinol Metab.* 1999;84(3):942-945. PMID: 10084575

Guitelman M, Garcia Basavilbaso N, Vitale M, et al. Primary empty sella (PES): a review of 175 cases. *Pituitary.* 2013;16(2):270-274. PMID: 22875743

3 ANSWER: B) Increase in polyuria and polydipsia

Cortisol and thyroid hormone deficiencies increase the sensitivity of vasopressin receptors to vasopressin. Thus, when these hormones are replaced, the small amount of vasopressin still being secreted in a patient with partial diabetes insipidus may no longer be sufficient to effect water reabsorption, and subclinical diabetes insipidus may manifest with polyuria and polydipsia (Answer B). The converse of excessive vasopressin secretion with hyponatremia (Answer A) is certainly not going to occur.

Although pharmacologic dosages of glucocorticoids can impair libido (Answer C) and erectile function, normal replacement dosages do not. Institution of steroids should not cause orthostatic hypotension (Answer D). Administration of levothyroxine alone without glucocorticoids could cause hypotension if it unmasks adrenal insufficiency.

Educational Objective

Explain the effects of thyroid hormone and cortisol on vasopressin action.

Reference(s)

Iida M, Takamoto S, Masuo M, Makita K, Saito T. Transient lymphocytic panhypophysitis associated with SIADH leading to diabetes insipidus after glucocorticoid replacement. *Intern Med.* 2003;42(10):991-995. PMID: 14606714

Huang CH, Chou KJ, Lee PT, Chen CL, Chung HM, Fang HC. A case of lymphocytic hypophysitis with masked diabetes insipidus unveiled by glucocorticoid replacement. *Am J Kidney Dis.* 2005;45(1):197- 200. PMID: 15696461

Sala E, Moore JM, Amorin A, et al. Natural history of Rathke's cleft cysts: a retrospective analysis of a two centres experience. *Clin Endocrinol (Oxf).* [Epub ahead of print] PMID: 29781512

Lin M, Wedemeyer MA, Bradley D, et al. Long-term surgical outcomes following transsphenoidal surgery in patients with Rathke's cleft cysts. *J Neurosurg.* 2018;130(3):831-837. PMID: 29775155

4 ANSWER: C) ⁶⁸Ga DOTATATE scan

Pituitary hormone excess syndromes are usually due to overproduction of these hormones in an unregulated fashion from pituitary adenomas. However, rare neuroendocrine tumors can produce hypophysiotropic hormones, such as corticotropin-releasing hormone and GHRH, resulting, respectively, in overproduction of ACTH (Cushing syndrome) and GH (acromegaly). In this circumstance, the pituitary becomes hyperplastic as a result of this overstimulation by hypothalamic-releasing hormone. Thus, in this patient with global pituitary gland enhancement and enlargement, along with lack of lateralization on inferior petrosal catheterization, the possibility of a neuroendocrine tumor producing ectopic corticotropin-releasing hormone, such as a bronchial carcinoid, should be considered. Therefore, imaging such as ⁶⁸Ga DOTATATE PET/CT (Answer C) should be performed to evaluate for an ectopic lesion. Other forms of imaging, such as MRI, could be performed as well to investigate the possibility of a bronchial carcinoid or pancreatic neuroendocrine tumor. Additionally, corticotropin-releasing hormone levels could be measured. If an ectopic tumor is not detected, then exploratory transsphenoidal surgery could be considered.

Performing a corticotropin-releasing hormone test (Answer A), a dexamethasone corticotropin-releasing hormone test (Answer B), or another inferior petrosal sinus sampling (Answer D) would not aid in diagnosis. A high-dose dexamethasone suppression test (Answer E) may be useful for evaluating causes of ACTH-dependent Cushing syndrome, but it does not reliably distinguish between pituitary and ectopic disease. Of note, transsphenoidal surgical exploration is a reasonable alternative, as there are cases of false-negative petrosal catheterizations, but it is very reasonable to search for ectopic disease first with imaging.

Educational Objective
Differentiate among the different causes of ACTH-dependent Cushing syndrome.

Reference(s)
Isidori AM, Kaltsas GA, Pozza C, et al. The ectopic ACTH syndrome: clinical features, diagnosis, management, and long-term follow-up. *J Clin Endocrinol Metab*. 2006;91(2):371-377. PMID: 16303835

Horvath E, Kovacs K, Scheithauer BW. Pituitary hyperplasia. *Pituitary*. 1999;1(3-4):169-179. PMID: 11081195

Newell-Price J, Bertagna X, Grossman AB, Nieman LK. Cushing's syndrome. *Lancet*. 2006; 367(9522):1605-1617. PMID: 16698415

5 ANSWER: D) Lymphocytic hypophysitis
The most likely lesion in this patient is lymphocytic hypophysitis (Answer D). The key historical point is that these lesions usually develop in the intrapartum or postpartum period and present as mass lesions towards the latter part of pregnancy. The diffuse enhancement with gadolinium of a symmetrically enlarged pituitary on MRI is characteristic of hypophysitis, often with extension up the stalk as in this case. ACTH insufficiency occurs in two-thirds of patients with these lesions and should be investigated and treated if found, as adrenal insufficiency is a major cause of death in this setting. In this patient, the progressive, severe fatigue and weight loss point to the possibility of ACTH deficiency. Expectant management will usually suffice for lymphocytic hypophysitis, as the size of most lesions decreases after delivery.

Nonsecreting and prolactin-secreting pituitary adenomas are far more common sellar lesions in women in this age group, but nonsecreting pituitary adenomas (Answer B) generally do not enlarge and cause symptoms during pregnancy. Prolactinomas (Answer A) can, of course, enlarge during pregnancy. However, this patient was previously well, had regular menses before pregnancy, and had no difficulty getting pregnant, implying that she had not been having difficulty with fertility as might be expected with a prolactinoma. The prolactin levels in this case are also helpful in that a patient with a macroprolactinoma should have prolactin levels exceeding 500 ng/mL (>21.7 nmol/L), but a patient with lymphocytic hypophysitis usually has prolactin levels less than 200 ng/mL (<8.7 nmol/L). Although craniopharyngiomas (Answer C) do occur in this age group, they are much less common, and there have been only 3 reports of a change in size during pregnancy. Pituitary apoplexy (Answer E) is usually due to hemorrhage into a preexisting tumor and has a dramatic presentation with sudden onset of severe headache, stiff neck, and often a decreased level of consciousness. Her presentation of gradually worsening headaches with lack of other CNS findings does not suggest a hemorrhage. The MRI findings are also not compatible with hemorrhage.

Educational Objective
Construct the differential diagnosis of mass lesions in pregnancy.

Reference(s)
Carmichael JD. Update on the diagnosis and management of hypophysitis. *Curr Opin Endocrinol Diabetes Obes*. 2012;19(4):314-321. PMID: 22543347

6 ANSWER: E) Continue to monitor clinical progress
This patient responded nicely to bromocriptine and stopped it appropriately when she became pregnant. She is now 34 weeks' gestation, she is has an increase in serum prolactin. Because serum prolactin increases during pregnancy, measuring prolactin is not useful for assessment of tumor status in this setting. Prolactinomas normally increase in size during pregnancy, and up to one-third of macroprolactinomas (as in this case) expand to the degree of causing chiasmal compression. In this case, the patient is asymptomatic (no headaches) and visual fields are normal. Therefore, restarting bromocriptine (Answer A), starting cabergoline (Answer C), delivering the baby (Answer B), and performing a pituitary-directed MRI scan (Answer D) are not indicated. The patient should continue to be

followed clinically (Answer E), with another visual field test during the last trimester of pregnancy.

Educational Objective

Manage prolactinoma during pregnancy.

Reference(s)

Molitch ME. Prolactinoma in pregnancy. *Best Pract Res Clin Endocrinol Metab.* 2011;25(6):885-896. PMID: 22115164

DeWilde JP, Rivers AW, Price DL. A review of the current use of magnetic resonance imaging in pregnancy and safety implications for the fetus. *Prog Biophys Mol Biol.* 2005;87(2-3):335-353. PMID: 15556670

7 ANSWER: A) Mifepristone

All of these treatment modalities can improve Cushing disease, and treatment during pregnancy is advocated because it results in better fetal outcomes. Transsphenoidal surgery (Answer C) has a cure rate of 80% to 90% in expert neurosurgical hands with very low complication and fetal loss rates when done in the second trimester. Metyrapone (Answer B) has been used safely in pregnancy in a few cases, but there is limited clinical experience. There is experience with only about 50 cases in which somatostatin analogues have been used to treat acromegaly during pregnancy, with relatively minor adverse effects. However, somatostatin analogues cross the placenta and have unknown effects on the fetus. There is no experience with pasireotide (Answer D) during pregnancy, and it would be expected to worsen glucose tolerance in this population susceptible to gestational diabetes. Although cabergoline (Answer E) is safe when stopped after conception, there is little experience when used throughout pregnancy, and its ability to normalize cortisol levels in Cushing disease is only modest. Neither pasireotide nor cabergoline is absolutely contraindicated during pregnancy.

Mifepristone (Answer A) was originally developed as a progesterone receptor blocker and is a potent abortifacient (RU486); therefore, its use in pregnancy is absolutely contraindicated.

Educational Objective

Identify which options are contraindicated in the treatment of Cushing disease during pregnancy.

Reference(s)

Marions L. Mifepristone dose in the regimen with misoprostol for medical abortion. *Contraception.* 2006;74(1):21-25. PMID: 16781255

Lindsay JR, Jonklaas J, Oldfield EH, Nieman LK. Cushing's syndrome during pregnancy: personal experience and review of the literature. *J Clin Endocrinol Metab.* 2005;90(5):3077-3083. PMID: 15705919

Cohen-Kerem R, Railton C, Oren D, Lishner M, Koren G. Pregnancy outcome following non-obstetric surgical intervention. *Am J Surgery.* 2005;190(3):467-473. PMID: 16105538

8 ANSWER: E) Decreased peak bone mass

The *transition period* refers to the time of life between the end of puberty and full maturation of bone, muscle, and body fat composition. Peak bone mass usually occurs by age 25 years, and GH deficiency during the transition period results in a failure to attain this peak bone mass (Answer E). Once GH is discontinued, there may be a change in body composition with a reduction in lean mass and an increase in fat mass, but overall weight does not increase significantly (Answer A). Mental functioning and energy levels may decrease when GH therapy is stopped, but this is not usually marked (Answer D). No data yet prove that GH treatment reduces the risk of mortality in patients with hypopituitarism, although findings from some recent studies suggest that this may be true. Thus, a reduced mortality rate (Answer C) is incorrect. GH therapy may result in insulin resistance and glucose intolerance (Answer B), but this is not usually seen when GH is discontinued.

Educational Objective

Discuss the effects of GH in the transition period (between the end of puberty and full maturation of bone, muscle, and body fat composition).

Reference(s)

Clayton PE, Cuneo RC, Juul A, Monson JP, Shalet SM, Tauber M; European Society of Paediatric Endocrinology. Consensus statement on the management of the GH-treated adolescent in the transition to adult care. *Eur J Endocrinol.* 2005; 152(2);165-170. PMID: 15745921

Radovick S, DiVall S. Approach to the growth hormone-deficient child during transition to adulthood. *J Clin Endocrinol Metab.* 2007;92(4):1195-1200. PMID: 17409338

Gaillard RC, Mattsson AF, Akerblad AC, et al. Overall and cause-specific mortality in GH-deficient adults on GH replacement. *Eur J Endocrinol.* 2012;166(6):1069-1077. PMID: 22457236

Hartman ML, Xu R, Crowe BJ, et al; International HypoCCS Advisory Board. Prospective safety surveillance of GH-deficient adults: comparison of GH-treated vs untreated patients. *J Clin Endocrinol Metab.* 2013;98(3):980-988. PMID: 23345098

ANSWER: C) Another MRI in 12 months

This 48-year-old patient has been found incidentally to have a microlesion of the pituitary gland. Because this is a microlesion without associated symptoms (eg, no diabetes insipidus), there is no indication for surgery (Answer B) or irradiation (Answers D). Appropriate management would simply be to perform serial monitoring and assess for a change in tumor size in 12 months with another MRI (Answer C). Tumors such as this one grow quite slowly (0.6 mm/y on average), so he is in no imminent danger from tumor growth. If the MRI had shown significant suprasellar extension with abutment of the optic chiasm, then visual field testing (Answer A) should have been performed; otherwise, it should not.

Educational Objective
Manage a pituitary incidentaloma.

Reference(s)

Molitch ME. Pituitary tumours: pituitary incidentalomas. *Best Pract Res Clin Endocrinol Metab.* 2009;23(5):667-675. PMID: 19945030

Freda PU, Beckers AM, Katznelson L, et al; Endocrine Society. Pituitary incidentalomas: an Endocrine Society clinical practice guideline. *J Clin Endocrinol Metab.* 2011;96(4):894-904. PMID: 21474686

ANSWER: D) Start hydrocortisone

This pregnant woman has pituitary enlargement presenting near term, and it is most likely to be lymphocytic hypophysitis. MRI shows diffuse pituitary enlargement, which is more compatible with hypophysitis than a tumor, and, had gadolinium been given, there would have been diffuse enhancement rather than focal enhancement. (No data show adverse effects of performing MRI or giving gadolinium during pregnancy, although it is recommended to withhold gadolinium during pregnancy.) One of the striking features of hypophysitis occurring during pregnancy is the high risk of ACTH deficiency. This patient had a morning serum cortisol concentration of 9.0 µg/dL (248.3 nmol/L), which does not seem very low. However, it should be remembered that cortisol production increases 3-fold during pregnancy and cortisol-binding globulin levels are also very high, resulting in normal morning cortisol levels well above 20 µg/dL (>551.8 nmol/L). Therefore, her cortisol level of 9.0 µg/dL is fairly low, and she most likely has adrenal insufficiency. Hydrocortisone should be started (Answer D).

Because dexamethasone (Answer A), unlike hydrocortisone, is not degraded by 11β-hydroxysteroid dehydrogenase type 2 in pregnancy, it should not be administered. Her prepregnancy history, indicating that she was well and had no problems conceiving, makes it very unlikely that this mass is a prolactinoma. Therefore, there is no indication for bromocriptine (Answer C). There is no reason to proceed with urgent cesarean delivery (Answer B), as she should be stabilized with adequate hormone replacement.

Educational Objective
Diagnose and treat lymphocytic hypophysitis in a pregnant woman.

Reference(s)

Rivera JA. Lymphocytic hypophysitis: disease spectrum and approach to diagnosis and therapy. *Pituitary.* 2006;9(1):35-45. PMID: 16703407

Molitch ME. Pituitary disorders during pregnancy. *Endocrinol Metab Clin North Am.* 2006;35(1):99-116. PMID: 16310644

Khare S, Jagtap VS, Budyal SR, et al. Primary (autoimmune) hypophysitis: a single centre experience. *Pituitary.* 2015;18(1):16-22. PMID: 24375060

11 ANSWER: D) Metastasis

The key features in this patient are the rapid growth of the mass, as well as the presence of diabetes insipidus. This is most consistent with a metastasis (Answer D). Diabetes insipidus occurs because the metastasis involves the posterior pituitary. The most common cancers causing such metastases are breast cancer in women and lung cancer in men. This patient's history of breast cancer makes this the most likely diagnosis.

Clinically nonfunctioning pituitary adenomas (Answer A) are usually slow growing and are rarely associated with diabetes insipidus. Prolactinoma (Answer B) is unlikely given the modestly elevated serum prolactin, the rapid increase in tumor size, and the presence of diabetes insipidus (rarely associated). Craniopharyngioma (Answer C) can also be associated with diabetes insipidus, but lesions are cystic and patients usually present at a younger age.

Educational Objective
Differentiate metastases from other pituitary mass lesions.

Reference(s)
Al-Aridi R, El Sibai K, Fu P, Khan M, Selman WR, Arafah BM. Clinical and biochemical characteristic features of metastatic cancer to the sella turcica: an analytical review. *Pituitary*. 2014; 17(6):575-587. PMID: 24337713

Ariel D, Sung H, Coghlan N, Dodd R, Gibbs IC, Katznelson L. Clinical characteristics and pituitary dysfunction in patients with metastatic cancer to the sella. *Endocr Pract*. 2013;19(6):914-919. PMID: 23757610

12 ANSWER: B) Perform a glucagon-stimulation test to assess GH levels

Because of her history of radiation therapy, this patient is at risk for hypopituitarism, including GH deficiency. The fatigue and forgetfulness may be symptomatic of GH deficiency, so further evaluation is recommended. A random GH level (Answer A) is not useful in the diagnosis of GH deficiency. An insulin tolerance test remains the gold standard for assessment of GH reserve, but caution is needed in a patient with previous cranial surgery because of concerns regarding possible seizure induction by hypoglycemia. This was not offered as an option. Therefore, a glucagon-stimulation test (Answer B) would be a reasonable alternative stimulation test. A novel, oral GH secretagogue, macimorelin, is an additional available option for GH-stimulation testing.

Because this patient has 3 pituitary hormone axes that are deficient, her chance of being GH deficient by any stimulation test would be about 96% if she had a lower IGF-1 level (<85 ng/dL [<11.1 nmol/L]). Because her IGF-1 level is higher than this cutoff, performance of a GH-stimulation test is indicated, as the IGF-1 level alone is insufficient to diagnose GH deficiency. Measuring IGF-1 again (Answer C) has no value. She has no clear contraindications to GH therapy, as she has no history of malignancy or relative contraindication of diabetes mellitus. Therefore, she is a candidate for GH therapy and assessment is indicated (thus, Answer D is incorrect).

Educational Objective
Select the most appropriate test to diagnose GH deficiency.

Reference(s)
Molitch ME, Clemmons DR, Malozowski S, Merriam GR, Vance ML; Endocrine Society. Evaluation and treatment of adult growth hormone deficiency: an Endocrine Society clinical practice guideline. *J Clin Endocrinol Metab*. 2011;96(6):1587-1609. PMID: 21602453

Ramos-Leví AM, Marazuela M. Treatment of adult growth hormone deficiency with human recombinant growth hormone: an update on current evidence and critical review of advantages and pitfalls. *Endocrine*. 2018;60(2):203-218. PMID: 29417370

Garcia JM, Biller BMK, Korbonits M, et al. Macimorelin as a diagnostic test for adult GH deficiency. *J Clin Endocrinol Metab*. 2018;103(8):3083-3093. PMID: 29860473

13 ANSWER: A) Ipilimumab

Ipilimumab (Answer A) is a monoclonal antibody used in the treatment of metastatic melanoma. Ipilimumab is an immune checkpoint inhibitor that enhances immune response by working through the cytotoxic T-lymphocyte–associated antigen 4 (CTLA-4). Hypophysitis has been reported in up to 17% of treated patients and often occurs within 6 to 8 weeks of treatment initiation, and corticotrophs and thyrotrophs are the most common cell types affected.

This form of hypophysitis is different from lymphocytic hypophysitis that occurs peripartum in women.

Bevacizumab (Answer B) is a vascular endothelial growth factor inhibitor that has been used to treat proliferative diabetic retinopathy, but it does not cause hypophysitis. Temozolomide (Answer C) is an alkylating agent used in the treatment of gliomas that has been useful in the treatment of some patients with pituitary carcinomas and very aggressive macroadenomas. Sunitinib (Answer D) is a tyrosine kinase inhibitor that has been used to treat thyroid cancer, among other cancers, but it has not been implicated as a cause of hypophysitis.

Educational Objective
Identify medications that can cause hypophysitis.

Reference(s)
Corsello SM, Barnabei A, Marchetti P, De Vecchis L, Salvatori R, Torino F. Endocrine side effects Induced by immune checkpoint inhibitors. *J Clin Endocrinol Metab*. 2013;98(4):1361-1375. PMID: 23471977

Faje AT, Sullivan R, Lawrence D, et al. Ipilimumab-induced hypophysitis: a detailed longitudinal analysis in a large cohort of patients with metastatic melanoma. *J Clin Endocrinol Metab*. 2014;99(11):4078-4085. PMID: 25078147

Albarel F, Gaudy C, Castinetti F, et al. Long-term follow-up of ipilimumab-induced hypophysitis, a common adverse event of the anti-CTLA-4 antibody in melanoma. *Eur J Endocrinol*. 2015; 172(2):195-204. PMID: 25416723

Faje AT, Lawrence D, Flaherty K, et al. High-dose glucocorticoids for the treatment of ipilimumab-induced hypophysitis is associated with reduced survival in patients with melanoma. *Cancer*. 2018;124(18):3706-3714. PMID: 29975414

Chang LS, Barroso-Sousa R, Tolaney SM, Hodi FS, Kaiser UB, Min L. Endocrine toxicity of cancer immunotherapy targeting immune checkpoints. *Endocr Rev*. 2019;40(1):17-65. PMID: 30184160

14 ANSWER: C) An adverse effect of cabergoline

Several studies have shown that dopamine agonists, both cabergoline and bromocriptine, can cause impulse control disorders, including hypersexuality compulsive behavior, in 15% to 20% of treated patients (Answer C). The effect appears to be somewhat dosage dependent, so lowering the dosage, if not discontinuing the dopamine agonist, may be helpful.

This patient's tumor is probably not large enough to cause substantial hypothalamic damage (Answer B). There are no reports substantiating that normalizing testosterone levels unmasks obsessive behavior (Answer A). While a behavior change unrelated to this tumor or treatment (Answer D) is possible, an adverse effect of cabergoline is the most likely explanation.

Educational Objective
Describe potential adverse effects of dopamine agonist treatment in patients with prolactinomas.

Reference(s)
Ioachimescu AG, Fleseriu M, Hoffman AR, Vaughan TB, Katznelson L. Psychological effects of dopamine agonist treatment in patients with hyperprolactinemia and prolactin-secreting adenomas. *Eur J Endocrinol*. 2019;180(1):31-40. PMID: 30400048

Bancos I, Nannenga MR, Bostwick JM, Silber MH, Erickson D, Nippoldt TB. Impulse control disorders in patients with dopamine agonist-treated prolactinomas and nonfunctioning pituitary adenomas: a case-control study. *Clin Endocrinol (Oxf)*. 2014;80(6):863-868. PMID: 24274365

Noronha S, Stokes V, Karavitaki N, Grossman A. Treating prolactinomas with dopamine agonists: always worth the gamble? *Endocrine*. 2016;51(2): 205-210. PMID: 26336835

15 ANSWER: D) Octreotide long-acting release

This patient has hyperthyroidism, a large multinodular goiter, and the unexpected finding of a TSH value that is not suppressed—an indication that a TSH-secreting tumor is the cause of her hyperthyroidism. Surgery would be the best option, but she prefers not to undergo this now.

Somatostatin inhibits both GH and TSH, and somatostatin analogues can inhibit TSH secretion from the tumor, as well as decrease tumor size. Given her history of coronary artery disease and congestive heart failure, control of the hyperthyroidism is the first step. Thus, octreotide long-acting release (Answer D), a somatostatin analogue, is the correct treatment to administer now. It is generally successful at normalizing thyroid hormone levels and can reduce the tumor size (which is important since it is invading the cavernous sinus). Surgery to debulk the pituitary tumor may be considered on an elective basis when she is clinically stable.

Methimazole (Answer B) could decrease thyroid hormone levels and help manage hyperthyroidism, but it will have either no effect on the size of the TSH-secreting tumor, or it could potentially facilitate tumor growth. Cabergoline (Answer A) has not been shown to be effective for TSH-secreting tumors. Although radioactive iodine (Answer C) could treat her hyperthyroidism, it will take months to work and would not treat her TSH-secreting pituitary tumor.

Educational Objective
Treat TSH-secreting tumors on the basis of the physiology and regulation of TSH secretion.

Reference(s)
Teramoto A, Sanno N, Tahara S, Osamura YR. Pathological study of thyrotropin-secreting pituitary adenoma: plurihormonality and medical treatment. *Acta Neuropathol.* 2004; 108(2):147-153. PMID: 15185102

Beck-Peccoz P, Persani L, Mannavola D, Campi I. TSH-secreting adenomas. *Best Pract Res Clin Endocrinol Metab.* 2009;23(5);597-606. PMID: 19945025

16 ANSWER: B) Decrease the GH dosage
Oral estrogens can act on the liver to decrease the responsiveness of the liver to GH with respect to IGF-1 production. Therefore, to maintain a steady level of IGF-1, the GH dosage may actually need to be decreased in this setting (thus, Answer B is correct and Answer C is incorrect). Interestingly, estrogens also stimulate hepatic thyroxine-binding globulin, so increases in levothyroxine dosages are sometimes needed and, presumably, the converse is also true (thus, Answer A is incorrect). Stopping estrogen has no effect on hydrocortisone dosage requirements (thus, Answers D and E are incorrect).

Educational Objective
Describe interactions among hormonal replacement therapies.

Reference(s)
Cook DM, Ludlam WH, Cook MB. Route of estrogen administration helps to determine growth hormone (GH) replacement dose in GH-deficient adults. *J Clin Endocrinol Metab.* 1999; 84(11):3956-3960. PMID: 10566634

Fleseriu M, Hashim IA, Karavitaki N, et al. Hormonal replacement in hypopituitarism in adults: an Endocrine Society clinical practice guideline. *J Clin Endocrinol Metab.* 2016;101(11):3888-3921. PMID: 27736313

17 ANSWER: C) Pasireotide
Of the somatostatin analogues, only pasireotide (Answer C) is effective in treating Cushing disease. Although lowering cortisol levels by pasireotide improves insulin resistance, pasireotide also inhibits insulin secretion to some extent and decreases GLP-1 and glucose insulinotropic peptide levels; the net effect is a worsening of glucose tolerance in most patients with the development of diabetes in many. Mifepristone (Answer D) blocks the glucocorticoid receptor, resulting in marked improvement in symptoms of hypercortisolism, including glucose levels. Metyrapone (Answer A) and ketoconazole (Answer B) decrease cortisol levels without any effect on insulin, GLP-1, or glucose insulinotropic peptide and thus decrease, rather than increase, glucose levels.

Educational Objective
Identify the adverse effects of medications used to treat Cushing disease.

Reference(s)
Colao A, Petersenn S, Newell-Price J, et al; Pasireotide B2305 Study Group. A 12-month phase 3 study of pasireotide in Cushing's disease. *N Engl J Med.* 2012;366(10):914-924. PMID: 22397653

Wallia A, Colleran K, Prunell JQ, Gross C, Molitch ME. Improvement in insulin sensitivity during mifepristone treatment of Cushing syndrome: early and late effects. *Diabetes Care.* 2013;36(9): E147-E148. PMID: 23970725

Molitch ME. Current approaches to the pharmacological management of Cushing's disease. *Mol Cell Endocrinol.* 2015;408:185-189. PMID: 25450859

18 ANSWER: C) Start tolvaptan

This patient has undergone 2 of the 3 phases of the triphasic response following pituitary surgery. She had immediate diabetes insipidus, followed by hyponatremia, which is usually due to syndrome of inappropriate antidiuretic hormone secretion. Diabetes insipidus in the subsequent phase would complete the 3 phases. This patient has severe hyponatremia, which occurred rapidly. Tolvaptan (Answer C) is an oral vasopressin receptor antagonist that is administered daily for up to 4 days, and it is very effective in the treatment of moderate to severe hyponatremia following pituitary surgery. A vasopressin receptor antagonist may facilitate recovery from syndrome of inappropriate antidiuretic hormone secretion in this setting. Tolvaptan administration (15 mg) will result in the most rapid normalization of sodium compared with the other listed options. Hypertonic saline can also be used in this setting. Given that the hyponatremia occurred rapidly, tolvaptan may be used to raise the sodium level quickly.

If fluid restriction is to be successful, it should be to less than 500 to 1000 mL/24 h. A 1500-mL limit (Answer A) is too high. Demeclocycline (Answer B) causes partial nephrogenic diabetes insipidus and can be useful for patients with chronic, symptomatic hyponatremia, such as that associated with malignancy; it is generally not used when hyponatremia develops acutely. Saline infusion with intermittent furosemide (Answer D) combines salt infusion with an increase in urinary excretion of water in excess of sodium. However, this form of sodium correction is slow and is minimally useful.

Educational Objective
Manage moderate to severe hyponatremia in the postoperative setting following transsphenoidal surgery.

Reference(s)
Verbalis JG, Goldsmith SR, Greenberg A, et al. Diagnosis, evaluation, and treatment of hyponatremia: expert panel recommendations. *Am J Med.* 2013;126(10 Suppl 1):S1-S42. PMID: 24074529

Jahangiri A, Wagner J, Tran MT, et al. Factors predicting postoperative hyponatremia and efficacy of hyponatremia management strategies after more than 1000 pituitary operations. *J Neurosurg.* 2013;119(6):1478-1483. PMID: 23971964

Woodmansee WW, Carmichael J, Kelly D, Katznelson L; AACE Neuroendocrine and Pituitary Scientific Committee. American Association of Clinical Endocrinologists and American College of Endocrinology disease state clinical review: postoperative management following pituitary surgery. *Endocr Pract.* 2015; 21(7):832-838. PMID: 26172128

19 ANSWER: D) Late-night salivary cortisol measurement

Following transsphenoidal surgery for Cushing disease, the recurrence rate is approximately 25% at 5 years. The degree of the cortisol decrease after surgery correlates with long-term remission. Therefore, it is important to perform serial evaluation for possible recurrence. Patients are often perceptive as to whether they may have had recurrence, and this information is useful in planning testing. The most accurate test for recurrence is late-night salivary cortisol measurement (Answer D). In recent studies, late-night salivary cortisol measurement had the highest predictive value compared with overnight dexamethasone testing and 24-hour urinary free cortisol excretion (Answer A).

Repeating an ACTH measurement (Answer E) is not useful for determining recurrence. Once recurrence has been confirmed, pituitary MRI (Answer B) should be performed to evaluate for a visible adenoma. A plan to perform serial monitoring (Answer C) with a follow-up appointment in 6 months is not an ideal option for this patient, as she does have some signs consistent with Cushing disease recurrence, so further testing should be performed now. In addition, an isolated serum cortisol measurement is not useful for determining recurrence.

Educational Objective
Assess patients with Cushing disease for recurrence following successful surgery.

Reference(s)

Patil CG, Prevedello DM, Lad SP, et al. Late recurrences of Cushing's disease after initial successful transsphenoidal surgery. *J Clin Endocrinol Metab.* 2008;93(2):358-362. PMID: 18056770

Hameed N, Yedinak CG, Brzana J, et al. Remission rate after transsphenoidal surgery in patients with pathologically confirmed Cushing's disease, the role of cortisol, ACTH assessment and immediate reoperation: a large single center experience. *Pituitary.* 2013;16(4):452-458. PMID: 23242860

Danet-Lamasou M, Asselineau J, Perez P, et al. Accuracy of repeated measurements of late-night salivary cortisol to screen for early-stage recurrence of Cushing's disease following pituitary surgery. *Clin Endocrinol (Oxf).* 2015; 82(2):260-266. PMID: 24975391

Amlashi FG, Swearingen B, Faje AT, et al. Accuracy of late-night salivary cortisol in evaluating postoperative remission and recurrence in Cushing's disease. *J Clin Endocrinol Metab.* 2015; 100(10):3770-3777. PMID: 26196950

20   ANSWER: C) Perform transsphenoidal surgery

This patient presents with a large sellar mass, with suprasellar extension and mild chiasmal compression. The relatively low serum prolactin concentration (less than 150 to 200 ng/mL [<6.5-8.7 nmol/L]) in this case is not consistent with a macroprolactinoma. Therefore, the lesion is most likely a nonfunctioning pituitary macroadenoma, and transsphenoidal surgery (Answer C) is indicated.

Given that the patient probably does not have a prolactinoma, neither higher-dosage bromocriptine (Answer A) nor cabergoline (Answer D) is indicated to reduce tumor size. Stereotactic radiosurgery (Answer E) is not indicated, as surgical resection with chiasmal decompression is necessary. Radiosurgery is unlikely to reduce tumor size and improve optic chiasmal function in a short timeframe. Further, radiosurgery is contraindicated when the tumor touches the chiasm, given risk of optic chiasmal injury. Somatostatin analogue therapy (Answer B) is generally not useful for these tumors, as there have been inconsistent results.

Educational Objective

Distinguish between hyperprolactinemia resulting from hypothalamic/stalk dysfunction and tumor production.

Reference(s)

Freda PU, Post KD. Differential diagnosis of sellar masses. *Endocrinol Metab Clin North Am.* 1999; 28(1):81-117. PMID: 10207686

Lucas JW, Zada G. Imaging of the pituitary and parasellar region. *Semin Neurol.* 2012;32(4):320-331. PMID: 23361479

Huang W, Molitch ME. Management of nonfunctioning pituitary adenomas (NFAs): observation. *Pituitary.* 2018;21(2):162-116. PMID: 29280025

21   ANSWER: B) Perform a macimorelin-stimulation test to assess GH levels

This patient is at risk for GH deficiency given his history of craniopharyngioma, sellar radiation therapy, and panhypopituitarism. He has signs and symptoms of GH deficiency, including increased abdominal girth, fatigue, and reduced short-term memory and attention span. In the setting of at least 3 deficient axes, the presence of a serum IGF-1 level less than 85 ng/dL (<15.1 nmol/L) is consistent with GH deficiency. However, IGF-1 can be normal or low normal in persons with GH deficiency. The next step would be to perform a provocative GH test, and of the listed answer choices, a macimorelin-stimulation test (Answer B) would be best. An insulin tolerance test would be another potential option, as would be use of glucagon.

Measuring a random GH level (Answer C) is not useful in the diagnosis of GH deficiency. Patients with GH deficiency may have mild depression, and although referral for psychiatry (Answer A) is not incorrect, addressing the underlying cause is a better first step. The patient's adequate free T_4 level suggests the current levothyroxine dosage is on target, so an increase in dosage (Answer D) is not indicated.

Educational Objective

Determine the most appropriate approach to diagnose GH deficiency.

Reference(s)

Molitch ME, Clemmons DR, Malozowski S, Merriam GR, Vance ML; Endocrine Society. Evaluation and treatment of adult growth hormone deficiency: an Endocrine Society clinical practice guideline. *J Clin Endocrinol Metab*. 2011;96(6):1587-1609. PMID: 21602453

Ramos-Leví AM, Marazuela M. Treatment of adult growth hormone deficiency with human recombinant growth hormone: an update on current evidence and critical review of advantages and pitfalls. *Endocrine*. 2018;60(2):203-218. PMID: 29417370

Garcia JM, Biller BMK, Korbonits M, et al. Macimorelin as a diagnostic test for adult GH deficiency. *J Clin Endocrinol Metab*. 2018;103(8): 3083-3093. PMID: 29860473

22   ANSWER: C) Add pegvisomant

Although studies do show that increasing the somatostatin analogue dosage (Answer A) may be beneficial, these regimens are not generally adopted. Cabergoline (Answer B) can be useful in the setting of modest acromegaly, and it may show benefit in combination with octreotide. However, this regimen is effective in less than half of patients and is unlikely to be effective in this patient with more active disease. Radiation therapy (Answer D) often takes a number of years to be effective and it is therefore unlikely to be effective within 6 months. Reoperation (Answer E) is unlikely to be effective in this case, as the tumor is in the cavernous sinus and is unlikely to be approachable surgically.

The addition of pegvisomant (Answer C) would be the most effective regimen in this timeframe. In this setting, pegvisomant is often prescribed weekly or twice weekly, in contrast to use of pegvisomant as monotherapy (prescribed daily). Because this patient has had some response to the somatostatin analogue with a partial reduction in IGF-1, it is reasonable to add the pegvisomant as combination therapy instead of switching to pegvisomant entirely.

Educational Objective

Recommend the best therapeutic approach in a patient with acromegaly who has had a partial response to adjuvant therapy with somatostatin analogue therapy.

Reference(s)

Katznelson L, Laws ER Jr, Melmed S, et al; Endocrine Society. Acromegaly: an endocrine society clinical practice guideline. *J Clin Endocrinol Metab*. 2014;99(11):3933-3951. PMID: 25356808

Giustina A, Chanson P, Kleinberg D, et al; Acromegaly Consensus Group. Expert consensus document: a consensus on the medical treatment of acromegaly. *Nat Rev Endocrinol*. 2014;10(4): 243-248. PMID: 24566817

Strasburger CJ, Mattsson A, Wilton P, et al. Increasing frequency of combination medical therapy in the treatment of acromegaly with the GH receptor antagonist pegvisomant. *Eur J Endocrinol*. 2018;178(4):321-329. PMID: 29371335

Lim DS, Fleseriu M. The role of combination medical therapy in the treatment of acromegaly. *Pituitary*. 2017;20(1):136-148. PMID: 27522663

23   ANSWER: A) Mifepristone

This patient has Cushing disease, with residual disease despite 2 attempts at transsphenoidal resection. Medical therapy is indicated. Mifepristone (Answer A) is a glucocorticoid receptor blocker that is effective in the treatment of patients with all forms of Cushing syndrome. Because it blocks the glucocorticoid receptor, cortisol and ACTH levels may actually rise during treatment (as is the case here). Mifepristone effectively improves the clinical manifestations of Cushing syndrome, as well as improves glucose control. Complications of mifepristone include edema and hypertension, most likely due to spill over of cortisol onto the mineralocorticoid receptor.

Ketoconazole (Answer B) is a steroidogenesis blocker, and it is useful for lowering cortisol. These patients are at risk for liver dysfunction, but hypertension and edema are not seen with ketoconazole. ACTH levels may rise with ketoconazole, but there is suggestion that ketoconazole may lead to stabilization of ACTH secretion. Pasireotide (Answer C) is a somatostatin analogue that can reduce ACTH secretion and lead to cortisol control in approximately 20% to 25% of patients, and it is not associated with edema and hypertension. Cabergoline (Answer D) is a dopamine agonist that may lower ACTH and cortisol in a subset of patients with Cushing disease, and it is not associated with edema and hypertension.

Educational Objective

Guide the use of mifepristone in the treatment of Cushing disease.

Reference(s)

Fleseriu M, Molitch ME, Gross C, Schteingart DE, Vaughan TB 3rd, Biller BM. A new therapeutic approach in the medical treatment of Cushing's syndrome: glucocorticoid receptor blockade with mifepristone. *Endocr Pract.* 2013;19(2):313-326. PMID: 23337135

Cuevas-Ramos D, Lim DST, Fleseriu M. Update on medical treatment for Cushing's disease. *Clin Diabetes Endocrinol.* 2016;2:16. PMID: 28702250

Fleseriu M, Biller BM, Findling JW, Molitch ME, Schteingart DE, Gross C; SEISMIC Study Investigators. Mifepristone, a glucocorticoid receptor antagonist, produces clinical and metabolic benefits in patients with Cushing's syndrome. *J Clin Endocrinol Metab.* 2012;97(6): 2039-2049. PMID: 22466348

24 ANSWER: D) ACTH

This patient is at risk for hypopituitarism given the history of radiation therapy to the sella, which results in hypopituitarism in approximately 30% to 40% of cases. She has hypothyroidism based on the low TSH and free T_4 levels, and levothyroxine replacement is indicated. This patient had a morning serum cortisol level of 9.6 µg/dL (264.8 nmol/L), which does not seem very low. However, it should be remembered that cortisol production increases 3-fold during pregnancy and cortisol-binding globulin levels are also very high, resulting in normal morning cortisol levels well above 20 µg/dL (>551.8 nmol/L). Therefore, her cortisol concentration of 9.6 µg/dL (264.8 nmol/L) is fairly low and she most likely has adrenal (ACTH) insufficiency (Answer D) and glucocorticoid replacement should be initiated. She has low gonadotropin levels, but she is taking an oral estrogen, so these values will be low accordingly. Thus, it is not possible to document hypogonadotropic hypogonadism (Answer A) at this time. She is at risk for GH deficiency. She has a low GH level, but this is not sufficient for a diagnosis of GH deficiency, and determination of a low IGF-1 value or peak GH value following a provocative test would be necessary to document GH reserve (Answer B). She does not have diabetes insipidus, so antidiuretic hormone (Answer C) is not deficient.

Educational Objective

Evaluate hypopituitarism in patients who have undergone radiation therapy.

Reference(s)

Zibar Tomšić K, Dušek T, Kraljević I, et al. Hypopituitarism after gamma knife radiosurgery for pituitary adenoma. *Endocr Res.* 2017;42(4): 318-324. PMID: 28537768

Pekic S, Popovic V. Diagnosis of endocrine disease: expanding the cause of hypopituitarism. *Eur J Endocrinol.* 2017;176(6):R269-R282. PMID: 28258131

25 ANSWER: A) Inability to lactate

This patient has Sheehan syndrome, referring to infarction of the pituitary gland after a complicated delivery with postpartum hemorrhage. The hemorrhage may be of sufficient severity to cause hypotension and require blood transfusion. When the blood loss results in hypotension and the diagnosis of Sheehan syndrome is considered, evaluation and treatment of adrenal insufficiency should be initiated. The serum cortisol level may not be severely low in such patients, as cortisol-binding globulin is elevated with pregnancy, resulting in measurement of a normal or higher total cortisol. When hypopituitarism is mild, there can be a delay in diagnosis for up to many years. When hypopituitarism is more severe, there is a failure to lactate (Answer A), which would be notable in the first days following delivery. Subsequently, menses may fail to resume (Answer D), and there may be loss of sexual hair. Affected patients may also describe fatigue, weight loss, and anorexia, possibly from adrenal insufficiency. Hypothyroidism can occur as well, although measurement of free T_4 (Answer B) and TSH may not reveal evidence of central hypothyroidism for several weeks. She will unlikely have vision loss (Answer C), as the mass does not impact the optic chiasm on imaging.

Educational Objective

Identify the endocrine sequelae of Sheehan syndrome.

Reference(s)

Diri H, Tanriverdi F, Karaca Z, et al. Extensive investigation of 114 patients with Sheehan's syndrome: a continuing disorder. *Eur J Endocrinol.* 2014;171(3):311-318. PMID: 24917653

Dökmetaş HS, Kilicli F, Korkmaz S, Yonem O. Characteristic features of 20 patients with Sheehan's syndrome. *Gynecol Endocrinol.* 2006; 22(5):279-283. PMID: 16785150

Thyroid Board Review

Elizabeth N. Pearce, MD, MSc

1 **ANSWER: B) Ultrasonography again in 12 months**

This patient has a nodule that was identified as sufficiently suspicious on ultrasound (according to the American College of Radiology TI-RADS system [Thyroid Imaging Reporting and Data System]), to require FNA biopsy. The TI-RADS system applies points to suspicious features. TI-RADS category 4 nodules (4-6 points) require FNA biopsy if they are larger than or equal to 1.5 cm. However, based on the image in this vignette, the individual who read the ultrasound has misinterpreted the echogenic foci as microcalcifications; without the microcalcifications, the nodule would be considered to be low suspicion under the TI-RADs system (TI-RADS 2) and would not require FNA biopsy. This illustrates the importance of reviewing ultrasound images rather than relying solely on reports. The TI-RADS system of classification is still relatively new, and poor interobserver reliability has been documented, particularly regarding echogenic foci other than macrocalcifications.

Colloid comets, the hyperechogenicities seen in the image, are defined by TI-RADS as echogenic foci with V-shaped echoes greater than 1 mm deep. They are associated with colloid and, when found within the cystic components of thyroid nodules, they are indicative of benign nodules. Punctate echogenic foci (microcalcifications) are smaller than macrocalcifications and may be shadowing or nonshadowing. In the solid components of thyroid nodules, they may correspond to the psammomatous calcifications associated with papillary cancers and are therefore considered highly suspicious. The TI-RADS white paper also notes that, "small echogenic foci may be seen in spongiform nodules, where they probably represent the back walls of minute cysts. They are not suspicious in this circumstance and should not add to the point total of spongiform nodules."

This nodule is most correctly classified as TI-RADS 2, for which monitoring (Answer B) would be more appropriate than FNA biopsy (Answer C). Using the American Thyroid Association criteria, similarly, this would be considered a very low suspicion nodule, which does not require FNA biopsy. Diagnostic thyroid lobectomy (Answer D) is overly aggressive. There is no indication for radioactive iodine uptake and scan (Answer A) because the patient's serum TSH level is normal.

Educational Objective

Summarize the American College of Radiology TI-RADS system for reporting thyroid ultrasound findings and identify features that are suspicious for malignancy on thyroid ultrasonography.

Reference(s)

Haugen BR, Alexander EK, Bible KC, et al. 2015 American Thyroid Association Management guidelines for adult patients with thyroid nodules and differentiated thyroid cancer: the American Thyroid Association Guidelines Task Force on Thyroid Nodules and Differentiated Thyroid Cancer. *Thyroid.* 2016;26(1):1-133. PMID: 26462967

Grant EG, Tessler FN, Hoang JK, et al. Thyroid ultrasound reporting lexicon: white paper of the ACR thyroid imaging, reporting and data system (TIRADS) committee. *J Am Coll Radiol.* 2015; 12(12 Pt A):1272-1279. PMIDL 26419308

Hoang JK, Middleton WD, Farjat AE, et al. Interobserver variability of sonographic features used in the American College of Radiology Thyroid Imaging Reporting and Data System. *AJR Am J Roentgenol.* 2018;211(1):162-167. PMID: 29702015

2 ANSWER: D) Measure serum TSH as soon as pregnancy is confirmed

Retrospective analyses suggest that pregnancy is most likely a mild stimulus to thyroid cancer growth, as evidenced by minor disease progression in some patients with known structural disease before pregnancy. However, pregnancy does not appear to cause thyroid cancer recurrence or progression in differentiated thyroid cancer survivors who have no structural or biochemical evidence of disease persistence at the time of conception.

The usefulness of following thyroglobulin values after lobectomy is more limited than after total thyroidectomy because thyroglobulin thresholds have not been defined in this patient population. However, this patient has a low and stable thyroglobulin value, with no evidence of disease on neck ultrasonography. In the absence of evidence of persistent cancer preconception, the likelihood that her cancer will progress during pregnancy is low. In general, goals for TSH suppression are not altered by pregnancy. In low-risk patients free of disease such as this one, TSH may be kept within the low-normal range in pregnancy. However, given increased thyroxine-binding globulin levels and more rapid metabolism of thyroid hormone in pregnancy, most pregnant women need levothyroxine dosage increases to maintain optimal TSH levels. Measuring serum TSH as soon as pregnancy is confirmed (Answer D) and then adjusting the levothyroxine dosage is reasonable.

TSH suppression (Answer B) is not indicated for this patient with low-risk cancer. Current guidelines recommend that neck ultrasound and thyroglobulin monitoring (Answer A) should be performed during pregnancy only in women diagnosed with well-differentiated thyroid cancer who have had a biochemically or structurally incomplete response to therapy, or in patients known to have active recurrent or residual disease. Increased frequency of fetal ultrasonography (Answer C) is not warranted on the basis of either hypothyroidism or thyroid cancer. Having a history of differentiated thyroid cancer should not inhibit an intended pregnancy (Answer E).

Educational Objective
Recommend appropriate thyroid cancer surveillance strategies in pregnant women.

Reference(s)
Haugen BR, Alexander EK, Bible KC, et al. 2015 American Thyroid Association Management guidelines for adult patients with thyroid nodules and differentiated thyroid cancer: the American Thyroid Association Guidelines Task Force on Thyroid Nodules and Differentiated Thyroid Cancer. *Thyroid*. 2016;26(1):1-133. PMID: 26462967

Alexander EK, Pearce EN, Brent GA, et al. 2017 guidelines of the American Thyroid Association for the diagnosis and management of thyroid disease during pregnancy and the postpartum. *Thyroid*. 2017;27:315-389. PMID: 28056690

Rakhlin L, Fish S. Pregnancy as a risk factor for thyroid cancer progression. *Curr Opin Endocrinol Diabetes Obes*. 2018;25(5):326-329. PMID: 29965867

3 ANSWER: A) TSH, high; free T_4, low; total T_3, low; TPO antibody, positive; TSH receptor antibody, negative (primary hypothyroidism with TPO antibody positivity)

Immune checkpoint inhibitors are cancer therapies that promote T-cell–mediated antitumoral responses. The currently available immune checkpoint inhibitors include monoclonal antibodies targeting CTLA-4 (ipilimumab, tremelimumab), PD-1 (nivolumab, pembrolizumab), and PD-L1 (durvalumab, atezolizumab, avelumab). Immune checkpoint inhibitor therapy has been associated with multiple different types of thyroid dysfunction, with rates of thyroid dysfunction as high as 35% on monotherapy and up to 65% with combination immune checkpoint inhibitor therapy, such as ipilimumab and nivolumab used in this patient. The most frequent form of immune checkpoint inhibitor–induced thyroid dysfunction is a painless destructive thyroiditis, in which transient thyrotoxicosis (typically asymptomatic) is rapidly followed by primary hypothyroidism (Answer A). TPO antibodies are positive in 54% to 80% of these patients. The thyrotoxic phase is typically mild and self-limited. In one case series, the median time from the start of immune checkpoint inhibitor therapy to thyrotoxicosis was 5.3 weeks (range, 0.6-19.6 weeks). Thyrotoxicosis lasted a median of 6 weeks (range 2.6-39.7 weeks). Hypothyroidism then developed in 84% of patients at a median of 10.4 weeks (range, 3.4-48.7 weeks) after starting immune checkpoint inhibitor therapy. The hypothyroidism may be permanent or transient; most patients will require levothyroxine therapy.

Central hypothyroidism (Answer B) from hypophysitis also occurs in up to 6% of patients treated with immune checkpoint inhibitors, but it is far less frequent than primary hypothyroidism and would not be expected to follow a thyrotoxic phase. Immune checkpoint inhibitor–induced central hypothyroidism may be either transient or permanent. Immune checkpoint inhibitor–induced Graves hyperthyroidism (Answer D) has been reported, but this is very rare. In addition, the T_3 to T_4 ratio less than 20 on the patient's initial presentation is more consistent with thyroiditis than with Graves disease. Euthyroidism (Answer C) is possible in this patient, but it is less likely than the rapid development of hypothyroidism. Given the high likelihood of immune checkpoint inhibitor–related thyroid dysfunction and the possibility of rapid evolution of thyrotoxicosis or subclinical hypothyroidism to overt hypothyroidism, close monitoring of thyroid function is recommended for all patients receiving immune checkpoint inhibitor treatment.

Educational Objective

Describe the most frequently observed thyroidal consequences of immune checkpoint inhibitor therapy.

Reference(s)

Chang LS, Barroso-Sousa R, Tolaney SM, Hodi FS, Kaiser UB, Min L. Endocrine toxicity of cancer immunotherapy targeting immune checkpoints. *Endocr Rev.* 2019;40(1):17-65. PMID: 30184160

Iyer PC, Cabanillas ME, Waguespack SG, et al. Immune-related thyroiditis with immune checkpoint inhibitors. *Thyroid.* 2018;28(10):1243-1251. PMID: 30132401

Patel NS, Oury A, Daniels GA, Bazhenova L, Patel SP. Incidence of thyroid function test abnormalities in patients receiving immune-checkpoint inhibitors for cancer treatment. *Oncologist.* 2018;23(10):1236-1241. PMID: 29769383

4 Answer C) Change the levothyroxine dosage to 875 mcg weekly in an observed setting

Most hypothyroid patients require a levothyroxine dosage of approximately 1.6 mcg/kg body weight daily to normalize serum TSH. When dosage requirements escalate, or when unusually high dosage requirements are observed, the cause should be investigated. Potential reasons for high levothyroxine requirements include concomitant use of other medications that can interfere with levothyroxine absorption (eg, calcium, iron, raloxifene, proton-pump inhibitors, cholestyramine), use of medications that increase thyroxine-binding globulin (eg, estrogen, selective estrogen receptor modulators), use of medications that increase levothyroxine metabolism (phenytoin, phenobarbital), malabsorption (celiac sprue, short bowel syndrome), or nonadherence to the treatment regimen. Occasionally, patients who report taking their levothyroxine consistently in fact have "pseudomalabsorption"—medication nonadherence to which they do not admit. Formal levothyroxine absorption testing can determine whether levothyroxine malabsorption is truly present. While optimal thresholds for normal levothyroxine absorption testing have not been validated, the literature suggests that when malabsorption is not present, serum free T_4 should peak 2 hours after ingestion of 1000 mcg of levothyroxine, often rising above the upper reference limit, as was the case in this patient. Taking a weekly, weight-based dose of levothyroxine in a supervised setting (Answer C) has been shown to be safe and to improve serum TSH values in patients with longstanding medication nonadherence.

Because testing has ruled out malabsorption as the cause of this patient's persistent TSH elevations, changing to a gluten-free diet (Answer D) is unlikely to improve her thyroid hormone levels. Increasing her levothyroxine dosage (Answer A) or adding liothyronine (Answer B) would most likely cause thyrotoxicosis if she actually took her thyroid hormone, but it would not change her TSH if she had continued nonadherence.

Educational Objective

Diagnose and treat levothyroxine pseudomalabsorption.

Reference(s)

Walker JN, Shillo P, Ibbotson V, et al. A thyroxine absorption test followed by weekly thyroxine administration: a method to assess non-adherence to treatment. *Eur J Endocrinol.* 2013; 168(6):913-917. PMID: 23554450

Srinivas V, Oyibo SO. Levothyroxine pseudomalabsorption and thyroxine absorption testing with use of high-dose levothyroxine: case report and discussion. *Endocr Pract.* 2010;16(6):1012-1015. PMID: 21041167

5 Answer A) Tumor size increase of at least 3 mm

In this vignette, a solitary microcarcinoma was identified. The patient has no evidence of metastatic disease. The risk of tumor persistence or recurrence in unifocal, intrathyroidal micropapillary carcinoma (tumor size ≤1 cm) is extremely low—on the order of 1% to 2%. The risk for tumor-related mortality is essentially zero. The American Thyroid Association guidelines recommend against FNA biopsy for nodules smaller than 1 cm. However, having diagnosed this patient's micropapillary carcinoma, there is a need to determine the best course of action. An active surveillance approach instead of immediate surgery can be considered in carefully selected patients and in appropriate settings. Ideal patients for this approach include euthyroid older individuals (since tumor progression is more likely in patients younger than 40 years) who have papillary microcarcinomas without known metastases or local invasion, and whose tumor is not adjacent to the thyroid capsule or the recurrent laryngeal nerve. Patients must be comfortable with the concept of following a low-risk cancer rather than pursuing immediate intervention, and must be willing to return for follow-up visits. The availability of high-quality neck ultrasonography is essential.

Cohort studies have demonstrated that among carefully selected patients undergoing active surveillance, clinically significant tumor growth occurs in only 10% to 15%. Protocols for active surveillance typically call for neck ultrasonography and TSH testing every 6 months, with the follow-up period extended to 12 months if the tumor size remains stable for 2 years. Proceeding to thyroid surgery is warranted for a tumor size increase of at least 3 mm (Answer A), new neck node metastases, a tumor size increase to at least 12 mm, or a tumor volume increase of at least 50% (not

100%, as in Answer B). Serum thyroglobulin values (Answers C and D) are not helpful in active surveillance protocols.

Educational Objective

Guide appropriate patient selection and strategies for active surveillance of micropapillary thyroid cancer.

Reference(s)

Tuttle RM, Fagin JA, Minkowitz G, et al. Natural history and tumor volume kinetics of papillary thyroid cancers during active surveillance. *JAMA Otolaryngol Head Neck Surg.* 2017;143(10):1015-1020. PMID: 28859191

Brito JP, Ito Y, Miyauchi A, Tuttle RM. A clinical framework to facilitate risk stratification when considering an active surveillance alternative to immediate biopsy and surgery in papillary microcarcinoma. *Thyroid.* 2016;26(1):144-149. PMID: 26414743

Kim TY, Shong YK. Active surveillance of papillary thyroid microcarcinoma: a mini-review from Korea. *Endocrinol Metab (Seoul).* 2017;32(4): 399-406. PMID: 29271613

6 ANSWER: E) Thyroid lobectomy

This patient has a thyroid nodule with indeterminate cytopathology that is known to be *RAS* positive. The *RAS* positivity confers an 80% probability of either a low-risk cancer or noninvasive follicular thyroid neoplasm with papillary-like nuclear features (NIFTP). Preoperatively, the FNA cytology of NIFTPs is most often read as Bethesda III (atypia of uncertain significance/follicular lesion of uncertain significance), Bethesda IV (follicular neoplasm/suspicious for follicular neoplasm), or Bethesda V (suspicious for malignancy). The most typical ultrasound findings in NIFTP are similar to those seen in this patient, with most nodules being wider-than-tall, hypervascular, isoechoic with smooth borders, and having no calcifications. On mutational analysis, NIFTP is most often positive for *RAS* and negative for *BRAF* V600E. However, ultrasonography, cytologic, and molecular marker testing cannot reliably distinguish NIFTP from the encapsulated/well-circumscribed follicular variant of papillary thyroid cancer. Diagnosis of NIFTP requires surgical resection with complete evaluation of the tumor capsule to exclude the presence of capsular invasion. Therefore, performing ultrasonography in 6 months (Answer D) is incorrect. Because *RAS*-associated thyroid malignancies (in the absence of additional mutations such as in the *TERT* gene) are typically relatively indolent, even if this were found to be a cancer, completion thyroidectomy might not be required and lobectomy (Answer E), rather than total thyroidectomy, is a reasonable choice despite the nodule size of greater than 4 cm.

Additional molecular marker testing (Answer A) will not provide a definitive diagnosis. Radioactive iodine scan (Answer B) would not help to distinguish between a benign or a malignant nodule in this patient and is not indicated. Flow cytometry (Answer C) is useful in the setting of suspected thyroid lymphoma, but it will not provide useful information here.

Educational Objective

Explain how the new diagnostic category of noninvasive follicular thyroid neoplasm with papillary-like nuclear features influences interpretation of cytopathology and molecular markers.

Reference(s)

Lloyd RV, Asa SL, LiVolsi VA, et al. The evolving diagnosis of noninvasive follicular thyroid neoplasm with papillary-like nuclear features (NIFTP). *Hum Pathol.* 2018;74:1-4. PMID: 29339178

Nishino M, Nikiforova M. Update on molecular testing for cytologically indeterminate thyroid nodules. *Arch Pathol Lab Med.* 2018;142(4):446-457. PMID: 29336606

Kim M, Jeon MJ, Oh HS, et al. BRAF and RAS mutational status in noninvasive follicular thyroid neoplasm with papillary-like nuclear features and invasive subtype of encapsulated follicular variant of papillary thyroid carcinoma in Korea. *Thyroid.* 2018;28(4):504-510. PMID: 29439609

7 Answer E) Perceived benefit of the change

About 10% of levothyroxine-treated hypothyroid patients report feeling unwell despite having normal serum TSH values. In overtly hypothyroid patients, the initiation of levothyroxine therapy is associated with modest weight loss that tends to be transient and is most likely largely due to diuresis rather than to changes in fat mass. Patients often anticipate that a levothyroxine dosage that results in lower TSH levels within the normal range may assist with weight loss or otherwise improve quality of life. A randomized controlled trial has demonstrated that patients were unable to detect differences in the symptoms associated with hypothyroidism when the levothyroxine dosage was changed by approximately 20%. More recently, another randomized clinical trial that examined the effects of variations in TSH within or just above the normal range in levothyroxine-treated patients concluded that body composition (including visceral and total fat [Answer B]), resting energy expenditure (Answer C), total energy expenditure, the thermic effect of food, physical activity energy expenditure, and daily energy intake did not vary by treatment group. The same trial did not report any differences in quality of life, mood (Answer A), or cognition (Answer D) based on target TSH group. Interestingly, although trial participants were blinded to their treatment and were unable to accurately determine how their levothyroxine dosages had been adjusted, they preferred levothyroxine dosages they perceived to be higher. Thus, levothyroxine-treated patients may prefer perceived higher levothyroxine dosages (Answer E) despite a lack of objective benefit. Current guidelines simply recommend targeting a serum TSH value within the reference range in levothyroxine-treated patients and note that additional research is needed to determine whether it is useful to adjust the levothyroxine dosage within the goal reference range for residual hypothyroid signs and symptoms.

Educational Objective

Counsel patients about anticipated clinical outcomes when levothyroxine dosages are adjusted to obtain TSH values within the reference range.

Reference(s)

Samuels MH, Kolobova I, Niederhausen M, Purnell JQ, Schuff KG. Effects of altering levothyroxine dose on energy expenditure and body composition in subjects treated with LT4. *J Clin Endocrinol Metab.* 2018;103(11):4163-4175. PMID: 30165520

Samuels MH, Kolobova I, Niederhausen M, Janowsky JS, Schuff KG. Effects of altering levothyroxine (L-T4) doses on quality of life, mood, and cognition in L-T4 treated subjects. *J Clin Endocrinol Metab.* 2018;103(5):1997-2008. PMID: 29509918

Jonklaas J, Bianco AC, Bauer AJ; American Thyroid Association Task Force on Thyroid Hormone Replacement. Guidelines for the treatment of hypothyroidism: prepared by the American Thyroid Association Task Force on Thyroid Hormone Replacement. *Thyroid.* 2014;24(12):1670-1751. PMID: 25266427

Walsh JP, Ward LC, Burke V, et al. Small changes in thyroxine dosage do not produce measurable changes in hypothyroid symptoms, wellbeing, or quality of life: results of a double-blind, randomized clinical trial. *J Clin Endocrinol Metab* 2006;91:2624-2630. PMID: 16670161

8 ANSWER: C) Treatment with ^{131}I, 30 mCI; initial TSH goal, 0.1-0.5 mIU/L

This patient has thyroid cancer that can be staged as American Joint Committee on Cancer 8th edition T3a(s)N1bMx or American Thyroid Association intermediate risk. She has a unifocal tumor larger than 4 cm with involvement of more than 5 cervical lymph nodules that are all smaller than 3 cm and has no evidence of distant metastases. Her risk for disease persistence or recurrence is approximately 20%.

Patients with intermediate-risk tumors are those with microscopic extrathyroidal extension, vascular invasion, aggressive histologic features, or, as is the case in this patient, metastases in the neck. The American Thyroid Association guidelines state that radioactive iodine therapy should be considered after total thyroidectomy in patients with intermediate-risk differentiated thyroid cancer. The primary goal of this treatment is to ablate any remaining normal thyroid tissue remnant, which will facilitate detection of recurrent or persistent disease. Although the evidence for benefit in patients with intermediate-risk cancer is less clear than that for patients with high-risk cancer, the literature suggests that radioiodine treatment may improve overall and disease-specific survival, as well as disease-free survival, in patients with nodal metastases who are 45 years or older and in those whose primary tumor is larger than 4 cm. Radioactive iodine ablation has been associated with decreased risk for both tumor recurrence and disease-specific mortality in patients with high-risk tumors (those with gross extrathyroidal extension, incomplete tumor resection, and known distant metastases or postoperative thyroglobulin levels suggesting distant metastasis). In patients determined to have low-risk tumors according to the American Thyroid Association criteria, radioactive iodine ablation has not been shown to reduce the risk for disease recurrence or mortality and is not routinely recommended.

An initial goal of mild TSH suppression (0.1-0.5 mIU/L) (Answer C) is typically recommended for patients with intermediate-risk disease, while patients who are at high risk should have full TSH suppression (TSH <0.1 mIU/L) (Answers D and E) as the initial goal of levothyroxine therapy. Patients with low-risk tumors do not require TSH-suppressive therapy, and the appropriate initial TSH goal in this group is in the low-normal range (0.5-2.0 mIU/L) (Answers A and B).

Answer C would provide an ablative dose of radioactive iodine and an appropriate level of initial TSH suppression for a patient with intermediate-risk disease. Answers D and E, with high-dose radioactive iodine treatment and full TSH suppression, are overly aggressive for this patient. While she does not absolutely require radioactive iodine treatment, she is at high enough risk to warrant mild TSH suppression.

Educational Objective
Manage American Thyroid Association intermediate-risk differentiated thyroid cancer postoperatively.

Reference(s)

Haugen BR, Alexander EK, Bible KC, et al. 2015 American Thyroid Association Management guidelines for adult patients with thyroid nodules and differentiated thyroid cancer: the American Thyroid Association Guidelines Task Force on Thyroid Nodules and Differentiated Thyroid Cancer. *Thyroid.* 2016;26(1):1-133. PMID: 26462967

Ruel E, Thomas S, Dinan M, Perkins JM, Roman SA, Sosa JA. Adjuvant radioactive iodine therapy is associated with improved survival for patients with intermediate-risk papillary thyroid cancer. *J Clin Endocrinol Metab.* 2015;100(4):1529-1536. PMID: 25642591

9 ANSWER: D) Vandetanib therapy

The tyrosine kinase inhibitors are a group of drugs that affect several proteins involved in the modulation of cell growth (*see table*). Receptor kinases are involved in both normal cellular function and pathologic processes such as oncogenesis, metastasis, tumor angiogenesis, and maintenance of the tumor microenvironment. Tyrosine kinase inhibitors are small, orally active molecules that inhibit phosphorylation of tyrosine molecules at key ATP-binding sites. Affected targets include VEGF receptors 2 and 3, platelet-derived growth factor receptor, Flt-3, c-kit, and RET. On the basis of phase III trials showing beneficial effects, 2 tyrosine kinase inhibitors, vandetanib (Answer D) and cabozantinib, have been approved for treatment of medullary thyroid cancer in patients with extensive local disease or distant metastases. Although complete remissions are very rare with these agents, disease stabilization and prolongation of progression-free survival have been found when compared with placebo (30.5 vs 19.3 months for vandetanib; 11.2 vs 4 months for cabozantinib in phase III trials). Palliative therapy is another option in this patient, given the limited, albeit improved, response duration for tyrosine kinase inhibitors.

There is no role for radioactive iodine therapy (Answer A) in medullary cancer. Cytotoxic chemotherapy (Answer B) has been applied to therapy for metastatic medullary thyroid cancer, with limited utility; most regimens involve dacarbazine combined with a second agent. Focal radiotherapy (Answer C) will not delay the systemic progression of metastatic disease in this patient. There is no role for somatostatin analogue therapy (Answer E) in this case.

TABLE. Tyrosine Kinase Inhibitors Currently Approved for Use in Advanced Thyroid Cancer.

Tyrosine Kinase Inhibitor	Type of Thyroid Cancer	Effectiveness: Progression-Free Survival Compared With Placebo*
Vandetanib	Medullary	30.5 vs 19.3 months
Cabozantinib	Medullary	11.2 vs 4 months
Sorafanib	Differentiated	10.8 vs 5.8 months
Lenvatinib	Differentiated	18.3 vs 3.6 months

*Note: enrolled populations were different; efficacy cannot be compared directly across studies. Many other multikinase inhibitors are currently being investigated for use in advanced thyroid cancer.

Larotrectinib, an inhibitor of neurotrophic receptor tyrosine kinase (NTRK) gene fusions, is newly approved by the US FDA for patients with an identified *NTRK* gene fusion in metastatic or unresectable solid tumors, without known resistance mutations, and who exhibit progression despite standard therapy. *NRTK* mutations may occur in 1% to 2% of papillary thyroid cancers.

Educational Objective
List indications for tyrosine kinase inhibitor therapy in advanced medullary thyroid cancer.

Reference(s)
Agrawal VR, Jodon G, Mushtaq R, Bowles DW. Update on multikinase inhibitor therapy for differentiated thyroid cancer. *Drugs Today (Barc).* 2018;54(9):535-545. PMID: 30303494

Wells SA Jr, Asa SL, Dralle H, et al; American Thyroid Association Guidelines Task Force on Medullary Thyroid Carcinoma. Revised American Thyroid Association guidelines for the management of medullary thyroid carcinoma. *Thyroid.* 2015;25(6):567-610. PMID: 25810047

Valerio L, Pieruzzi L, Giani C, et al. Targeted therapy in thyroid cancer: state of the art. *Clin Oncol (R Coll Radiol).* 2017;29(5):316-324. PMID: 28318881

Drilon A, Laetsch TW, Kummar S, et al. Efficacy of larotrectinib in TRK fusion-positive cancers in adults and children. *N Engl J Med.* 2018;378(8):731-739. PMID: 29466156

10 ANSWER: A) <3%

The image shows a spongiform nodule with clearly defined margins. This ultrasound pattern strongly suggests that the nodule is benign. Because of the low risk for malignancy in these nodules, current American Thyroid Association guidelines recommend consideration of FNA biopsy for spongiform nodules 2 cm or larger, but note that these can also be observed without proceeding with FNA biopsy. Intermediate suspicion patterns (Answer B) associated with a 10% to 20% risk of malignancy include hypoechoic nodules with smooth margins but without microcalcifications, extrathyroidal extension, or a taller-than-wide shape. Nodules with a high risk of malignancy (Answer D) include those that are hypoechoic with irregular margins, microcalcifications, a taller-than-wide shape, or evidence of extrathyroidal extension. There is no currently defined ultrasonographic pattern associated with a 20% to 40% risk for malignancy (Answer C).

Educational Objective

Interpret the malignancy risk associated with different thyroid ultrasonographic patterns.

Reference(s)

Haugen BR, Alexander EK, Bible KC, et al. 2015 American Thyroid Association Management guidelines for adult patients with thyroid nodules and differentiated thyroid cancer: the American Thyroid Association Guidelines Task Force on Thyroid Nodules and Differentiated Thyroid Cancer. *Thyroid.* 2016;26(1):1-133. PMID: 26462967

Brito JP, Gionfriddo MR, Al Nofal A, et al. The accuracy of thyroid nodule ultrasound to predict thyroid cancer: systematic review and meta-analysis. *J Clin Endocrinol Metab.* 2014;99(4): 1253-1263. PMID: 24276450

11 ANSWER: B) Stop liothyronine and increase the levothyroxine dosage to 150 mcg daily

This patient's recent prepregnancy TSH value was normal. However, most women require an increase of 25% to 30% in thyroid hormone dosages with pregnancy, due largely to increased thyroxine-binding globulin levels. The goal of therapy in the first trimester is a TSH concentration less than 2.5 mIU/L. Whether the levothyroxine/liothyronine combination therapy improves quality of life in selected patients remains controversial. However, levothyroxine/liothyronine combination therapy is not recommended for pregnant women because it is primarily maternal T_4, not T_3, which crosses the placenta. Therefore, normalizing maternal TSH on combination therapy could potentially result in fetal hypothyroxinemia (thus, Answers A, C, and D are incorrect). In converting from levothyroxine/liothyronine to levothyroxine therapy (Answer B), it is important to remember that liothyronine is approximately 3 times more potent metabolically than levothyroxine.

Educational Objective

Recommend appropriate thyroid hormone replacement in early pregnancy.

Reference(s)

Jonklaas J, Bianco AC, Bauer AJ, et al. Guidelines for the treatment of hypothyroidism: prepared by the American Thyroid Association task force on thyroid hormone replacement. *Thyroid.* 2014; 24(12):1670-1751. PMID: 25266247

Yassa L, Marqusee E, Fawcett R, Alexander EK. Thyroid hormone early adjustment in pregnancy (the THERAPY) trial. *J Clin Endocrinol Metab.* 2010;95(7):3234-3241. PMID: 20463094

Calvo RM, Jauniaux E, Gulbis B, et al. Fetal tissues are exposed to biologically relevant free thyroxine concentrations during early phases of development. *J Clin Endocrinol Metab.* 2002; 87(4):1768-1777. PMID: 11932315

12 ANSWER: C) Thyroid lobectomy

All of the options provided could achieve euthyroidism in this patient with a toxic adenoma. However, if she opts for therapy with antithyroid medication (Answer B) she will be committed to lifelong treatment since toxic nodules do not remit. Thyroid lobectomy for toxic adenoma (Answer C) results in a high cure rate (treatment failure of <1%) with only a 2% to 3% risk for postoperative hypothyroidism. Radioactive iodine treatment for toxic adenoma (Answer A) results in a higher risk for hypothyroidism than does thyroid lobectomy, with progressively increasing rates of hypothyroidism that approach 60% at 20 years. The risk for posttreatment hypothyroidism is higher in patients with underlying thyroid autoimmunity, as is the case in this patient who is TPO antibody positive. Ethanol injection (Answer D) is not routinely recommended as a treatment for toxic adenoma because of high rates of thyroid pain and other complications. Finally, radiofrequency ablation (Answer E) is potentially appealing for this patient due to low reported complication rates and a very low risk for permanent hypothyroidism. However, this technique is relatively new and is not routinely being used in the United States.

Educational Objective

Summarize factors in decision-making regarding available treatment modalities for toxic nodules.

Reference(s)

Bonnema SJ, Hegedüs L. Radioiodine therapy in benign thyroid diseases: effects, side effects, and factors affecting therapeutic outcome. *Endocr Rev.* 2012;33(6):920-980. PMID: 22961916

Ross DS, Burch HB, Cooper DS, et al. 2016 American Thyroid Association guidelines for diagnosis and management of hyperthyroidism and other causes of thyrotoxicosis. *Thyroid.* 2016;26(10):1343-1421. PMID: 27521067

13 ANSWER: A) Start propranolol

The key to this question is recognizing that the case represents thyroid hormone resistance and that because of variable tissue sensitivity to thyroid hormone in this setting, the patient has symptomatic cardiac effects, which are amenable to treatment with a β-adrenergic blocker (Answer A). Thyroid hormone resistance occurs in approximately 1 in 40,000 live births. Thyroid hormone effects are seen at the cellular level through interaction with nuclear receptors including THR-α and THR-β. Patients with thyroid hormone resistance most frequently are heterozygous for a defect in THR-β, which presents with elevated serum TSH, free T_4, and free T_3 levels. Symptoms are due to a combination of low thyroid hormone action in predominantly THR-β–expressing tissues (such as the liver) and TH overexposure in THR-α–expressing tissues (such as the heart, skeletal muscle, and brain). Goiter and tachycardia, as seen in this patient, are common presenting symptoms (*see table*).

This disorder presents with discordant TSH and free T_4 values, but there is a differential diagnosis to be considered, which includes a TSH-secreting pituitary adenoma; TSH or free T_4 assay interference; and medications such as amiodarone, which this patient is not taking. In this vignette, the α-subunit to TSH molar ratio less than 1.0 favors thyroid hormone resistance rather than a TSH-producing pituitary tumor (the MRI is also normal and most TSH-secreting tumors are macroadenomas). Heterophile antibodies may cause a falsely elevated TSH value in a patient with thyrotoxicosis, but this interference was eliminated by the test results provided.

The goals of treatment for patients with resistance to thyroid hormone are to improve the symptoms that are caused by excessive THR-α signaling, while minimizing symptoms caused by deficient THR-β signaling. Of the options provided in this case, the best is to proceed with treatment with β-adrenergic blockade to reduce the palpitations. Other approaches such radioiodine (Answer C) and thyroidectomy (Answer D) would not be beneficial. They would cause hypothyroidism, which would be challenging to treat because the supraphysiologic levothyroxine dosing that would be required to achieve euthyroidism in THR-β–sensitive tissues would cause hyperthyroidism in the THR-α–sensitive tissues. Use of methimazole (Answer B) would most likely improve palpitations, but it would worsen symptoms caused by deficient THR-β signaling.

Because he has symptomatic cardiac involvement, no treatment (Answer E) is also incorrect.

TABLE. Clinical Features of Thyroid Hormone Resistance

Sign or Symptom	Frequency
Thyroid	
Goiter	66%-95%
Heart	
Tachycardia	33%-75%
Nervous system	
Emotional disturbance	60%
Attention deficit	40%-60%
Hearing loss	10%-22%
Growth and development	
Short stature	18%-25%

Data derived from Refetoff S, Dumitrescu AM. Syndromes of reduced sensitivity to thyroid hormone: genetic defects in hormone receptors, cell transporters and deiodination. *Best Pract Res Clin Endocrinol Metab*. 2007;21(2):277-305.

Educational Objective

Diagnose thyroid hormone resistance and treat variable tissue sensitivity.

Reference(s)

Dumitrescu AM, Refetoff S. The syndromes of reduced sensitivity to thyroid hormone. *Biochim Biophys Acta*. 2013;1830(7):3987-4003. PMID: 22986150

Refetoff S, Dumitrescu AM. Syndromes of reduced sensitivity to thyroid hormone: genetic defects in hormone receptors, cell transporters and deiodination. *Best Pract Res Clin Endocrinol Metab*. 2007;21(2):277-305. PMID: 17574009

14 ANSWER: C) Suppressed serum TSH level

Drug-induced thyrotoxicosis, which occurs in up to 5% of patients treated with amiodarone, can present both diagnostic and therapeutic challenges. The diagnostic uncertainty is due to the dramatic effects that amiodarone has on thyroid function, even in euthyroid patients. A large iodine load is delivered with each dose (74 mg total iodine, 7.4 mg of free iodine per 200-mg tablet). Further, amiodarone inhibits both peripheral and central (intrapituitary) conversion of T_4 to T_3 through its action on type 1 deiodinase (DIO1) and type 2 $5'$-monodeiodinase (DIO2) enzymes, respectively. Amiodarone also has T_3 antagonistic effects at the nuclear level. The common pattern seen in euthyroid patients is a high free T_4, high total T_4, low-normal T_3, and high-normal TSH. Because of the potent inhibition of DIO2 and DIO1, either a suppressed TSH level or an elevated (rather than low) T_3 level is suggestive of amiodarone-induced thyrotoxicosis. An undetectable TSH value in this patient (Answer C) would be the most accurate indicator of thyrotoxicosis. An elevated total T_4 level (Answer A) or free T_4 level (Answer B), as noted, can occur in euthyroid individuals. The radioactive iodine uptake (Answer D) is expected to be lower than normal even in a euthyroid patient on amiodarone because of the large iodine load. The free T_4 level is higher than expected (in the mid- to high-normal range), but this is not as helpful as the undetectable TSH value. Clinical signs and symptoms (Answer E) are insufficiently specific to make this diagnosis.

Educational Objective

Identify the pattern of thyroid function test results in patients with amiodarone-induced thyrotoxicosis.

Reference(s)

Trohman RG, Sharma PS, McAninch EA, Bianco AC. Amiodarone and the thyroid physiology, pathophysiology, diagnosis and management. *Trends Cardiovasc Med*. 2019;29(5):285-295. PMID: 30309693

Basaria S, Cooper DS. Amiodarone and the thyroid. *Am J Med*. 2005;118(7):706-714. PMID: 15989900

15 ANSWER: E) Increase the levothyroxine dosage to 88 mcg daily

This patient has central hypothyroidism due to her previous pituitary surgery. It is important to recognize that patients with central hypothyroidism may secrete a bioinactive form of TSH; in this case, serum free T_4 is low and TSH is either normal or slightly elevated. In such patients, the serum TSH may drop precipitously when even low-dosage levothyroxine is initiated. The goal of therapy in central hypothyroidism is a free T_4 value in the upper half of the reference range. Discontinuing or reducing the levothyroxine dosage (Answers A and B) is incorrect because this patient's hypothyroidism is already undertreated. In the single study examining this topic to date, there was no added benefit of combination levothyroxine/liothyronine therapy (Answer C) in patients with secondary hypothyroidism when compared with outcomes of patients treated with adequate dosages of levothyroxine alone. Continuing the current levothyroxine dosage and increasing the hydrocortisone dosage (Answer D) would not adequately treat her underlying hyperthyroidism.

Educational Objective

Use free T_4 values rather than TSH values for therapeutic targets in the management of central hypothyroidism.

Reference(s)

Persani L. Clinical review: central hypothyroidism: pathogenic, diagnostic, and therapeutic challenges. *J Clin Endocrinol Metab.* 2012;97(9): 3068-3078. PMID: 22851492

Chaker L, Bianco AC, Jonklaas J, Peeters RP. Hypothyroidism. *Lancet.* 2017;390(10101): 1550-1562. PMID: 28336049

Jonklaas J, Bianco AC, Bauer AJ, et al; American Thyroid Association Task Force on Thyroid Hormone Replacement. Guidelines for the treatment of hypothyroidism: prepared by the American Thyroid Association Task Force on Thyroid Hormone Replacement. *Thyroid.* 2014; 24(12):1670-1751. PMID: 25266247

16 ANSWER: B) Repeated blood tests after stopping biotin for 7 days

The recommended daily intake for biotin is 300 mcg daily, but dosages that are orders of magnitude higher than requirements are available in many nutritional supplements. The use of biotin supplements can cause artifactual interference with commonly used biotin-streptavidin immunoassays for TSH, thyroid hormone, and TSH receptor antibodies. High circulating biotin levels cause falsely low measurements in immunometric sandwich assays (such as that for TSH), but falsely high measurements for competitive immunoassays (such as those for free T_4, T_3, and thyroid-stimulating immunoglobulin [Answer D]). Thus, euthyroid patients taking biotin may have laboratory results identical to those found in Graves hyperthyroidism. Artifactual thyroid function results have been reported in patients taking at least 1500 mcg of biotin daily. Test results normalize 2 to 7 days after stopping the biotin. Therefore, the best next step is to repeat blood tests after stopping biotin for 7 days (Answer B).

Radioactive iodine uptake and scan (Answer A) would be diagnostic if this patient truly had Graves disease, but it would not be warranted if his blood tests normalize after ceasing biotin. Finally, starting methimazole (Answer C) will not be indicated if this patient's laboratory values normalize once off biotin.

Educational Objective

Describe the potential for biotin interference with thyroid function assays.

Reference(s)

Kummer S, Hermsen D, Distelmaier F. Biotin treatment mimicking Graves' disease. *N Engl J Med.* 2016;375(7):704-706. PMID: 27532849

Elston MS, Sehgal S, Du Toit S, Yarndley T, Conaglen JV. Factitious Graves' disease due to biotin immunoassay interference-a case and review of the literature. *J Clin Endocrinol Metab.* 2016;101(9):3251-3255. PMID: 27362288

17 ANSWER: C) TSH, 0.2 mIU/L; total T_4, 2.5 µg/dL (SI: 31.2 nmol/L); total T_3, 25 ng/dL (SI: 0.4 nmol/L); free T_4, 0.5 ng/dL (SI: 6.4 pmol/L)

This patient has been admitted to the intensive care unit for sepsis and multiorgan failure and his condition is deteriorating. He would be expected to have the classic changes in thyroid hormone levels that occur as a result of an acute nonthyroidal illness of this severity. The most prevalent and pronounced change of thyroid function during nonthyroidal illness is a low T_3 level, present in 70% or more of hospitalized patients, and it may be considered, with a few notable exceptions, the sine qua non of euthyroid sick syndrome. Total T_4 is frequently low in patients with severe nonthyroidal illness and a very low T_4 portends a poor prognosis. Free T_4 generally remains in the normal range, but may be frankly low in gravely ill or moribund patients, such as the patient in this case. TSH is frequently normal early in illness, but it may also be suppressed in critical illness and then elevated during the recovery stages (generally it is <20 mIU/L). Using the process of elimination, only Answers B and C have a low T_3 value. Answer B has a slightly elevated serum TSH level, which can be seen in the recovery stage after a nonthyroidal illness, but this patient is unfortunately not recovering. Answer C, with more severe alterations in T_3, as well as depressions in both total and free T$_4$, is a better fit for this particular moribund patient.

Educational Objective

Identify expected thyroid function test patterns in the recovery from severe nonthyroidal illness.

Reference(s)

Farwell AP. Nonthyroidal illness syndrome. *Curr Opin Endocrinol Diabetes Obes.* 2013;20(5):478-484. PMID: 23974778

Van den Berghe G. Non-thyroidal illness in the ICU: a syndrome with different faces. *Thyroid.* 2014;24(10):1456-1465. PMID: 24845024

18   ANSWER: B) Figure B

The sample presented in Figure B (Answer B) shows typical features of papillary thyroid cancer, including nuclear overlap and inclusions. Figure A shows a colloid nodule, Figure C shows adenomatous hyperplasia, and Figure D shows cystic fluid with macrophages. Cytopathology of papillary cancers typically demonstrates large, nonuniform cells with sparse or absent colloid. Nuclei are large and may contain clefts or holes ("Orphan Annie eyes") due to intranuclear cytoplasmic inclusions. The cytoplasm has a "ground-glass" appearance. Psammoma bodies, small laminated calcifications, may be present. Benign nodules (Answer A, Bethesda I) typically include abundant colloid, which stains blue on a Papanicolaou stain. Cells in benign nodules generally have a uniform appearance and are not crowded; microfollicles and macrofollicles may be present. Cyst fluid (Answer D) typically contains relatively few cells, but cellular debris and hemosiderin-laden macrophages may be seen. Adenomatous hyperplasia (Answer C) is characterized by the presence of abundant colloid and a variable number of follicular cells; the follicular cells are predominately arranged in flat sheets with a honeycomb configuration. Nuclei have a uniform appearance and there is minimal nuclear overlapping and crowding.

Educational Objective

Explain classic features of papillary carcinoma on thyroid cytopathology.

Reference(s)

Papanicolaou Society of Cytopathology. Online Image Atlas. Available at: http://www.papsociety.com/atlas.html.

19   ANSWER: A) Repeat thyroid function tests in 6 months

Subclinical hyperthyroidism, in which serum TSH values are low but peripheral thyroid hormone is normal, is relatively common, affecting approximately 1.5% of the US adult population. About 5% of patients progress to overt hyperthyroidism, an outcome that is more likely when TSH is fully suppressed. Up to one-third of patients with subclinical hyperthyroidism spontaneously become euthyroid again; this is most common when the underlying cause of their hyperthyroidism is Graves disease and when the baseline TSH level is between 0.1 and 0.4 mIU/L. Subclinical hyperthyroidism has been associated with increased risk for all-cause and cardiovascular mortality, atrial fibrillation, osteoporosis, and fracture. However, there is currently limited evidence for treatment benefit, particularly in younger individuals, and treatment confers some risks. Current guidelines recommend observation (Answer A) rather than treatment (Answers C, D, and E) for asymptomatic patients younger than 65 years who do not have cardiac disease or osteoporosis in whom the TSH is persistently lower than normal but 0.1 mIU/L or greater. β-adrenergic blockade (Answer B) might be useful in the setting of hyperthyroid symptoms or tachycardia, but this patient has neither.

Educational Objective

List indications for treatment of subclinical hyperthyroidism.

Reference(s)

Ross DS, Burch HB, Cooper DS, et al. 2016 American Thyroid Association guidelines for diagnosis and management of hyperthyroidism and other causes of thyrotoxicosis. *Thyroid.* 2016;26(10):1343-1421. PMID: 27521067

Carle A, Andersen SL, Boelaert K, Laurberg P. Management of endocrine disease: subclinical thyrotoxicosis: prevalence, causes and choice of therapy. *Eur J Endocrinol.* 2017;176(6):R325-R337. PMID: 28274949

Vadiveloo T, Donnan PT, Cochrane L, Leese GP. The Thyroid Epidemiology, Audit, and Research Study (TEARS): the natural history of endogenous subclinical hyperthyroidism. *J Clin Endocrinol Metab.* 2011;96(1):E1-E8. PMID: 20926532

20 ANSWER: C) Familial dysalbuminemic hyperthyroxinemia

Familial dysalbuminemic hyperthyroxinemia (Answer C) is the most common inherited form of hyperthyroxinemia. It is found in 0.1% to 1.8% of individuals and is most common in Hispanic populations. Patients with familial dysalbuminemic hyperthyroxinemia are frequently overlooked with the widespread measurement of TSH alone to screen for thyroid dysfunction. Although free T_4 by equilibrium dialysis yields normal values in patients with familial dysalbuminemic hyperthyroxinemia, many free T_4 assays that are more susceptible to binding-protein changes give spurious elevations in free T_4, due to the altered protein binding (*see figure*).

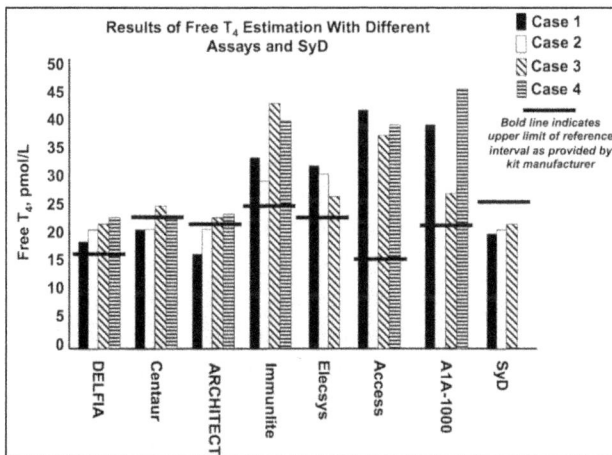

Reproduced from Cartwright D, O'Shea P, Rajanayagam O, et al. Familial dysalbuminemic hyperthyroxinemia: a persistent diagnostic challenge. *Clin Chem.* 2009;55(5):1044-1046, permission conveyed through Copyright Clearance Center, Inc.

Familial dysalbuminemic hyperthyroxinemia is transmitted in an autosomal dominant fashion and is the result of gain-of-function pathogenic variants in the *ALB* gene encoding albumin that enhance the affinity of albumin for T_4, but generally not for T_3. As a result, reliance on total T_4 (elevated) or free T_4 index (also elevated, since this is a product of a normal T_3 resin and an elevated T_4) testing may be misleading.

A defect in 5'-monodeiodination due to selenium deficiency (Answer A) is much less common than familial dysalbuminemic hyperthyroxinemia. This patient does not have a TSH-secreting pituitary adenoma (Answer E) given that he is clinically euthyroid and T_3 levels are normal. This is not thyroid hormone resistance (Answer D) nor familial thyroxine-binding globulin excess (Answer B) because the total T_3 level is normal rather than elevated—an elevated total T_3 level would be expected in each of these disorders.

Educational Objective
Diagnose familial dysalbuminemic hyperthyroxinemia on the basis of clinical findings and thyroid function test results.

Reference(s)
Pappa T, Ferrara AM, Refetoff S. Inherited defects of thyroxine-binding proteins. *Best Pract Res Clin Endocrinol Metab.* 2015;29(5):735-747. PMID: 26522458

Pannain S, Feldman M, Eiholzer U, Weiss RE, Scherberg NH, Refetoff S. Familial dysalbuminemic hyperthyroxinemia in a Swiss family caused by a mutant albumin (R218P) shows an apparent discrepancy between serum concentration and affinity for thyroxine. *J Clin Endocrinol Metab.* 2000;85(8):2786-2792. PMID: 10946882

21 ANSWER: D) Thyroidectomy from collar incision

The CT shows a substernal goiter with mass effect on the trachea. The patient is symptomatic, with positional dyspnea, most likely due to compression of her trachea by the asymmetrically enlarged thyroid when she lies on her side. More than 90% of substernal goiters can be "delivered" through a collar incision (Answer D).

The remaining therapeutic options listed are less helpful. Specifically, this euthyroid patient's thyroid mass is unlikely to respond significantly to levothyroxine suppressive therapy (Answer A). Recombinant human TSH treatment (Answer B) with radioiodine in a patient with an intact thyroid is potentially dangerous due to a release of thyroid hormone from the gland under the influence of recombinant human TSH. Thermal ablation (Answer C) would not prove useful in reducing the size of this very large substernal goiter. No intervention (Answer E) would be inappropriate given her symptomatic disease.

Educational Objective
Devise an approach to a symptomatic substernal goiter.

Reference(s)
Bahn RS, Castro MR. Approach to the patient with nontoxic multinodular goiter. *J Clin Endocrinol Metab.* 2011;96(5):1202-1212. PMID: 21543434

Fast S, Nielsen VE, Bonnema SJ, Hegedüs L. Dose-dependent acute effects of recombinant human TSH (rhTSH) on thyroid size and function: comparison of 0.1, 0.3 and 0.9 mg of rhTSH. *Clin Endocrinol (Oxf).* 2010;72(3):411-416. PMID: 19508679

Bonnema SJ, Hegedüs L. Radioiodine therapy in benign thyroid diseases: effects, side effects, and factors affecting therapeutic outcome. *Endocr Rev.* 2012;33(6):920-980. PMID: 22961916

22 Answer C) Thyroid-stimulating immunoglobulin level

Overall, without considering individual risk factors, the chance of remission after 12 to 18 months of antithyroid drug therapy is 30% to 50%. Men, persons older than 40 years, individuals with large goiters, cigarette smokers, and those with higher baseline thyroid hormone levels are less likely to achieve remission (thus, Answers A, D, and E are incorrect). After 12 to 18 months of antithyroid drug treatment, thyroid-stimulating immunoglobulin levels (Answer C) can be used to refine estimates for the likelihood of remission. Patients with negative thyroid receptor antibodies after 18 months of antithyroid drug treatment are more likely to remit than those in whom thyroid receptor antibodies remain detectable. In this patient who is euthyroid on methimazole but whose thyroid-stimulating immunoglobulin level remains high, the likelihood of long-term remission is only approximately 15%. TPO antibody titer (Answer B) is not associated with the probability of remission.

Educational Objective
List predictors of remission in Graves hyperthyroidism.

Reference(s)
Franklyn JA, Boelaert K. Thyrotoxicosis. *Lancet.* 2012;379(9821):1155-1166. PMID: 22394559

Barbesino G, Tomer Y. Clinical review: clinical utility of TSH receptor antibodies. *J Clin Endocrinol Metab.* 2013;98(6):2247-2255. PMID: 23539719

Carella C, Mazziotti G, Sorvillo F, et al. Serum thyrotropin receptor antibodies concentrations in patients with Graves' disease before, at the end of methimazole treatment, and after drug withdrawal: evidence that the activity of thyrotropin receptor antibody and/or thyroid response modify during the observation period. *Thyroid.* 2006;16(3):295-302. PMID: 16571093

23 ANSWER: D) Referral for total thyroidectomy

In the Bethesda classification system for reporting thyroid cytopathology, nodules with indeterminate results, which include Bethesda class III (atypia of uncertain significance/follicular lesion of uncertain significance [AUS/FLUS]) and class IV (follicular neoplasm/suspicious for follicular neoplasm [FN/SFN]) are sometimes selected for molecular testing. Testing using a small panel of pathogenic variants known to be associated with thyroid cancer is most helpful when a mutation or rearrangement is present (higher positive predictive value) and is generally not helpful when no mutation is identified (lower negative predictive value) because many cancers do not contain the limited set of abnormalities sought in the test. In this patient with a large nodule (>4 cm), a follicular neoplasm on FNA biopsy and a positive finding of a *RET/PTC* rearrangement, there is a high enough risk of thyroid cancer (80%-90%) that total thyroidectomy (Answer D) is recommended. However, bilateral neck dissection (Answer E) is not warranted given the absence of suspicious lymph nodes on ultrasonography. The *RET/PTC* gene rearrangement, found in 20% to 70% of papillary thyroid cancers, causes constitutive activation of transcription of the RET tyrosine-kinase domain in follicular cells, leading to uncontrolled cell proliferation.

Cytologic Diagnosis	AUS/FLUS		FN/SFN		SMC	
Cancer Risk Based on Cytology Only	14% ↓		27% ↓		54% ↓	
Testing for Panel of Mutations (*BRAF, RAS, RET/PTC, PAX8/PPARγ*)	↗ ↘		↗ ↘		↗ ↘	
Mutational Status	Positive	Negative	Positive	Negative	Positive	Negative
Cancer Risk	88%	5.9%	87%	14%	95%	28%
Clinical Management	Total thyroidectomy	Lobectomy vs. observation +/- repeat FNA	Total thyroidectomy	Lobectomy	Total thyroidectomy	Lobectomy

Reproduced with permission from Nikiforov YE, Ohori NP, Hodak SP, Carty SE, LeBeau SO, Ferris RL, et al. Impact of mutational testing on the diagnosis and management of patients with cytologically indeterminate thyroid nodules: a prospective analysis of 1056 FNA samples. *J Clin Endocrinol Metab.* 2011;96(11):3390-3397.

Another form of molecular testing—a gene expression classifier (uses a microarray of a large panel of genes associated with either benign or malignant thyroid nodules)—is currently only available from a single source. Limited data for this molecular classifier suggest that it is associated with a higher negative predictive value such that, in general, if negative, no surgery would be recommended. No study to date has examined the tandem use of both technologies, although the cost of this approach could be prohibitive.

Lobectomy (Answer C) is inappropriate because of the high risk of malignancy. Given that his nodule is larger than 4 cm, a completion thyroidectomy would most likely be required when pathologic examination confirms a malignant nodule. Performing thyroid ultrasonography (Answer A) or FNA biopsy (Answer B) again in 6 months would incorrectly avoid thyroid surgery.

Educational Objective
Apply molecular testing to thyroid nodule evaluation.

Reference(s)
Steward DL, Carty SE, Sippel RS, et al. Performance of a multigene genomic classifier in thyroid nodules with indeterminate cytology: a Prospective blinded multicenter study. *JAMA Oncol.* 2018 [Epub ahead of print] PMID: 30419129

Alexander EK, Kennedy GC, Baloch ZW, et al. Preoperative diagnosis of benign thyroid nodules with indeterminate cytology. *N Engl J Med.* 2012; 367(8):705-715. PMID: 22731672

Nikiforov YE. Role of molecular markers in thyroid nodule management: then and now. Endocr Pract. 2017;23(8):979-988. PMID: 28534687

Nikiforov YE, Ohori NP, Hodak SP, Carty SE, LeBeau SO, Ferris RL, et al. Impact of mutational testing on the diagnosis and management of patients with cytologically indeterminate thyroid nodules: a prospective analysis of 1056 FNA samples. *J Clin Endocrinol Metab.* 2011;96(11): 3390-3397. PMID: 21880806

24 ANSWER: B) Serum thyroglobulin measurement

The differential diagnosis for patients with thyrotoxicosis and low radioactive iodine uptake includes painless and postpartum thyroiditis, subacute thyroiditis, struma ovarii (with low radioactive iodine uptake in the neck, but uptake in the pelvis on whole-body scan), factitious or iatrogenic thyroiditis, amiodarone use, and recent high-dose iodine exposure. In this male patient, struma ovarii and postpartum thyroiditis are not possibilities. He is not taking amiodarone. Subacute thyroiditis is unlikely given the lack of a viral prodrome, fever, or thyroid tenderness, so assessing his erythrocyte sedimentation rate (Answer C) is incorrect. The urinary iodine concentration is not consistent with recent excessive iodine exposure, so repeating the radioactive iodine uptake following a low-iodine diet (Answer A) is unlikely to change results. In this patient, the most likely diagnoses are either factitious thyrotoxicosis or painless thyroiditis. Graves disease has already been ruled out by the low radioactive iodine uptake, so thyroid-stimulating immunoglobulin measurement (Answer E) is incorrect. Thyroid ultrasonography with color Doppler (Answer D) would show absent hypervascularity with both of these entities. However, the serum thyroglobulin concentration (Answer B) in this thyroglobulin antibody–negative patient would be elevated in painless thyroiditis but low in factitious thyrotoxicosis.

Educational Objective
Construct the differential diagnosis for low radioiodine uptake thyrotoxicosis.

Reference(s)
De Leo S, Lee SY, Braverman LE. Hyperthyroidism. *Lancet.* 2016;388(10047):906-918. PMID: 27038492

Ross DS, Burch HB, Cooper DS, et al. 2016 American Thyroid Association Guidelines for Diagnosis and Management of Hyperthyroidism and Other Causes of Thyrotoxicosis. *Thyroid.* 2016;26(10):1343-1421. PMID: 27521067

25 ANSWER: B) Repeated thyroglobulin and thyroglobulin antibody measurements in 6 weeks using the same radioimmunoassay

This patient has an elevated serum thyroglobulin value shortly after undergoing thyroidectomy for thyroid cancer. Thyroglobulin measurement is a sensitive tool for thyroid cancer surveillance, especially in thyroglobulin antibody–negative patients such as this one, but it is important to be aware of its limitations. In this case, it is simply too soon to measure the serum thyroglobulin postoperatively; values tend to be elevated in the first few days to weeks after surgery given serum thyroglobulin elevations caused by the surgical manipulation of the thyroid gland and the serum half-life of thyroglobulin. It is generally recommended to wait 6 weeks after thyroidectomy or 3 months after radioactive iodine ablation before the initial postoperative thyroglobulin measurement. If the measurements are repeated in 6 weeks (Answer B), it is likely that the thyroglobulin level will be substantially lower.

Ideally, thyroglobulin should be measured with the same assay over time due to substantial intra-assay variability (as much as 40%-60%) between methods. Repeating the measurement immediately with a different assay (Answers A and D) will still most likely result in an uninterpretable value because of timing. Measuring thyroglobulin in serially diluted sera (Answer C) can determine whether thyroglobulin is artifactually elevated (or, less frequently, artifactually decreased) due to the presence of heterophile antibodies. Such antibodies can form a bridge between capture and detection antibody leading to a false thyroglobulin measurement in immunometric assays. However, heterophile antibodies are unlikely to have caused an artifactual thyroglobulin elevation in this patient, since thyroglobulin was measured by radioimmunoassay. The patient has a low-risk tumor based on surgical pathology, so radioactive iodine ablation (Answer E) is not indicated.

Educational Objective
Identify common pitfalls with the use of serum thyroglobulin for thyroid cancer surveillance.

Reference(s)
Giovanella L, Clark PM, Chiovato L, et al. Thyroglobulin measurement using highly sensitive assays in patients with differentiated thyroid cancer: a clinical position paper. *Eur J Endocrinol.* 2014;171(2):R33-R46. PMID: 24743400

Haugen BR, Alexander EK, Bible KC, et al. 2015 American Thyroid Association management guidelines for adult patients with thyroid nodules and differentiated thyroid cancer: the American Thyroid Association Guidelines Task Force on Thyroid Nodules and Differentiated Thyroid Cancer. *Thyroid.* 2016;26(1):1-133. PMID: 26462967

26 ANSWER: E) Repeated surveillance testing in 1 year

This patient has microscopic local invasion of tumor and positive central compartment lymph node disease. According to the AJCC-8 staging system (American Joint Committee on Cancer, 8th edition), her tumor is classified as T3,N1,M0, stage I. After surgery and radioiodine therapy, the patient has persistent elevation of serum thyroglobulin, but this is down-trending over time. According to current recommendations for restratification of risk on the basis of response to initial therapy, she has had an acceptable response to therapy, with unstimulated thyroglobulin less than 1.0 ng/mL (<1.0 µg/L) and stimulated thyroglobulin less than 10 ng/mL (<10 µg/L). Numerous studies have demonstrated progressive spontaneous decreases in thyroglobulin over years after initial therapy. The best option in this patient is to continue to monitor without intervention or additional unnecessary testing (Answer E).

PET-CT (Answer B) can be considered in patients with cancer who are at high risk and have elevated serum thyroglobulin (>10 ng/mL [>10 µg/L]) and a negative whole-body scan. However, such imaging is not indicated in this patient who has low and declining serum thyroglobulin values. Noncontrast chest CT (Answer C) is the most sensitive test for small lung metastases and may be obtained in patients with cancer who are at high risk and have elevated or rising serum thyroglobulin values. Neck MRI (Answer D) is occasionally useful for visualization of metastatic disease not well visualized by ultrasonography or contrast neck CT, but this is not the case here. There is no evidence for spurious thyroglobulin measurements, and assessing serum thyroglobulin over time in the same assay is preferred due to intra-assay variability (thus, Answer A is incorrect).

Educational Objective
Recommend an appropriate surveillance strategy for differentiated thyroid cancer.

Reference(s)
Yim JH, Kim WB, Kim EY, et al. The outcomes of first reoperation for locoregionally recurrent/persistent papillary thyroid carcinoma in patients who initially underwent total thyroidectomy and remnant ablation. *J Clin Endocrinol Metab*. 2011;96(7):2049-2056. PMID: 21508143

Al-Saif O, Farrar WB, Bloomston M, Porter K, Ringel MD, Kloos RT. Long-term efficacy of lymph node reoperation for persistent papillary thyroid cancer. *J Clin Endocrinol Metab*. 2010; 95(5):2187-2194. PMID: 20332244

Haugen BR, Alexander EK, Bible KC, et al. 2015 American Thyroid Association management guidelines for adult patients with thyroid nodules and differentiated thyroid cancer: the American Thyroid Association Guidelines Task Force on Thyroid Nodules and Differentiated Thyroid Cancer. *Thyroid*. 2016;26(1):1-133. PMID: 26462967

27 Answer A) Perform FNA biopsy

This patient presents with thyrotoxicosis and neck pain with low radioactive iodine uptake, consistent with subacute thyroiditis. She has been treated with prednisone with little improvement. Over a period of only 3 weeks she has had progressive asymmetric thyroid enlargement, now accompanied by compressive symptoms. The diagnosis in this patient was anaplastic thyroid cancer with thyrotoxicosis due to a destructive thyroiditis. There have been numerous reports of this unusual presentation of anaplastic thyroid cancer in the medical literature, and some patients have been treated with prolonged courses of corticosteroids before a correct diagnosis has been made. These patients typically have exceptionally aggressive disease and very limited survival. Although this is an atypical presentation, very rapid thyroid enlargement in an older patient should always prompt concern for anaplastic thyroid cancer. FNA biopsy (Answer A) would determine her underlying diagnosis.

Glucocorticoid therapy may help with the pain from her thyroid inflammation. However, switching to a different corticosteroid (Answer C), starting methimazole (Answer B), or performing contrast CT of the neck (Answer D) would all fail to determine the underlying diagnosis. In addition, methimazole is generally not useful in the management of low iodine uptake inflammatory thyroiditis, since thyroid hormone synthesis is not increased. Thyroidectomy (Answer E) should not be performed in the absence of a definitive diagnosis.

Educational Objective
Recognize low radioactive iodine uptake thyrotoxicosis and neck pain with rapid thyroid growth and no response to steroids as anaplastic cancer.

Reference(s)
Kumar V, Blanchon B, Gu X, et al. Anaplastic thyroid cancer and hyperthyroidism. *Endocr Pathol*. 2005;16(3):245-250. PMID: 16299408

Heymann RS, Brent GA, Hershman JM. Anaplastic thyroid carcinoma with thyrotoxicosis and hypoparathyroidism. *Endocr Pract*. 2005;11(4):281-284. PMID: 16006301

Smallridge RC, Ain KB, Asa SL, et al; American Thyroid Association Anaplastic Thyroid Cancer Guidelines Taskforce. American Thyroid Association guidelines for management of patients with anaplastic thyroid cancer. *Thyroid*. 2012; 22(11):1104-1139. PMID: 23130564

28 ANSWER: B) TSH, 0.1 mIU/L; free T$_4$ index, 4.2; total T$_3$, 350 ng/dL (5.4 nmol/L)

The goal of antithyroid drug therapy for Graves disease during pregnancy is to keep the serum TSH suppressed and the free T$_4$ high-normal to mildly elevated. The rationale for these targets is to minimize the amount of antithyroid drug exposure to the fetus by administering the lowest effective dosage, since the fetal thyroid is more susceptible than the maternal thyroid to the effects of antithyroid drugs. Both methimazole and propylthiouracil can cross the placenta and affect the fetal thyroid. The values in Answer B are within recommended targets for this patient. Answer A is incorrect because these values are consistent with overt hyperthyroidism, which is associated with an increased risk of intrauterine growth retardation and fetal demise. Answers C, D, and E each would be associated with higher dosages of antithyroid drug than the minimally effective dosage. As an aside, it is important to note that the total T_3 level, like the total T_4 level, is affected by the increases in thyroxine-binding globulin that occur during pregnancy.

Educational Objective

Explain the goals of therapy for Graves disease in pregnancy.

Reference(s)

Alexander EK, Pearce EN, Brent GA, et al. 2017 guidelines of the American Thyroid Association for the diagnosis and management of thyroid disease during pregnancy and the postpartum. *Thyroid*. 2017;27(3):315-389. PMID: 28056690

Pearce EN. Management of thyrotoxicosis: pre-conception, pregnancy, and the postpartum period. *Endocr Pract*. 2019;25(1):62-68. PMID: 30289300

29 ANSWER: D) Levothyroxine, 70 mcg intravenously once daily

Intravenous levothyroxine dosing is generally started at 50% to 75% of the patient's usual oral therapy dosing (Answer D). The remaining choices are either too high (Answers A and B) or inappropriately substitute lio-thyronine (Answer E). Although case studies have been published describing successful use of intramuscular levothyroxine (Answer C), the US FDA has not approved this route of administration, and the dosage listed is incorrect.

Educational Objective

Guide the transition from oral to intravenous levothyroxine in a patient with hypothyroidism.

Reference(s)

Hays MT. Parenteral thyroxine administration. *Thyroid*. 2007;17(2):127-129. PMID: 17316114

30 Answer E) Orbital decompression surgery

This patient is at risk for permanent vision loss due to ischemic neuropathy, and high-dosage glucocorticoid therapy has already failed. She should undergo urgent orbital decompression surgery (Answer E).

Teprotumumab (Answer D) is a monoclonal antibody that inhibits the IGF-1 receptor and has recently been shown to effectively improve symptoms of active moderate-to-severe Graves ophthalmopathy, but this would not take effect rapidly enough to prevent threatened vision loss. Strabismus surgery (Answer C) may ultimately be needed, but it would be premature to perform this while the Graves eye disease is still active and evolving, and it would not reduce her risk for imminent vision loss. There are conflicting clinical trial data regarding the efficacy of rituximab (Answer B) in patients with moderate-to-severe Graves eye disease, but, even if it were effective, it would not work rapidly enough to be an appropriate choice in this clinical setting. Similarly, orbital radiotherapy (Answer A) is effective in about half of patients with moderate-to-severe eye disease, but the effects would not be rapid enough for this to be an appropriate response to sight-threatening disease.

Educational Objective

List indications for orbital decompression surgery in Graves orbitopathy.

Reference(s)

Bartalena L, Tanda ML. Clinical practice. Graves' ophthalmopathy. *N Engl J Med*. 2009;360(10): 994-1001. PMID: 19264688

Wiersinga WM. Advances in treatment of active, moderate-to-severe Graves' ophthalmopathy. *Lancet Diabetes Endocrinol*. 2017;5(2):134-142. PMID: 27346786

Smith TJ, Kahaly GJ, Ezra DG, et al. Teprotumumab for thyroid-associated ophthalmopathy. *N Engl J Med*. 2017;376(18):1748-1761. PMID: 28467880

www.ingramcontent.com/pod-product-compliance
Lightning Source LLC
Chambersburg PA
CBHW061324190326
41458CB00011B/3883